S. Johnson

W9-BOC-214

S. Johnson

Introduction to
Veterinary
Pathology

SECOND EDITION

Editorial Board

Mark Ackermann DVM PhD
Ames, Iowa

Claire Andreasen DVM PhD
Ames, Iowa

Dominique Brees DVM PhD
Frythe, England

Joseph Haynes DVM PhD
Ames, Iowa

Olaf Hedstrom DVM PhD
Corvallis, Oregon

Vince Meador DVM PhD
Indianapolis, Indiana

Derek Mosier DVM PhD
Manhattan, Kansas

Ronald Myers DVM PhD
Ames, Iowa

Tim O'Brien DVM PhD
St. Paul, Minnesota

Introduction to
Veterinary
Pathology

SECOND EDITION

NORMAN F. CHEVILLE

IOWA STATE UNIVERSITY PRESS / AMES

Norman F. Cheville, DVM, PhD, is Chief of the Pathology Research Laboratory, National Animal Disease Center, Ames, Iowa, and Professor of Veterinary Pathology, Iowa State University.

© 1999 Iowa State University Press
All rights reserved

Iowa State University Press
2121 South State Avenue, Ames, Iowa 50014
Orders: 1-800-862-6657
Office: 1-515-292-0140
Fax: 1-515-292-3348
Web site: www.isupress.edu

☺ Printed on acid-free paper in the United States of America

No part of this book may be reproduced in any form or by any electronic or
mechanical means, including information storage and retrieval systems,
without permission in writing from the copyright holder, except for brief
passages quoted in review.

First edition, 1988

International Standard Book Number: 0-8138-2496-6

Library of Congress Cataloging-in-Publication Data

Cheville, Norman F.
Introduction to veterinary pathology / Norman F. Cheville. * 2nd ed.
        p.   cm.
    Includes bibliographical references.
    ISBN 0-8138-2496-6
    1. Veterinary pathology. I. Title.
SF769.C473   1999   99-22664
636.089′607—dc21   CIP

The last digit is the print number: 9 8 7 6 5 4 3 2 1

For Beth
. . . who makes it all possible

Contents

Preface

Introduction to Veterinary Pathology, Second Edition, is constructed for the beginning student in veterinary pathology—to introduce new scientific information on mechanisms of general tissue injury into the language of pathology. The discipline of pathology is divided into anatomic pathology and clinical pathology. Microscopic examination of tissue taken at the necropsy (postmortem examination) after death or from a biopsy specimen obtained in the clinic tells the anatomic pathologist about the nature and extent of the disease process. Examination of blood and other body fluids during life leads the clinical pathologist to the same conclusion, although by different methods. In some difficult cases, lesions are detectable only by microscopy and in others only by biochemical methods. For every chemical change in a cell, there is a corresponding structural change. The challenge to the pathologist lies in finding it.

General pathology, which deals with basic reactions of cells and tissues to etiologic agents, is our beginning point in the study of pathology. Here we deal with diseases of vertebrate animals. Occasionally disease processes in humans or nonvertebrate species will be considered when they provide useful models for a basic process. Although the spontaneous diseases of these species are not mirrors of their counterparts in vertebrate animals, the biologic processes are similar and at the level of the cell may even be identical. One of the most exciting eras of pathology began with observations on the inflammatory response of the water flea.

In doing the necropsy, careless observation and sampling can result in useless, and sometimes harmful, information. Those who do postmortem exams in this manner run risks, for to bypass fundamental changes in tissue can be costly to both pocketbook and intellectual development. An understanding of molecular biology is viewed by some as not necessary for the practicing veterinarian. To refute that, the difference between the scientific and technical faces of veterinary medicine can be cited. Acceptance of the title "Doctor" is acceptance of the responsibility for understanding disease, not merely knowing how to deal with it technically. One cannot condone planners of curricula who, while insisting on rigorous preprofessional courses in mathematics and physics, constrict the curriculum that provides the very foundation of medical knowledge.

As a student, you will become aware of the special burden of the veterinarian—the lifelong need to keep one foot in science and one in clinical medicine. It is your responsibility to distill new science into clinical practice. This not only will enrich your professional life but also will benefit your patients and protect you legally.

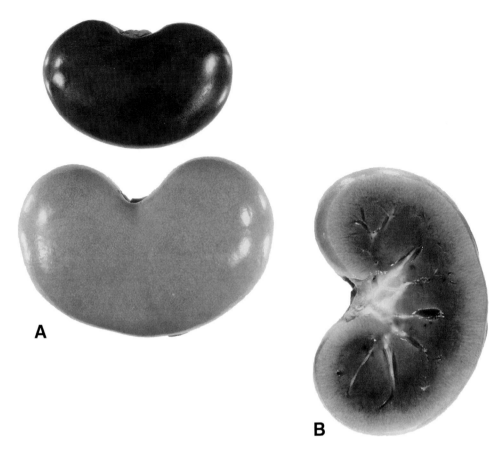

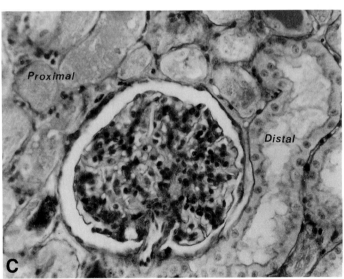

A. Normal kidney (*top*) and large pale kidney with diffuse cell swelling and necrosis, oxytetracycline toxicity. Kidneys are from twin kids of the same age, one treated and one not treated. The marked increase in size and color developed 5 days after initial antibiotic therapy. B. Cross section of necrotic kidney. C. Histology with necrosis of proximal convoluted tubular epithelium and sparing of epithelium of distal tubules.

PART 1

Introduction to Pathology

PATHOLOGY, IN THE BROADEST SENSE, is abnormal biology. As a science, it encompasses all abnormalities of body structure and function. It involves the study of cells, tissues, organs, and body fluids and is the link between basic sciences and clinical studies. Pathology is essentially the study of cellular and tissue responses to injury. The goal of pathology is to understand the disease process sufficiently to provide a diagnosis. A **diagnosis** is a conclusion regarding cause and pathogenesis, especially with a view to distinguishing one disease from another. The components of the disease process that form the foundation of pathology are

- Lesions
- Pathogenesis
- Etiology
- Clinical consequences

Lesions are abnormal structural and functional changes that occur in the body. The lesions that you observe in injured tissue may be gross, microscopic, or biochemical, and each observation tells you something about the disease process. The renal lesion of swelling and necrosis in the frontispiece directs us to a group of possible causes of injury.

The **morphologic diagnosis** (or "lesion" diagnosis) is based on the dominant lesions in the tissues of the animal. Gross and microscopic examination of lesions establishes the basic tissue response and provides clues to the cause of disease. The morphologic diagnosis tells the clinician about the extent, duration, distribution, and type of lesions.

Pathogenesis is the developmental process of a disease, the sequence of events involved in the cellular and tissue response to injury. Pathogenesis extends from the initial cellular injury to the complete manifestation of the disease that is seen in the clinic. To fully understand the pathogenesis of a disease, you must identify both causal agent and host response, as well as their changing relationships as disease progresses. Determination of cause and tissue reaction must be followed by an interpretation of their significance; that is, are the causal agent and lesions that have been identified the primary cause and effect, or are they secondary to some more dangerous process that remains hidden?

Etiology is the study of the cause of disease. An **etiologic diagnosis** provides the precise cause of a disease. Toxic doses of oxytetracycline caused the renal lesion in the frontispiece. An **etiologic agent** induces cell and tissue injury and causes lesions to develop. This, in turn, leads to the clinical manifestations of disease.

Etiologic agent → lesions → clinical signs

Combining the clinical signs with data from the study of lesions in cells and tissue, we work backward to determine the etiologic agent, and then piece together the pathogenesis of the disease in order to determine the clinical consequences.

Your success as a veterinarian will depend in great part on your ability to observe—to detect by sight, touch, and sound the evidence of disease in the patient. In making a pathologic diagnosis, you must observe deviations in size, color, texture, and location from normal organs and tissues. Examine again the kidneys in the frontispiece. **Nephritis** (inflammation of the kidney) was the clinical diagnosis in the goat whose kidney was affected. At necropsy, the marked enlargement, softness, pallor, and increased intracapsular pressure of the kidney suggest the pathologic changes to be **acute cell swelling and necrosis** (death of cells in the living animal), and this conclusion leads to a search for the cause of acute toxic injury. The microscopic lesions of tubular epithelial necrosis are consistent with oxytetracycline toxicity, a known cause of acute renal failure. When excessive oxytetracycline therapy is found in the clinical history of an animal with swelling and necrosis of the kidneys, the etiologic diagnosis can be established.

The **differential diagnosis** is a listing of which diseases may be involved in a sick patient, and a determination of which disease is responsible for illness. The differential diagnosis for the swollen kidney in the frontispiece would include oxytetracycline toxicity, other nephrotoxins, bacterial infections of the kidney (especially leptospirosis), and renal amyloidosis. The differential diagnosis is developed by systematically comparing clinical and pathologic findings. It provides a framework for analysis. A highly developed capacity to connect what appear to be unrelated clinical signs and lesions leads to success in the clinic.

It is traditional to begin the study of general pathology by examining basic categories of tissue response. The processes we examine here are necrosis, inflammation, circulatory disorders, growth defects, and neoplasia. In the clinic, you will see that these processes are sometimes linked, but here we look closely at how the process develops, and the consequences that each process has for the animal. A clear understanding of pathogenesis of these processes allows a **prognosis**, a statement regarding the expected outcome of the disease.

In examining abnormal tissue, the first step is to answer the question, What is the basic process? You should be directed to identifying the tissue response. To interpret an abnormal mass in tissue, you must consider all types of host responses. Did the lesion in question arise from a congenital defect or from an inflammatory process? Is the mass that you see in tissue an abscess, a cyst, a neoplasm, or a focus of necrosis? The postmortem examination (necropsy) is an important event in establishing a diagnosis. Evaluation of gross lesions tells the pathologist what type of disease process has occurred and to what extent it has damaged specific organ systems. The methodical examination of the dead animal may be called either **necropsy** (Gr. *necros,* dead body, plus *opsis,* sight) or **autopsy** (Gr. *autopsia,* seen by oneself). *Necropsy* is preferred by veterinary pathologists; *autopsy* is used in medical pathology.

FOCUS

Origins of Veterinary Pathology

PATHOLOGY IS ROOTED in the anatomical theaters of the Italian Renaissance. In Padua, the chair of anatomy was occupied by a succession of great scientists: Vesalius, Malpighi, and Valsalva. Morgagni began the modern era of pathology with *Seats and Causes of Disease* in 1761, one year before the first veterinary school was founded in Lyon, France. The correlation of clinical signs with lesions was the turning point from ancient to modern medicine. Before Morgagni, physicians spoke of imbalanced mixtures of humors, and after him, of changes in organs that were constant for specific diseases. William Harvey studied in Padua and returned to London to discover the circulation of blood. His legacy of experimental pathology extended into John Hunter's treatises on vascular pathology and William Osler's discovery of platelets in the 1800s. Hunter was on the founding board of the Royal Veterinary College in London, and Osler was a staff member of the Montreal Veterinary College.

▶

Medical pathology ascended in the German-speaking world with a group around Johannes Müller in Berlin in the 1880s. Using the newly invented achromatic objective on the light microscope, Rudolf Virchow introduced systematic histologic analysis of lesions. His book *Cellular Pathology* (1848) laid the foundations of medical and veterinary pathology. Involved in public health, Virchow advocated postmortem examinations of farm animals as a form of meat inspection. He was influential in the establishment of the first chair of veterinary pathology in Berlin in 1870, and his techniques spread throughout the world.

In the early 1900s, William Welsh at Johns Hopkins brought systemic pathology to North America. He and his students had great influence on veterinary pathologists, many of which were trained in large medical institutes such as the Rockefeller Institute, Armed Forces Institute of Pathology, and Mayo Clinic. From the latter came William Feldman, an outstanding veterinary pathologist and first president of the American College of Veterinary Pathologists. Founded in 1948 by pathologists from the U.S. and Canada, this organization—along with its counterpart, the European College of Veterinary Pathologists (1995)—have guided much of the scientific development of veterinary pathology.

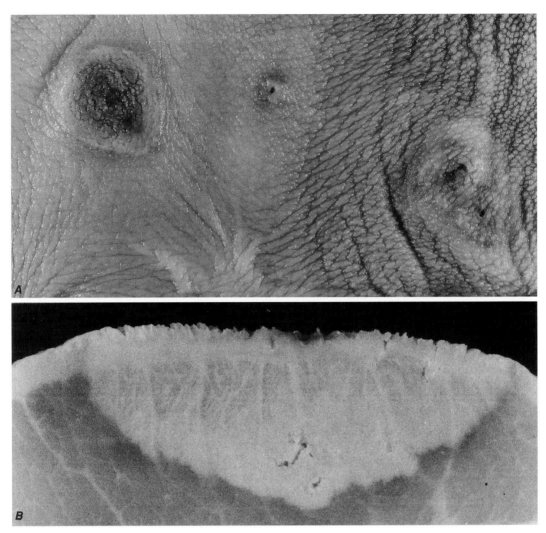

FIGURE 1.1. Degeneration and necrosis. Rumen of a cow, lesions caused by *Fusobacterium necrophorum*. A. Three foci of necrosis at different stages of development. B. Enlarged cross section of one necrotic focus. Necrosis extends into muscle layers of the rumen wall. The causal bacteria are at the advancing edge of the necrotic lesion. Preservation of tissue architecture in the necrotic mass is typical of coagulation necrosis.

▦ CHAPTER 1

Lethal Injury and Cell Death

Death of an animal is based on irreversible cessation of activity in heart, lungs, or brain. Absence of function in any of these organs will cause sudden collapse and somatic death (death of the body). After death, body fluids become so acidic and devoid of oxygen that the cells rapidly die. Even so, some cells may live for several hours. When the death process is short, as in the action of cyanide on the mitochondrial enzyme cytochrome oxidase, the microscopic evidence of cellular injury is subtle and beyond the scope of routine methods of detection. At the other end of the spectrum, when dying extends over a long time, lesions are often so extensive, multiple, and interrelated that they are difficult to interpret. In these cases, the excitement of discovering and integrating these pieces of evidence toward an acceptable thesis on the cause of death is the reward of thorough pathologic examination.

The process of dying is complex, and many terminal events—those involved in shutdown of body systems—may mask or override the primary disease process. Kidney failure induced by oxytetracycline leads to death, yet determining the dying process is a demanding intellectual exercise and involves effects of nitrogenous wastes, endogenous toxic peptides, and imbalances in electrolytes and acid-base equilibrium. The effects of these substances on brain centers for respiration and cardiovascular action—or directly on lungs, kidney, and heart—are responsible for death.

NECROSIS

Necrosis (Gr. *nekrosis,* deadness) is death of cells and tissues in the living animal. Necrotic tissue appears grossly as a pale, coagulated mass of dead tissue that stands out against the darker color of the normal organ. It lacks the texture of adjacent normal tissue. Although cellular detail is distorted, tissue architecture is preserved, and the outline of tissue structures can usually be seen (Fig. 1.1). Common causes of necrosis are ischemia and a variety of exogenous agents, including physical agents (burns and trauma), chemical poisons, viruses, and other microorganisms and their toxins.

Classically, necrosis has been defined as "the sum of the morphologic changes indicative of cell death and caused by the progressive degradative action of enzymes." Later we will more clearly define death at the cellular level. Mechanisms that lead to cell death include a spectrum from direct, lethal injury that interrupts critical metabolic pathways to the activation of suicide genes that lead to a controlled, programmed cell death.

In describing necrosis in tissues at the necropsy or in biopsy specimens, it is important to be precise about the distribution of the lesions. In **diffuse necrosis**, the entire organ or tissue is affected. In the diffuse renal swelling and necrosis caused by oxytetracycline toxicity (see Frontispiece, Part 1), the necrotic process affects all parts of the renal tubule. The severe swelling suppresses blood flow to the kidney, causing the necrotic tissue to be pale.

Focal necrosis is used to describe a single, clearly defined focus of necrosis. The necrotic focus is commonly caused by bacteria, fungi, and viruses, and evidence of these etiologic agents can be found in histologic analysis of tissue.

If several foci of necrosis are present in an organ, the distribution is called **multifocal** (Fig. 1.2). If the entire organ contains many, randomly distributed small foci of necrosis, the lesions are **disseminated**. The appearance of the necrotic tissues depends not only on the type of cellular degeneration but also on the extent of injury to surrounding vascular and connective tissues.

The animal body tends to surround foci of necro-

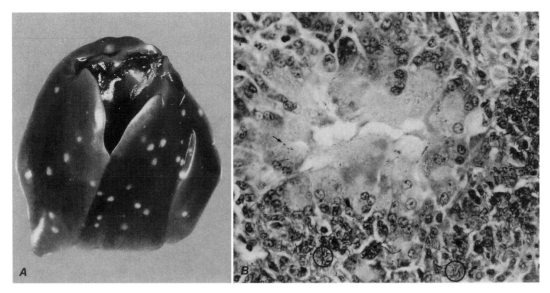

FIGURE 1.2. Focal necrosis of liver. A. Pale foci of necrosis in the liver. B. Histology of a necrotic focus surrounded by zone of macrophages. *Eubacteria* sp. *(circles)* are associated with macrophages at the lesion periphery. Tiny cocci *(Staphylococcus aureus)* have superinfected the necrotic tissue *(arrow)*. (Photographs: Larry Arp, *Vet Pathol* 20:80, 1983)

sis with a zone of inflammation to "wall off" the area and sequester the causal agent. Thus, the necrotizing process is typically tied to an inflammatory process, and these lesions may be described according to their inflammatory component (e.g., diffuse "necrotizing" purulent laryngitis).

Special types of necrosis

Gangrene

Superimposition of growth of saprophytic bacteria on necrotic tissue results in gangrene, a variant of coagulation necrosis. **Gangrenous necrosis** may occur because of bacterial invasion of an infarct or as a result of restriction of blood supply in an established bacterial infection, especially where there is collection of fluid and intravascular clotting.

The term *gangrene* is also applied to necrosis of tissues in an extremity in which vascular occlusion has resulted in coagulation necrosis. When pus-producing bacterial infection does not occur, the tissue mummifies and the condition is called **dry gangrene** (Fig. 1.3). Affected tissue is cool, dry, and discolored. There is a sharp demarcation of inflammatory tissue, preventing systemic infection. When pus-producing organisms invade, the combination of ischemia and infection produces putrefactive, foul-smelling tissues, a lesion called **moist gangrene**.

Infarcts

An **infarct** is a local area of necrosis caused by ischemia due to obstruction in the arterial supply or venous drainage. Infarction is a special manifestation of coagulation necrosis. Infarcts can be caused both by damage to the vascular supply to a tissue or organ, and by any obstructive mass that moves through the vascular system to lodge itself in a way

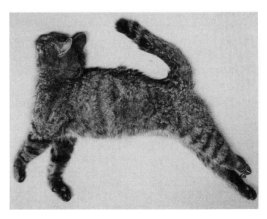

FIGURE 1.3. Tetanus, cat. Gangrene of the left hind leg (trap injury) provided the focus for growth of *Clostridium tetani.* Rigidity is due to tetanic spasm (note tail, paws, and ears) caused by the neurotoxin tetanospasmin.

that deprives tissues of oxygen. The most common causes of infarction are clots and other emboli.

Infarcts have a characteristic irregular appearance on surfaces of solid organs. On cross sections of kidney and spleen, infarcts are wedge shaped; the base of the wedge is at the periphery with the occluded vessel at the apex (see Fig. 7.7). The margins of the infarct may be irregular, a reflection of the vascular supply from adjacent, nonaffected tissue (Fig. 1.4). Initially, infarcts are commonly red because of hyperemia, but by 48 hours most become progressively more pale. At necropsy, infarcts of the kidney are usually white (ischemic) and are clearly demarcated from the surrounding normal tissue.

In organs that have collateral arterial supplies, such as the lungs and the gastrointestinal tract, infarcts are typically red (hemorrhagic). Extensive gastric necrosis is a complication of uremia, the systemic manifestation of end-stage renal disease (see Fig. 2.10). Uremia is associated with arteriopathy (a disease process in the artery) in the gastric mucosa, and arteriopathy leads to infarction. The gastric mucosa with massive infarction in prolonged canine uremia appears velvety and red black, with manifestations of swelling, edema, and hemorrhage.

Caseation necrosis

Caseation necrosis is a variant of coagulation necrosis in which dead tissue has a firm, dry, cheesy consistency. Caseation necrosis occurs when dead tissue is converted into a granular friable mass resembling cottage cheese. Caseation is characteristic of specific chronic bacterial diseases such as tuberculosis. Other examples are the lesions of caseous lymphadenitis of sheep and tularemia in primates. The chronicity of the cellular reaction and the presence of special lipids prevents liquefaction or resolution of these lesions.

Enzymatic necrosis of fat

Enzymatic necrosis of fat is a common sequela of steatitis and of other inflammatory lesions that occur in or are surrounded by adipose tissue. Grossly, the affected area loses the yellow translucent nature of fat and changes to a hard, white, opaque mass. The change is initiated by lipases that split neutral fats, releasing fatty acids that then undergo saponification. Histologically, these degraded lipids impart a granular eosinophilic appearance to the fat cell. Fat necrosis is a common finding in acute pancreatic necrosis and pancreatitis; enzymes released from damaged pancreatic acinar cells activate lipases in fat cells, which cause autodigestion of triglyc-

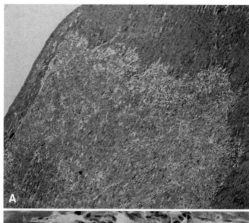
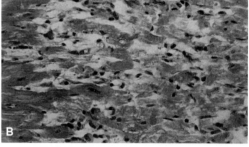

FIGURE 1.4. Infarction, heart. A. Low-power view showing irregular margins of the infarct. B. Necrotic myocytes (coagulation cell death) at the margins of the infarct.

erides. Fat necrosis is also seen in trauma of adipose tissue—for example, in the peripelvic fat after a difficult parturition of cows and other ruminants.

Liquefactive necrosis

Rapid enzymatic dissolution of the cell that results in complete destruction is referred to as **liquefactive necrosis**. Examples include pus and necrosis of the brain. A special form of liquefactive necrosis known as **malacia** appears as foci of softening in the brain and spinal cord. Brain tissue responds to severe toxic and hypoxic injury with characteristic focal dissolution of the neuropil.

Pus. Pus is a thick, opaque creamy fluid matter composed of an exudate of leukocytes, tissue debris, and microorganisms. Pus formation is sometimes referred to as suppuration. Pus develops in bacterial infections when proteolytic enzymes released from neutrophils convert dead leukocytes and cellular debris into a liquid amorphous material. Histologic examination of pus reveals dark, contracted, agranular neutrophils with varying amounts of tissue debris, fibrin, and plasma proteins. Pus is common in abscesses, ulcers, and empyema.

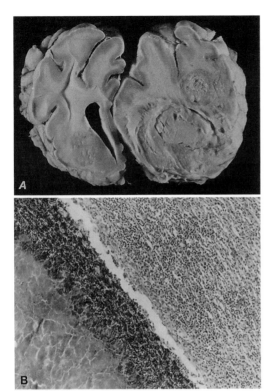

FIGURE 1.5. A. Abscesses in the brain of a cow. B. Abscesses consist of central area of homogeneous necrotic debris *(bottom left),* margin of degenerate neutrophils, and capsule of inflammatory cells and connective tissue *(top right).*

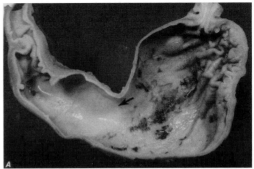

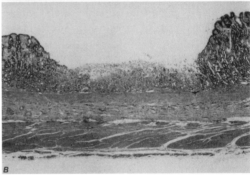

FIGURE 1.6. Gastric ulcers, aged dog with uremia. A. Ulcers occur largely in fundus and body of the stomach. Affected areas are clearly demarcated from the normal pylorus *(arrow).* B. Histology: ulcer involves necrosis and erosion of the mucosa but does not extend into the deep layers of the gastric wall.

Abscess. An **abscess** is a localized collection of liquefaction necrosis caused by suppuration deep in tissues. Abscesses start as focal collections of neutrophils in spaces created by necrosis and are nearly always produced by pyogenic bacteria. Abscess formation is an integral component of the inflammatory response. Abscesses are of great clinical importance when they obstruct critical blood vessels or ducts in organs such as the brain and lung (Fig. 1.5). **Empyema** is pus in a body cavity. Used unqualified, this term typically means thoracic empyema, since pus in the thorax is a common sequel to pyogenic infections of the thoracic cavity.

Ulcer. An **ulcer** is a local defect or excavation of a cutaneous or mucosal surface that is produced by sloughing of necrotic tissues. Focal necrosis on epithelial surfaces typically produces ulcers. Ulcers are common lesions in the skin, oral cavity, and gastrointestinal tract (Fig. 1.6). Ulcers are typically surrounded by inflammatory tissue. Acute ulcers are surrounded by a vascularized connective tissue barrier, and other components of acute inflammation.

Chronic ulcers will have fibroblastic proliferation at their bases and margins with scarring and infiltrates of lymphocytes and plasmacytes.

Postmortem changes

Interpretation of lesions is often clouded by tissue changes that have taken place between the time of death and the necropsy. Postmortem changes vary in the rapidity with which they occur, depending on environmental temperature and humidity and the condition of the animal (Table 1.1). For example, layers of fat, hair, or feathers act as insulators against heat loss after death.

Postmortem autolysis of cells is due to anoxia. When the heart stops, then blood circulation ceases and oxygen levels drop rapidly, so that cellular metabolism is shut down and autolysis begins. Autolytic changes mimic early ischemic change. Immediately after death, muscle cells show a massive uncontrolled burst of glycolysis. Uncoupled to oxidative phosphorylation, this energy is dissipated as heat. The body temperature (if measured in deep

TABLE 1.1. Postmortem changes

Algor mortis (cooling)—aids in estimating time of death
Rigor mortis (rigidity)—begins 2–4 hours after death
Postmortem clotting (thrombi are antemortem)
Hypostatic congestion (dependent lividity)—due to gravity
Pseudomelanosis (Fe + S → FeS)—green and black
Autolysis—involves no inflammatory response
Putrefaction—ruptures and displacement of organs
Emphysema—due to gas-producing bacteria
Biliary imbibition—green in liver around gall bladder

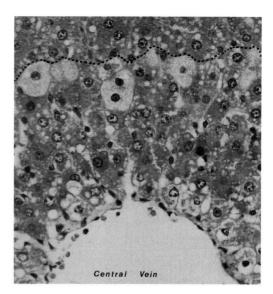

FIGURE 1.7. Centrolobular liver necrosis, rat, experimental carbon tetrachloride toxicity. Differences in pattern of cell death are related to the path of blood flow from portal triad *(top)* to the central vein *(bottom)*. Dotted line marks the border between midzone and centrolobular zone. Areas of effect: early degeneration *(top)*, hydropic degeneration (large foamy hepatocytes), coagulation necrosis, and cell lysis.

muscle masses) can be very high for a few minutes after death. This effect is transient, and the body cools rapidly to the ambient temperature.

Within the autolyzing cell, mitochondria are first affected by the accumulation of lactic acid and the precipitous drop in pH. Postmortem autolysis is characterized by relatively uniform destruction of the cell and all of its neighbors. In the cytoplasm, protein disintegrates into small granules and is distributed through the cell.

Rigor mortis

Rigor mortis, or stiffening of muscles, occurs 2–4 hours after death. Immediately after the circulation of blood ceases, there is a massive burst of metabolic activity as substrates are depleted. Much heat is produced in this period, and there is a progressive decrease in the pH of muscle. Oxygen, ATP, and creatine phosphate are also decreased. Muscle fibers shorten as they pass into rigor. This movement resembles contraction: it is initiated by Ca^{2+} efflux from sarcoplasmic reticulum of the muscle cell, it uses ATP as energy, and the structural changes that occur resemble those of contraction.

Rigor begins earliest in cardiac muscle and expresses the blood from the left ventricle. Failure to do this indicates antemortem degeneration in the heart. Of the skeletal muscles, the head and neck are first affected in most species, with progression to the extremities. Rigor disappears as putrefaction begins, a matter of 1–2 days, depending on external factors. Rigor mortis is enhanced by high metabolic activity and temperature before death and in diseases such as strychnine poisoning. It is delayed by starvation, cachexia, and cold.

Putrefaction

Putrefaction occurs when dead tissue is invaded by anaerobic, saprophytic organisms that digest proteins and form gas. Bacteria in the genus *Clostridium*, which are normally present in feces, are common in putrefaction. Foul-smelling substances formed during putrefaction include ammonia, hydrogen sulfide, indole, skatole, putrescine, and ca-

daverine. Tissue turns green and brown from breakdown of hemoglobin and formation of hydrogen sulfide.

CELL DEATH: MORPHOLOGY AND MECHANISMS

Here we examine death at the cellular level. Somewhat artificially, the mechanisms by which cells die have been placed in three patterns: coagulation cell death, cell lysis, and programmed cell death (referred to by some as "apoptosis"). Each of these patterns has unique mechanisms by which the death process is initiated, and cells dead of each type have distinct histologic characteristics. Some pathologists separate cell death into two types: "necrosis and apoptosis," but this is biologically unsound and is not consistent with the morphologic evidence of cell death.

The three patterns of cell death are not mutually exclusive and can develop concurrently. For example, in acute toxic injury of the liver, hepatocytes of centrolobular zones typically die by coagulation cell death, yet some cells die by lysis and, in liver tissue surrounding centrolobular zones, by programmed cell death (Fig. 1.7). In all of these patterns, the dying cell undergoes changes that are common to all mechanisms. These include the following:

- Depletion of ATP
- Acidification (drop in pH)
- Rise in Ca^{2+}
- Activation of lytic enzymes

Each of the above events affects normal cellular structure and function, and the extent to which each event develops determines the manifestations of cell death. Potent lytic enzymes (including proteases, phospholipases, and endonucleases) are activated in cell death, and differential activation of the enzymes in this spectrum underlies the differences in how the cell is killed.

Coagulation cell death (coagulation necrosis)

Histologic analysis of coagulation cell death (or coagulation necrosis) reveals that cells have collapsed into dense amorphous eosinophilic masses. Here the contraction of denatured proteins has caused loss of basophilia, and the abnormal cytoplasmic proteinaceous debris stains intensely with eosin. Calcium may be deposited in the dying cell because of marked ionic imbalances. Nuclei of necrotic cells are shrunken, and chromatin is condensed to solid, structureless masses, a condition called **pyknosis**. Chromatin clumping is a consequence of both protease activity and a decrease in cellular pH (which occurs as lactate builds up in the degenerating cell).

Coagulation cell death can be caused by many exogenous agents and mechanisms of injury that arise from within the animal, including these:

- Ischemia and other forms of anoxia and hypoxia
- Free-radical injury
- Blockade of DNA synthesis and transcription
- Blockade of pathways of peptide synthesis

FOCUS

Acute Cell Swelling

ACUTE CELL SWELLING that arises from lytic agents includes a spectrum of cellular changes that begins with proteolysis and water intake and ends with diffuse disintegration of soluble cytoplasmic proteins. With time, cells continue to swell uniformly, and this leads directly to cellular lysis. Acute cell swelling in surface epithelium is especially revealing because acute swelling of epithelial cells often underlies the formation of blisters, ulcers, or other diagnostically useful lesions.

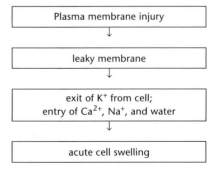

▶

▶

Histologic examination reveals that cells with acute swelling bulge from their normal limits. Swollen cells press on one another, and normal tissue architecture is distorted. In the **cytoplasm**, swelling of organelles causes a granular, cloudy appearance. Tiny granules of protein debris accumulate, and the cytoplasm becomes blurred and disorganized. **Nuclei** may undergo **karyolysis**, with disappearance of chromatin and other proteins. However, if lytic injury is rapid, nuclei shrink and move to the periphery of the cell.

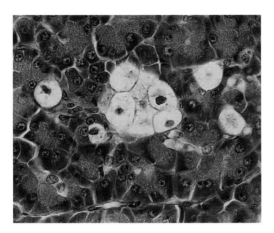

Vacuolar degeneration is a generic term indicating the presence of vacuoles in the cytoplasm. In acute injury of some cells, water and proteins are sequestered in cytoplasmic vacuoles. Membrane-bound pumps rapidly move ions and water out of the cytosol and into the cisternae of the endoplasmic reticulum, which expands to create large fluid-filled cytoplasmic vacuoles. Vacuolar degeneration tends to occur in cells with large amounts of membranes that actively pump ions.

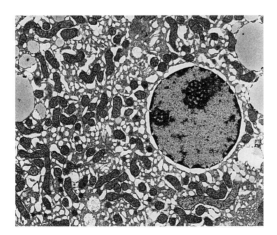

Pathogenesis of coagulation cell death

Early phase of cell degeneration: acute cell swelling. Acute cell swelling is expansion of cell volume due to loss of control of water intake. It is a fundamental expression of acute cellular injury and is to the dying cell what electrolyte imbalance is to the dying animal, a basic killing mechanism over which are superimposed many other degenerative phenomena. Acute cell swelling begins with a subtle accumulation of water in the cytosol and cisternae of endoplasmic reticulum. With time, cells continue to swell uniformly, or water may be sequestered in vacuoles formed by degenerating cytoplasmic organelles.

End stage of degeneration: collapse and shrinkage. In the cascade to cell death after injury, degenerating cells suffer indirect injury because of the interdependency of cell structures and functions. Secondary factors that amplify the cascade of degeneration into death include **pressure changes** of swelling, **lower pH** as lactate accumulates (acidosis), **increased metabolic rates** due to fever-induced temperature elevation, and **hypoxia**, which often results from decreased blood flow and directly affects mitochondria and energy production. Whatever the complicating events, they ultimately lead to depletion of ATP, the common energy currency of the cells. In the end, all energy-requiring processes are halted, and degeneration becomes necrosis.

Cell death: entry of Ca^{2+} kills the cell. When cell permeability is altered, Ca^{2+} rushes in from higher amounts present in interstitial fluids. Ca^{2+} is especially toxic to the cell and acts in three major ways: (1) Ca^{2+} normally regulates permeability of gap junctions between cells, and in the presence of high Ca^{2+}, rapid **uncoupling of gap junctions** isolates the injured cell from its neighbors, an attempt to prevent the spread of injury or infection. (2) Increased Ca^{2+} in the cytoplasm leads to **depolymerization of the cytoskeleton**; filaments and microtubules in the cell periphery disappear and cannot function in cell movement, phagocytosis, and secretion. (3) Ca^{2+} stimulates **activation of endogenous phospholipases** that are present in cell membranes, which leads to a cascade of reactions that cause membrane breakdown in the cell. Specific phospholipid molecules are present in the membrane in an asymmetric pattern and are maintained by an aminophospholipid translocase that moves specific phospholipids between the lipid bilayer leaflets. Loss of energy causes the phospholipid pattern to become symmetric, and this signals processes for cell death.

Proteins and enzymes leak from the injured cell. As cells die, proteins and other large molecules normally present in the cell escape into the interstitium and then into circulating blood. These proteins can be detected in circulating blood by the clinical pathologist and provide evidence of necrosis. When cell death occurs in the heart, skeletal muscle, and liver, specific enzymes appear in the blood and are assayed to assess the extent of necrosis. In **myocardial infarction**, for example, the rapid rise of serum creatine phosphokinase is useful in predicting the extent of necrosis of cardiac muscle cells. Massive damage to skeletal muscle leads to progressively increasing concentrations of muscle enzymes in plasma.

Energy deficit injury: oxygen deficit

Oxygen is required for production of the common energy currency of the cell, ATP. In turn, mitochondrial ATP production underlies all energy-requiring processes. When ATP production is blocked, all critical metabolic pathways in the cell are stopped.

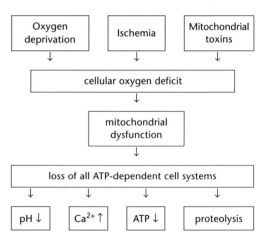

Oxygen deficiency, one of the most common causes of tissue injury, may be partial (**hypoxia**) or total (**anoxia**). When combined with increased body temperature, hypoxia becomes a potent cause of death. Oxygen deficit may be due to one or a combination of mechanisms that prevents oxygen from reaching its ultimate destination, the mitochondrion.

Three types of mechanisms that cause anoxia are **anoxic anoxia** (inadequate oxygen in the presence of adequate blood supply), **ischemic anoxia** (decrease of arterial flow and pressure, with stagnation and decrease in oxygen delivery), and **cytotoxic anoxia** (interference with oxygen utilization by the cell) (Table 1.2).

TABLE 1.2. Mechanisms of anoxia in cellular injury

Type	Mechanism	Example
Anoxic	Circulatory failure	Shock
	Erythrocyte deficiency	Anemia
	Respiratory failure	Pneumonia
Ischemic	Arterial blockade	Infarction
Cytotoxic	Mitochondrial lesion	Cyanide poisoning

Cellular changes that result from hypoxia vary according to the tissue affected and to the severity of the oxygen deficiency. The consequences are greater in visceral organs such as brain, heart, liver, and kidney, whose parenchymal cells are metabolizing to a high degree. These organs have elaborate vascular systems with shunts, anastomoses, and double blood supplies that protect them from some hypoxia. They are vulnerable, however, to severe hypoxia and anoxia.

The duration and form of oxygen deficit are important determinants of cellular injury. In death due to oxygen deficiency from asphyxiation (suffocation), **hypoxia** develops more slowly and many tissues are injured. Conversely, cyanide quickly causes death of the animal by the rapid inhibition of cytochrome oxidase in mitochondria of neurons. **Anoxia** develops because there is interference with utilization of oxygen, which results in damage to neurons and white matter.

When **anoxia** occurs, cell ATP values approach zero within seconds. As a result of loss of energy production, cell water volume control is lost and pumping of sodium into extracellular spaces cannot occur. Crucial morphologic changes develop in mitochondria (the sites of ATP generation) and in the cytocavitary network (which accumulates water). Calcium homeostasis is especially important for cell survival. As the level of calcium ions rises in the cytoplasm (because of a leaky cell membrane), widespread disintegration of cell cytoplasmic organelles occurs (Table 1.3).

Heart. Cardiac muscle extracts oxygen from blood efficiently. Mammalian skeletal muscle uses about 40% of the oxygen in the blood that circulates through the muscle. In contrast, cardiac muscle uses nearly 100% of the oxygen in the blood circulating through the myocardial capillaries. This high oxygen demand makes myocardium susceptible to systemic hypoxia. Shock and other diseases that severely compromise blood pressure and circulation are associated with small random foci of necrosis of the ventricular muscle.

FOCUS

The Reflow Injury Phenomenon

BLOCKAGE OF THE ARTERIAL SYSTEM of the heart leads to myocardial infarction. Cardiac muscle cells are killed and release their proteins into circulating blood. Much of the injury to the ischemic heart occurs not at the time of injury but after **reflow of blood** begins. Oxygen-induced resumption of ATP production by mitochondria provides energy for contraction. One of the earliest manifestations of hypoxia in myocardium is a "sensitization" to oxygen. When blood flow (and reoxygenation) to the hypoxic myocardium resumes, contraction of muscle cells occurs, and contraction of hypoxic cardiac myocytes is associated with increased plasma membrane permeability.

As hypoxic cardiac muscle cells become energy depleted, calcium and sodium levels rise and activate contractile proteins. With reoxygenation, the sudden increase in ATP induces cell contraction before ionic pumps can reestablish ionic equilibrium. Damage caused by calcium repletion is called the **calcium paradox** and is attributed to calcium overload due to uncontrolled entry of Ca^{2+} into the cells. Injury results from the multiple effects of Ca^{2+}, including the strong contracture of myofilaments, which causes sarcolemmal membrane defects.

TABLE 1.3. Cellular changes in anoxia

Mitochondrial shutdown
   Enzyme depletion
   Calcium pools altered
   Phospholipase activation
   β-Oxidation of fatty acids inhibited
Ion shifts in cytoplasm
   Entry of sodium
   Entry of calcium
   Loss of potassium
Metabolic shifts
Membrane lysis

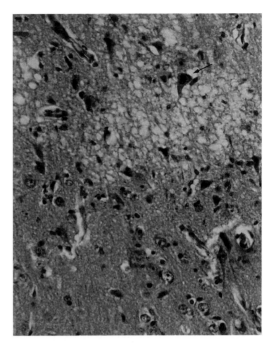

FIGURE 1.8. Brain damage (vacuolation and demyelination), dog with severe systemic anoxia during a prolonged epileptic seizure.

Myocardial infarction occurs when the arterial blood supply to the heart is blocked. Massive infarcts cause extensive myocardial necrosis and death.

Liver. Necrosis from oxygen deficit develops in centrolobular areas of the hypoxic liver. In mammals, ischemic hepatic necrosis occurs in cardiac failure, severe anemia, and shock with prolonged low circulatory flow rates. Necrosis is especially severe in combinations of these disorders. Hepatocytes in the centrolobular zone of the liver are preferentially affected because they are at the end of the sinusoid, a site where blood is hypoxic relative to cells in the other hepatic zones. In young animals, anoxic liver damage is more apt to result from severe anemia, especially when coupled with agonal cardiac insufficiency and reduced hepatic blood flow. Although the liver is supplied by both the portal vein and the hepatic artery, it remains susceptible to hypoxic injury because of its intense rate of metabolism. Blockage of the hepatic artery or portal vein (although this rarely happens clinically) can lead to hepatic necrosis.

Kidney. The renal cortex is highly sensitive to hypoxia, especially the proximal convoluted tubules, which are often affected in ischemic injury. Hypoxic injury is dependent on the ion transport rate in the proximal convoluted tubules and Henle's loop. That is, the consequences of hypoxia are influenced by energy demand and oxygen utilization.

The thick ascending limb of Henle's loop is selectively vulnerable to oxygen deficiency because of its high transport activity plus its meager oxygen supply. Thus hypoxia results in necrosis of the tubular segment of the nephron. This is such a distinctive lesion that this pattern of tubular necrosis is called **hypoxic (or ischemic) renal tubular necrosis**.

The renal medulla and papillary regions are also sensitive to hypoxia because it is there that blood pressure is lowest. In the severely hypoxic mammal, degeneration and necrosis preferentially occur in tubules at the corticomedullary junction. As hypoxia develops in the kidney, prostaglandins are synthesized and released by renal tissue, to cause vasodilation and increased blood flow. Drugs that decrease the production of prostaglandins, especially in the sick animal with poor circulation or dehydration, will exacerbate renal hypoxic damage, particularly in the papillary areas of the kidney. Some analgesic drugs (such as ibuprofen) cause **renal papillary necrosis** by depressing the enzymes that catalyze prostaglandin formation.

Brain. The brain is markedly sensitive to hypoxia. Newborn mammals suffer brain damage with transient asphyxia during birth in as little as 12 minutes. The cerebellum, precentral gyrus of the cerebral cortex, and auditory colliculus are selectively injured (Fig. 1.8). Hypoxic neurons become necrotic, astrocytes swell and show evidence of dissolution of chromatin, and myelin swells to form pale areas in the neuropil. In neurosurgery, cytopathic changes are produced in neurons even by temporary clamping of the larger cerebral arteries. When reflow of blood to the brain is reestablished, neuronal mitochondria swell and water accumulates in the cytoplasm.

Free radical injury

Mammalian cells, like the cells of all aerobic organisms that derive energy from the reduction of oxygen, are susceptible to cellular injury from free radicals. Free radicals are volatile and tissue-destructive molecules. The important free radicals and toxic intermediate compounds in mammalian cells are superoxide anion radical ($O_2^{\bullet-}$), hydroxyl radical ($OH^{\bullet}$), and hydrogen peroxide (H_2O_2), and all are generated during the metabolism of oxygen. The mitochondrial electron transport system is the major source of $O_2^{\bullet-}$. Cells generate energy aerobically by reducing oxygen to water. The cytochrome c oxidase–catalyzed reaction involves transfer of electrons to oxygen, a reaction that releases partially reduced oxygen species. As many as 5% of electrons in the respiratory chain lose their way, most ending as $O_2^{\bullet-}$. Any toxin that decreases the coupling efficiency of electron transport increases the production of superoxides. Superoxide is also generated enzymatically in the cytosol by xanthine oxidase or other oxidases:

$$O_2 \xrightarrow{\text{oxidase}} O_2^{\bullet-}$$

The presence of superoxide anion radicals leads to a protective cascade that is initiated by the enzyme superoxide dismutase (SOD):

$$2O_2^{\bullet-} + 2H^+ \xrightarrow{\text{SOD}} H_2O_2 \rightarrow OH^{\bullet}$$

The excessive accumulation of free radicals in the cell (due to imbalance of free radical generation and removal) is referred to as **oxidative stress**. The three radicals $O_2^{\bullet-}$, $OH^{\bullet}$, and H_2O_2, together with unstable intermediates of lipid peroxidation, are called **reactive oxygen species** (**ROS**). These radicals react with lipid membranes, proteins, and carbohydrates to induce cell damage. The lack of an electron in the free radical makes it oxidize proteins, membranes, genetic material, and any other cellular component.

Reactive oxygen species are a major cause of injury. However, free radical damage can also develop from unpaired electrons associated with nitrogen and carbon. Nitric oxide (NO) in excess acts like a free radical and can be converted to highly reactive **peroxynitrite anion** ($ONOO^-$), $NO_2^{\bullet}$, or NO_3^-. Peroxynitrite, the reaction product of nitric oxide and superoxide radical, $O_2^{\bullet-} + NO \rightarrow ONOO^-$, causes nitration of tyrosine residues as it is broken down. Aberrant addition of a nitrate group to the ortho position of tyrosine is one outcome of cellular oxidative stress that renders nitrated proteins dysfunctional.

Carbon-directed free radical injury is important in some toxins and is exemplified by the conversion of carbon tetrachloride to its toxic intermediate: $CCl_4 \rightarrow CCl_3^{\bullet} + Cl^-$. This reaction is driven by the P-450 mixed-function oxidases of the smooth endoplasmic reticulum (SER), the main detoxification organelle of the cell. Rapid destruction of SER membranes and formation of small vacuoles occur when $CCl_3^{\bullet}$ causes auto-oxidation of fatty acids of phospholipid molecules that make up the membrane (lipid peroxidation).

Iron is especially important in injury caused by ROS. Superoxide reduces ferric iron (Fe^{3+}) to ferrous iron (Fe^{2+}), which is required for iron to participate in the formation of hydroxyl radicals that enhance tissue injury:

$$H_2O_2 + Fe^{2+} \rightarrow Fe^{3+} + OH^{\bullet}$$

Membranes, DNA strands, and proteins are the cellular structures and organelles most affected by free radical–induced injury, in the following ways:

- Lipid peroxidation of **membrane** damage throughout the cell
- Random breakage of **DNA strands** in the nucleus
- Oxidation and cross-linking of **proteins**

Radiation kills cells by free radical injury. Lethal ionizing radiation induces formation of free radicals, either by direct ionization or indirectly by action of radiolytic products. In acute radiation injury, radiolysis of water in the cell leads to formation of highly toxic hydroxyl radicals, superoxide anions, and hydrogen peroxide. All of these react with membrane phospholipids to cause lipid peroxidation.

Toxins that block DNA, RNA, and peptide pathways

Toxins may produce selective injury to any segment of the pathways of protein synthesis, from transcription of genes, through translation of mRNA in the ribosome, to secretion of proteins from the cell. Toxins that act on DNA or on the polymerases that transcribe its genetic code tend to produce the most rapid and widespread changes. Cyclophosphamide, which is used clinically to treat cancer, causes necrosis in tissues with high mitotic rates by alkylating DNA nucleotides (guanosine is most markedly alkylated). Cells are killed if they are unable to repair the injury before they enter mitosis.

Cellular lysis (cytolysis)

Histologic examination of **cell lysis** reveals cells that are large, pale, transparent, and relatively

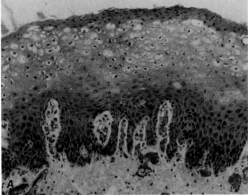

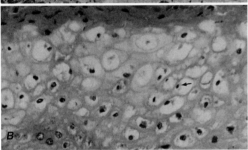

FIGURE 1.9. Acute cell swelling (hydropic degeneration) caused by a poxvirus (bovine papular stomatitis), oral mucosa, cow. A. Swollen cells are in the upper squamous layers. B. Ballooning of cytoplasm is accompanied by pyknosis and eccentricity of nuclei *(arrow)*.

structureless (Fig. 1.9). These characteristics are brought about by lytic destruction of cytoplasmic proteins, fragmentation of membranes, and acute swelling. Cells die from the effects of potent lytic toxins that act on proteins and membrane phospholipids. If proteases extend to the nucleus, there is also a pale structureless nucleus. Lysis of nuclear chromatin and disappearance of nuclear remnants are referred to as **karyolysis.**

To cause lysis, an etiologic agent must either have the properties of a potent protease or membrane toxin or have the capacity to in some way activate endogenous proteases of the cell. Most causal agents damage the plasma membrane barrier that controls water and electrolyte transport at the cell surface. In cellular lysis, the plasma membrane becomes leaky, sodium (Na^+) and calcium (Ca^{2+}) enter the cell, potassium (K^+) is lost, and water enters the cell and dilutes the cytoplasm. In contrast to coagulation necrosis, in which the architecture of the dead cell is preserved, lysed cells leave only small fragments remaining in affected tissue. The following are some of the important causes of cell lysis:

- Phospholipase toxins of bacteria, snake venoms
- Pore-forming bacterial toxins that insert into plasma membranes
- Complement (the attack sequence of complement, C5–C9)
- Viral infections that activate endogenous proteases or phospholipases
- Ca^{2+} entry from any cause (Ca^{2+} activates endogenous phospholipases)

Hydropic degeneration is a form of severe acute cell swelling in which free water dilutes the cytoplasm. Protease activation leads to proteolysis that clears the cytoplasm. In epithelium, this pattern of degeneration is common to many injuries and is called ballooning degeneration (see Fig. 1.9). Epithelial hydropic degeneration is often associated with blisters and is caused by etiologic agents as diverse as burns, bacterial toxins, and epitheliotropic viral diseases. Hydropic degeneration also occurs in sunburn injury to tongue epithelium, and ruminal epithelium of sheep and cattle that develop ruminal acidosis shows diffuse hydropic degeneration early in the disease.

Activation of endogenous proteases

By inhibiting metabolic processes on which the plasma membrane depends for its integrity, damage to **membrane ATPases** leads to swelling. Depression of electrolyte-pumping ATPases results in acute cell swelling. Depletion of cellular ATP by the blocking of oxidative phosphorylation in mitochondria is a common cause and most often occurs through anoxia, the deficit of oxygen (Table 1.4). Some toxins react specifically with cell surface ATPases to cause acute cell swelling; for example, digitalis acts on membrane ATPases of the cardiac myocyte. In the brain, the toxin triethyl tin inhibits

TABLE 1.4. Cellular damage in acute cell swelling caused by membrane damage

1. Plasma membrane barrier is broken—membrane becomes leaky with
    a. loss of potassium
    b. entry of sodium and calcium
2. ATP deficit—decrease in ion-pumping ATPases
3. Cells move more fluid by increasing the number of membrane pumps
4. Entry of calcium ions rises and
    a. uncouples gap junctions
    b. depolymerizes the cytoskeleton
    c. activates endogenous phospholipases in cell membranes
5. Plasma proteins enter the cell
6. Enzymes leak from the injured cell into the plasma

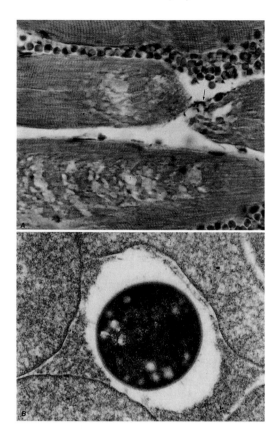

FIGURE 1.10. Muscle necrosis caused by *Clostridium septicum,* lamb: severe edema, gas production, and hemorrhage. A. Dissection of gas and fluid throughout degenerate muscle fibers; bacteria *(arrow).* B. Ultrastructure of bacterium surrounded by a zone of lysis and lysed, extravasated erythrocytes (hemorrhage).

ATPases on astrocyte foot processes, causing astrocytes to swell.

Membrane lysis from phospholipases

Direct destruction of cellular membranes by potent phospholipases is a common cause of cell lysis. The enzymatic attack is specifically directed to phospholipid molecules of membranes, and the most lethal effects are in membranes that make up the cell surface. **Exogenous phospholipases** are found in venoms, bacterial toxins, and other biologic toxins that hydrolyze membrane phospholipids at specific sites according to the nature of the attacking enzyme.

Extensive skeletal muscle necrosis occurs in **clostridial myositis** of sheep and cattle (Fig. 1.10). In this disease, bacteria of the genus *Clostridium* secrete powerful phospholipases that degrade membranes to cause massive lysis of myocytes, erythro-

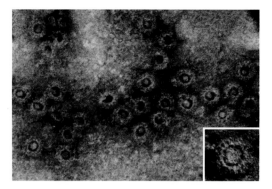

FIGURE 1.11. Complement components in plasma assemble on surfaces of an erythrocyte. Holes formed by complement complexes are seen on the surface of a lysed cell, negative staining. Rings, or annuli, are outlined by the stain. Intermediate lines in some annuli appear as globular stain deposits in radiating patterns. (Photographs: J. Tranum-Jensen, *Scand J Immunol* 7:45, 1978)

cytes, and blood vessels. Intracellular enzymes appear in circulating blood as they are released from the dying myocytes, and are an index for the extent of necrosis.

Lysis of membranes is also produced by **endogenous phospholipases**—for example, phospholipase A_2, which under an inappropriate stimulus is activated in ductular epithelial cells of the pancreas to produce acute pancreatic necrosis.

In **exertional rhabdomyolysis** of racing greyhounds, soluble enzymes released by damaged myocytes appear in plasma early in the disease (larger myoglobin molecules leak from the cell only after necrosis occurs). Flow of proteins also goes from plasma and interstitial fluid to cell. When cardiac myocytes are killed by anoxia, for example, they can be shown to contain albumin and, in severe injury, even globulin and fibrinogen.

Lysis from pore-forming toxins

Microbial pore-induced lysis. Cells are lysed when certain exogenous proteins localize and aggregate on the membrane to form protein complexes that are then inserted directly into the plasma membrane. These channels, called **porins**, function as pores to transmit ions and water, causing the cell to become leaky (Fig. 1.11). Porins are major mechanisms of virulence in bacterial and protozoal diseases and include leishporin of leishmaniasis, α-toxin of staphylococcal infection, perfringolysin of clostridial myositis, and α-hemolysin and enterohemolysin of infections caused by *Escherichia coli*. Secreted directly onto target cell surfaces, these potent porins cause lysis of host cells. Studies of ion conductance during pore formation on artificial membranes suggest that, with the appearance of each new pore, a discrete amount of current crosses the membrane. This change in current reflects the progressive incorporation of single channels into the lipid bilayer that makes up the plasma membrane.

Killer lymphocytes. Natural killer (NK) cells and certain cytotoxic T cells destroy microorganisms and other host cells by releasing **perforin**, a peptide that aggregates to form pores on target cell surfaces. The aggregated perforin molecules embed in the plasma membrane, causing the cell to become leaky. Cellular ion balances are disrupted, acute cell swelling develops, and the cell is lysed. In cell-mediated immune responses, protein antigens on surfaces of target cells attract T-cytotoxic cells and NK cells, which then secrete tiny perforins into the surface of the target cell. Some attacking lymphocytes also appear to inject a serine protease, granzyme B, through the perforin molecule into the cell to block specific metabolic pathways in or-

FOCUS

Hyperthermia and Rhabdomyolysis in Racing Greyhounds

FOCAL RHABDOMYOLYSIS (lysis of skeletal muscle cells) and myoglobinuria can occur after severe, prolonged exercise, especially in hot climates. Potassium ions (K^+) are released from contracting skeletal muscle fibers and dilate arterioles. When K^+ release is subnormal, a relative ischemia may develop, and tiny foci of necrosis develop in the hardest-working muscle groups.

Focal rhabdomyolysis is a problem in racing greyhounds. Typically, a winning dog is returned to the kennel, fed, and watered. Over the next 48 hours the dog develops stiffness, anorexia, and excessive thirst. Urine is apt to be voided in excess and is often slightly pink. Mucous membranes are dry and rose or purple. The epaxial muscles are swollen, often more severely on the right side (because of the running pattern of the track). Such dogs are frequently destroyed because they rarely return to top racing form. At necropsy, foci of rhabdomyolysis are common, and the lungs are congested.

Blood taken before death in one case had the following values in clinical pathology tests. These results reveal that glucose has been depleted and that ions and proteins have been released from dying cardiac muscle cells into the bloodstream.

Test	Hyperthermic dog	Normal
Glucose	10.0	70–110 mg/dl
Blood urea nitrogen	83.0	5–28 mg/dl
Alkaline phosphatase	274.0	10–100 IU
ALAT[a]	101.0	0–40 mU/ml
ASAT[b]	194.0	4–66 mU/ml
LDH	4,234.0	100 mU/ml
CPK	14,028.0	8–60 mU/ml
Sodium	88.8	140–155 mEq/l
Potassium	5.9	3.6–5.6 mEq/l

[a]Aspartate aminotransferase (SGOT).
[b]Aminotransferase (SGPT).

der to kill the target cell. Granzyme B from T cells also kills target cells by inducing apoptosis (see Programmed Cell Death, below).

Complement. Complement components are a circulating system of proteins that interact to bring about different protective functions. The complement **membrane attack sequence**, the last five components of complement (C5 through C9), act together. C5–C8 are required for C9 monomers to aggregate and polymerize. As the C9 molecule changes conformation, it is inserted into the plasma membrane, creating the 100-nm-diameter pores that cause the cell to lyse (Fig. 1.12). The pores allow sodium and calcium to enter the cell, cell water balance is destroyed, and the cell is lysed.

Programmed cell death

Programmed cell death (PCD) is a genetically controlled homeostatic mechanism that deletes cells that are no longer needed or that in some way would be damaging to the animal. In PCD, "death genes" encode for proteins that flow through the cytoplasm to collectively bring about cell death. These proteins direct other executioner molecules to break chromosomes, depolymerize the cytoskeleton, and cause mitochondria to dump cytochrome *c*—all events that kill and fragment the cell in a controlled manner.

In PCD, degenerative cellular changes evolve in orderly and reproducible sequences because genetic codes contain specific instructions for death. PCD occurs without clinical sequelae because the dying cell's function has been fulfilled. In contrast to other forms of cell death, cells dying in PCD do not release panic signals of impending death. There is no increase in surface molecules or release of cytokines that attract leukocytes or activate endothelial cells to initiate inflammation or repair. PCD is not accompanied by concomitant vascular injury, the major cause of inflammation in other types of necrosis.

Cellular change in programmed cell death

The following cellular characteristics appear to be unique for PCD and collectively are sometimes referred to as **apoptosis**:

- Nuclear chromatin aggregates and support fibrils (lamins) disconnect
- Cytoskeleton depolymerizes
- Cell junctions disengage, and cells become round
- Cytoplasmic blebs and pyknotic nuclei are shed from the cell
- Mitochondria are preserved, then suddenly disintegrate

Nuclei, which tend to be preserved until death occurs, either undergo karyorrhexis (rupture of the nuclear envelope with release of nuclear fragments) or are ejected from the cell. The round, homogenous, anuclear remnants of the dead cell that remain are called **apoptotic bodies**.

Processes in which PCD is critical

PCD plays an essential role in these processes:

- Gene-directed cell deletion in **embryogenesis**
- Cell loss in remodeling and involution of **atrophy**
- Removal of **neoplastic cells** or other cells with lethal mutations
- Deletion of cells damaged by some **toxins** and **infectious agents**

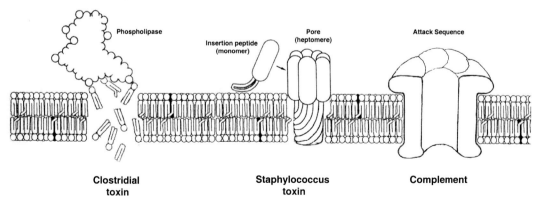

Membrane Lysis   **Membrane Pores**

FIGURE 1.12. Cell lysis. Different patterns of injury of the plasma membrane: membrane lysis (enzyme), pore formation (toxin), and channel formation (complement).

In **embryogenesis**, growth is controlled by normal genes in the chromosome that are activated and, in turn, activate death genes; the process is truly "programmed," being initiated and stopped by controlling genes. In **neoplastic mutation**, abnormal cells that have lethal mutations (often genes that are designed to control the cell cycle) are able to trigger PCD and thus prevent cancer from developing. In **acute cell injury**, cellular signals are generated when specific molecules bind to receptors at the cell surface, activating signal molecules that flow to the nucleus to activate death genes. In all cases—embryogenesis, cancer, and acute cell injury—the products of these death genes travel to the nuclei, mitochondria, and cell surfaces, where they control a regulated process of cell shutdown and death.

Much of the cellular change in PCD is brought about by a family of protein-cleaving enzymes known as **caspases** (for cysteine-containing aspartate specific protease). Caspases, which cleave their substrates at specific aspartic acid segments, play the critical roles in two phases of programmed cell death—**signaling** and **execution**. "Initiator caspases" (caspases 8 and 10) respond to death signals and activate the second group, the "executioner caspases" (caspases 3, 6, and 7), enzymes that make specific cuts in key proteins that are required for cell survival.

Initiation: signals control programmed cell death

Signals that initiate the process of PCD may be **extracellular** or **intracellular**. In embryogenesis, the initiating signal arises from within the cell. In contrast, signals from outside the cell can initiate PCD by binding to cell surface receptors. The pathways that lead to PCD include the following:

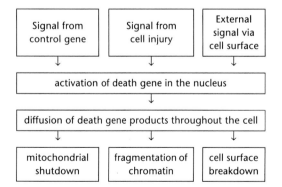

Genetic control. PCD is critical for **embryogenesis** because it permits the deletion of lineages of cells that are no longer required or that might in some way be destructive. In normal embryogenesis,

PCD is initiated by controlling genes in the nucleus. Gene-controlled PCD is also a significant mechanism in the tissue remodeling that accompanies **atrophy**—for example, involution of the uterus (after birth), mammary gland, and other organs in which previously functioning cells must be deleted without inciting other host cellular responses. PCD also plays a major role in **neoplasia** and other pathologic processes including inflammation.

Pathologic cellular processes. Cellular injury can initiate the terminal pathway of programmed cell death. In **sublethal injury**, cells are not killed directly but may be damaged in a way that is deleterious to the animal. In these pathologic processes, the cell can trigger PCD as a mechanism to remove the dead cell and repair injured tissue.

Genetic mutation in somatic cells occurs sporadically over the life span of an animal, and these abnormal cells are removed by PCD. The mutant gene codes for an abnormal protein, which, because it is abnormal, can trigger PCD. In the tissue proliferative responses, this deletion of mutant cells by PCD helps to prevent malignant cells from developing. This capacity is often missing in **cancer**, and it is known that any suppression of PCD diminishes the ability to control cell proliferation and increases the risk for development of cancer. The failure of the developing cancer cell to trigger PCD leads to the continued replication of the mutant cell.

External activation. Toxins, drugs, cytokines and steroid hormones can all initiate PCD via specific signaling events that occur at the cell surface. When a PCD-inducing toxin attaches to a critical receptor molecule embedded in the plasma membrane, a specific signal is conveyed to the nucleus to activate death genes. Potent cytokines such as **tumor necrosis factor-α** can trigger PCD in target cells by activating PCD. **Fas–Fas ligand signaling** is an important mechanism for PCD via external signaling. Binding of Fas to FasL activates PCD. That is, binding of Fas, a membrane-spanning protein on one cell, to FasL on the cell membrane of another cell, is a stimulus for PCD to begin.

Execution: the final pathway— the "caspase cascade"

The final death event centers on the ratio of the protein products of two families of genes: *Bax* genes that lead to cell death, and the *Bcl-2* genes, which are death repressor genes. It is this ratio of agonist to antagonist that determines whether or not the cell will respond to signals for PCD. *Bax* (and a related gene *Bak*) encode proteins that induce PCD.

FOCUS

Fas Signaling

ONE OF THE MOST IMPORTANT MECHANISMS for programmed cell death via external signaling is **Fas–Fas ligand (FasL) signaling**. Binding of Fas on one cell to FasL of another cell is the stimulus for PCD to begin. Fas-FasL signaling controls the killing of target cells in T cell–mediated cytotoxicity. When FasL binds to Fas (its receptor), it induces death in Fas-bearing cells. Many cells express Fas, whereas only activated T cells express FasL. In PCD via Fas binding, the first signal is caspase 8 activation at the cell surface, at the site where the Fas extends through the plasma membrane into the cytoplasm. FasL on the lymphocyte surface binds to the Fas protein on a target cell, causing Fas molecules to form surface clusters. An adapter protein called FADD (for "Fas-associated death domain") then binds to the clustered Fas-FasL molecules. Because FADD also contains a caspase-binding domain, it recruits inactive precaspase 8 molecules, which then auto-activate to initiate the caspase cascade.

Target Cell

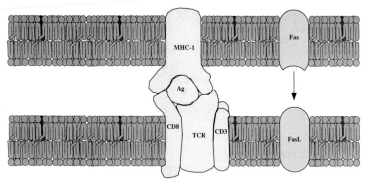

Cytotoxic T Cell

1. Antigen presented by target cell MHC-1 to T cell receptor
2. TCR-CD8 transduces signals for granule exocytosis and FasL transcription
3. Fas-FasL binding initiates cell death

Fas signals between lipid bilayer members of killer and target cells.

Lymphocyte death in **thymic atrophy** of young animals, particularly in the thymic destruction caused by viruses, may follow a similar type of PCD. Destruction of antigen-reactive T cells in virus-infected patients appears to occur through activation of similar mechanisms. CD4$^+$ and CD8$^+$ cells become unresponsive to antigen stimulation and, in this anergic or hyperactive state, may be programmed for cell death much as thymocytes are in the depletion of T cells in thymic atrophy. Deletion of lymphocytes in feline immunosuppressive virus infection (like human HIV infection) may be a response to binding of virus to lymphocyte CD4 surface antigens.

Abnormal Fas systems are associated with lymphoproliferative disorders and accelerated autoimmune disease.

In contrast, PCD is prevented by the Bcl proteins that function as death repressor molecules. If *Bcl-2* is inactivated or deleted from a cell, PCD is initiated. Bcl-2 family proteins exert potent effects on mitochondria, probably by inserting as pores or ion channels in the outer mitochondrial membrane.

Bcl-2 blocks the release of cytochrome *c* from mitochondria, possibly by blocking ionic imbalances that lead to mitochondrial swelling. Bcl proteins also appear to directly bind to Apaf-1 (see Mitochondrial Shutdown, below) to prevent caspase activation. *Bcl* genes are particularly important in neoplasia; excess amounts of Bcl-2 can contribute to cancer by making cells unresponsive to death signals.

Mitochondrial shutdown. In the caspase cascade, the final pathway to programmed cell death, mitochondria play a critical role, and the initial event involves the loss of permeability in mitochondrial membranes. Cytochrome *c* released from mitochondria binds to a critical protein, **apoptotic protease activating factor-1** (Apaf-1), which in turn binds to and activates caspase 9:

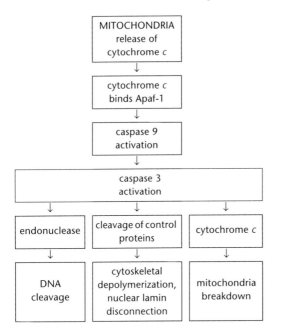

Dysfunction of mitochondria, which kills the cell, is associated with a phenomenon called **mitochondrial permeability transition**. The collapse of normal membrane permeability, represented by $\Delta\Psi\mu$, is due to abnormal opening of mitochondrial transition pores, which in turn leads to a host of changes that include collapse of $\Delta\Psi\mu$, uncoupling of the respiratory chain, depletion of NAD(P)H, reduced glutathione, generation of superoxide anion, cessation

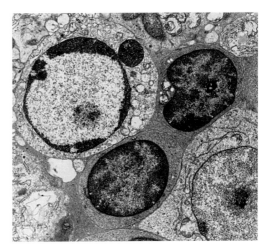

FIGURE 1.13. Programmed cell death, lymph node, brucellosis. Lymphocyte death with aggregation of chromatin at the periphery of the nucleus and degeneration of cytoplasmic organelles.

of ATP synthesis, outflow of matrix Ca^{2+}, and dumping of cytochrome *c* and other membrane proteins into the cytosol—all changes associated with death of the cell.

Endonuclease activation and DNA cleavage. One of the early events in PCD is the cleavage of DNA into uniform nucleosomal fragments that aggregate into dense clumps of chromatin (Fig. 1.13). Microscopic examination of cells in PCD shows masses of dense chromatin in crescentic aggregates along the inner nuclear envelope. Biochemists show that a characteristic DNA fragmentation appears clearly on gel electrophoresis of pooled DNA extracts—for example, a unique ladder of nucleosomal DNA fragments. Histochemical studies with in situ labeling of DNA breaks in nuclei in tissue sections reveal that chromatin cleavage is initiated at the periphery of the nucleus and is relatively short and that cell death occurs in clusters.

Cytoskeletal degradation. The morphologic evidence of cell death includes a peculiar rounding of the cell. This change, when accompanied by karyorrhexis and loss of internal structure, is called single-cell necrosis and is now thought to be a prototypic manifestation of PCD. Cell rounding is due to multiple breaks in the cytoskeleton, particularly depolymerization of actin microfilaments and loss of their connections to the plasma membrane. Like small hernias, the loss of cytoskeletal support allows formation of cytoplasmic blebs at the cell surface. Bleb formation, a general prelude to cell death, is not restricted to PCD.

CELL PROTECTION AND RECOVERY

In response to injury, cells rapidly shift metabolic pathways, synthesizing unique proteins and altering the spectrum of pumps and receptors on the cell surface. All of these events are directed to removing damaged components and neutralizing toxic compounds that have entered the cell. To do this, the cell must trigger genes that control these processes. The genetic control of cell repair and recovery tells us much about survival, and defines how the host response to disease occurs (Table 1.5).

Production of antioxidant enzymes

Superoxide anions ($O_2^{\bullet-}$) are formed nonenzymatically in all aerobic cells from the autoxidation of components of the mitochondrial electron transport chain (small amounts of $O_2^{\bullet-}$ are also formed from enzymatic reactions involving xanthine oxidase and other oxidases in the cytosol). In mitochondria, the electron transport system is designed to produce water as the sole product of oxygen reduction. Large-scale production of $O_2^{\bullet-}$, hydrogen peroxide, and hydroxyl radicals ($OH^{\bullet}$) are thereby avoided. However, finite quantities of these reactive

TABLE 1.5. Cell mechanisms for recovering from injury

1. Antioxidants that counteract free radicals increase
   a. superoxide dismutase
   b. glutathione peroxidase
   c. ubiquitins to degrade abnormal proteins
2. Energy production shifts to anaerobic glycolysis
3. Protein synthesis is redirected to form stress proteins
4. Membrane pumps and receptors are altered
   a. ATPases (sodium pumps) increase
   b. P-glycoprotein (toxin pump) increases
   c. surface receptors shift
5. Detoxifying enzymes increase in smooth endoplasmic reticulum
6. Gap junctions between cells shut down
7. Genes that control the external environment are activated
   a. hypoxia inducible factor gene (vasodilation, erythropoiesis)
   b. genes for DNA repair
   c. synthesis and release of cytokines, which stimulate acute phase proteins
8. Genes that modulate cell activities are activated to produce proteins
   a. p53, which blocks DNA synthesis in the cell cycle
   b. Bcl-2, which blocks programmed cell death

intermediates are produced in aerobic organisms by minor pathways of oxygen utilization and, when they accumulate, can result in hazardous consequences. Inside the cell, $O_2^{\bullet-}$ reacts with proteins, DNA, and lipids. The best known of these reactions is the interaction of toxic $O_2^{\bullet-}$ with amino acids, a cause of significant damage to cellular proteins.

All cells that operate in an aerobic environment contain **superoxide dismutases** (SODs), enzymes that protect against toxic effects of the toxic oxygen metabolite, superoxide anion ($O_2^{\bullet-}$). SODs are found in the mitochondrial matrix and in the cytosol—the sites where most superoxide anion is generated. SODs catalyze the conversion of potentially harmful superoxide free radicals to hydrogen peroxide and oxygen:

$$2O_2^{\bullet-} + 2H^+ \xrightarrow{\text{SOD}} H_2O_2 \rightarrow O_2$$

Increased amounts of SOD have been found in chronic toxicity; for example, in human alcoholics, SODs prevent some of the sequelae of alcohol toxicity. In animals and microorganisms, tolerance of high environmental oxygen is closely correlated with increased cellular levels of superoxide dismutase.

Hydrogen peroxide produced by SOD is reduced to water by two enzymes: **catalase** in peroxisomes and **glutathione peroxidase**, an enzyme in the cytosol and mitochondria. The oxygen-oxygen bond of hydrogen peroxide can be split by a reaction involving iron (the Fenton reaction) to yield the innocuous hydroxide anion (OH^-) and the very reactive hydroxyl radical ($OH^{\bullet}$).

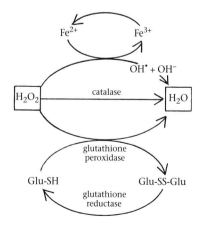

Glutathione peroxidase catalyzes the oxidation phase, and the cyclic oxidation and reduction of glutathione provide a major antioxidation phenomenon in the cell.

$$\text{Glutathione (reduced)} + H_2O_2 \rightarrow$$
$$\text{glutathione disulfide} + H_2O$$

Peroxides are destroyed by this reaction immediately after they are generated during the interaction of membranes with free radical groups. Glutathione peroxidase is protective in normal cellular catabolism and is highly protective in most types of oxidative injury. It is especially important in myocardium, which has less SOD and catalase than do liver and other tissues. The cell's capacity to detoxify oxygen radicals is reflected by the ratio of oxidized glutathione (Glu–SS–Glu) to reduced glutathione (Glu–SH).

Selenium is a cofactor of glutathione peroxidase. Dietary Se is essential for survival, even in embryos, largely because selenoproteins play such a critical role in antioxidant defense. Pathogenic bacteria, eukaryotes, and even one virus (poxvirus) use selenoproteins for protection against cytotoxicity of hydrogen peroxide and toxic oxygen radicals.

Vitamin E is a strong biologic antioxidant molecule. It is lipid soluble and is an antioxidant in lipid environments, particularly in and near cellular membranes. Vitamin A and ascorbic acid are other antioxidants that block or inactivate free radicals.

Anaerobic shift of glycolysis

When a cell is deprived of oxygen, mitochondrial function rapidly ceases. ATP-utilizing processes such as membrane transport of Na^+, filament contraction, and phagocytosis continue for a short time, but ATP is rapidly depleted, leaving excesses of ADP and inorganic phosphate. Depletion of ATP results in activation of phosphofructokinase, which leads to this progression: fructose-1,6-diphosphate formation, pyruvate kinase activation, pyruvate accumulation. Pyruvate is converted to lactate with a fall in cell pH and an increase in H^+ concentration. These events represent the **anaerobic shift** to glycolysis and are the hallmark of the anoxic cell. Glycogen is rapidly broken down, and calcium accumulates. The shift from aerobic respiration in mitochondria to the more transient and inefficient anaerobic glycolysis may prevent irreversible damage. Ultimately, for the cell to survive, other mechanisms to prevent cell degeneration are required.

The effect of the anaerobic shift depends on continued availability of glucose. Resistance to ischemia of cardiac muscle cells of starved animals (which accumulate myocardial glycogen) illustrates the value of glycogen. Ligation of coronary arteries of rabbits produces myocardial necrosis, but if rabbits had been starved before ligation, cell degeneration was less severe.

Shift in protein synthesis: stress proteins

A major response to injury is a shift in protein synthesis. The machinery for production of new proteins is shifted away from normal proteins designed for export and is redirected to **stress proteins**, unique molecules that protect the cell by binding to other, abnormally folded or denatured proteins. Stress proteins appear rapidly in the injured cell and accumulate in the cytoplasm. Cells that produce stress proteins survive an otherwise lethal amount of injury; conversely, cells in which the capacity to produce stress proteins has been destroyed are much more susceptible to heat than normal cells. In cell cultures, addition of these proteins will prevent necrosis from an otherwise lethal dose of toxins.

Families of stress proteins have been identified that not only function in protein degradation but also control and stabilize peptide chains that are held in the cell for an appropriate time for assembly into larger proteins. The prototype stress protein BiP binds transiently to normal peptides (but permanently to malfolded peptides) to control assembly into protein chains; for example, in plasmacytes, BiP binds to immunoglobulin heavy chains within the rough endoplasmic reticulum until they can complex with appropriate light chains to form the immunoglobulin molecule.

Increase in membrane pumps

Increasing the numbers of channels and ion pumps on the cell surface is a strategy used for survival. As more ion pumps are placed on the plasma membrane, cytoplasmic fluids are moved out of the cell. In the initial stages of acute swelling, cells increase ion transport by increasing the number of Na-K-ATPase pumps and by expanding pump-bearing surface membranes. In the colon of animals deprived of sodium, epithelial cells show marked expansion of basolateral surfaces and increased ATPase activity. The new membrane surfaces are a response to move more Na^+ into the body from gut fluids. Thyroid hormone causes increased amounts of ATPase pumps, and this mechanism underlies the increased cellular activity in hyperthyroidism. Epinephrine also suppresses cell swelling by regulating ATPase pumping on cell surfaces.

Increasing plasma membrane channels that expel toxins from the cell is a major protective mechanism. One of the most important membrane channel proteins, called **P-glycoprotein**, functions as a "hydrophobic vacuum cleaner" to excrete hydrophobic drugs, anesthetics, and toxins. P-glycoprotein is especially important in secretory cells of the renal tubular epithelium.

Cytoplasmic proteolysis: autophagy and ubiquitinization

Autophagy is the uptake and degradation of damaged cellular organelles into cytoplasmic vacuoles. Microscopically, these autophagic vacuoles can be seen to arise by budding from membranes of the endoplasmic reticulum and fusing with lysosomes to acquire enzymes that degrade the damaged cellular components. Autophagy is part of normal metabolism in the cell, but it is markedly increased in cellular injury. In fact, cellular injury of any kind is a stimulant for autophagy to begin.

Ubiquitinization is another proteolytic process that is used in normal cells to selectively degrade unwanted proteins. Attachment of ubiquitin to abnormal peptides allows their recognition by a proteolytic complex that degrades the substrate protein. The process is controlled by the specificity of ubiquitin. The proteosome, a granular complex found in all eukaryotic cells, is the structural site of the proteolytic complexes of ubiquitinization. It is a hollow cylinder with multiple catalytic sites that carry out the events of ubiquitinization.

Microbial pathogens alter the ubiquitin system as a means of surviving in the host, and they use

FOCUS

Cellular Ions and the Sodium Pump

NORMALLY, WATER TRAVERSES THE CELL passively by diffusion equilibrium. Intracellular water is regulated by modification of electrolyte composition, chiefly Na^+ and K^+, thereby regulating cell volume. The ionic concentrations (in mEq) in the cell are Na^+ 12 and K^+ 155; in extracellular fluid the concentrations are Na^+ 145 and K^+ 4. This unequal distribution across the plasma membrane is maintained by the enzyme Na-K-ATPase (sodium-potassium-dependent adenosine triphosphatase). Na-K-ATPase is an integral protein embedded in the lipid bilayers of membrane; it functions at the cell surface and on internal membranes of the cell. As Na-K-ATPase interacts with ATP (its energy source), the configuration of the molecule changes to permit Na^+ to be pumped out of the cell; this again changes the molecule so that K^+ can flow into the cell in the same operation. Na-K-ATPase is called the sodium-potassium pump because the movement of ions is linked in actively pumping Na^+ out of and K^+ into the cell.

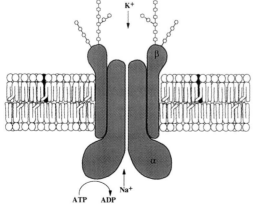

Sodium-potassium pump (Na-K-ATPase) embedded in the phospholipid bilayer of the cell's plasma membrane.

proteosomes and the ubiquitin system to replicate. For example, the papilloma E6 gene binds to the tumor suppressor p53 and induces its ubiquitinization and degradation. Levels of p53 are thereby reduced, increasing the chances of oncogenicity.

DNA repair

DNA molecules are not permanent but slowly undergo decay. This requires mechanisms of repair that, after toxic or irradiation injury to DNA, maintain normal cellular genomes. These elaborate procedures to protect the DNA molecule against mutagenesis include two major pathways: (1) the altered part of the molecule may be repaired in situ (with or without enzymes), or (2) a damaged segment of DNA and replacement with newly synthesized DNA units can occur by a complex enzymatic process called excision, or "cut-and-patch" repair. This process involves endonucleases (for incision of damaged DNA segments), exonucleases (for subsequent degradation), polymerases (for initiation of DNA replication for repair), and ligases (for rejoining of the new segment into the DNA molecule). DNA repair is critically important in radiation injury. Radiation kills cells by breaking DNA in the presence of oxygen. Damage is mediated by free radicals that cause single-strand damage; that is, injury is oxygen mediated and free-radical induced.

Activation of genes to protect the cell

Hypoxia is a strong signal for energy conservation

Hypoxic cells sense diminished oxygen levels well before their ATP pools are depleted, responding with a program to curb energy use by shutdown of nonessential cellular functions. Hypoxia triggers expression of genes involved in the protective response, including isoforms of glycolytic enzymes and glucose transporters that function best in a low-oxygen environment. Many of these responses arise through hypoxia-induced activation of genes that function both to change cellular metabolism and to cause changes in the cell's environment. The **hypoxia inducible factor 1** (HIF-1) gene is a pivotal regulator of hypoxic gene expression, and the responses to hypoxia include adaptation to anaerobic metabolism and stimulation of angiogenesis, vasodilation, and erythropoiesis.

The *Bcl-2* gene encodes a death repressor molecule

The *Bcl-2* gene encodes for a 25-kd integral membrane protein that is localized in mitochondria, the nuclear envelope, and endoplasmic reticulum. The *Bcl-2* product prevents PCD, and when it is blocked or inactivated, cell death ensues. *Bcl-2* was discovered as an oncogene in human follicular B-cell lymphoma that carries the chromosomal translocation (14;18)(q32;q21) in which *Bcl-2* sequences are juxtaposed to immunoglobulin heavy chains on chromosome 14. Translocation leads to the marked overexpression of *Bcl-2*.

The *p53* gene controls the cell cycle

The gene *p53* plays critical roles in programmed cell death by blocking the cell cycle and stimulating DNA repair. This gene encodes p53, a protein that holds cells in the G_1 phase of the cell cycle for repair. Acting as a transcription factor, p53 binds to and controls other genes. Acting as a "guardian of the genome," p53 blocks the cell cycle to provide time for DNA repair and, if injury is too severe, to trigger programmed cell death. Any injury to DNA induces the expression of *p53* and the product of *p53* rises in cells with DNA damage.

ADDITIONAL READING

Necrosis

Bouchard PR, et al. 1994. Uremic encephalopathy in a horse. *Vet Pathol* 31:111.

Chen CS, et al. 1997. Geometric control of cell life and death. *Science* 276:1425.

Griffiths IR, et al. 1994. Autonomic neurons from horses with grass sickness contain serum proteins. *Vet Rec* 135:90.

O'Brien TD, et al. 1986. Hepatic necrosis following halothane anesthesia in goats. *J Am Vet Med Assoc* 189:1591.

Cell death

Chervonsky AV, et al. 1997. The role of Fas in autoimmune diabetes. *Cell* 89:17.

Farber JL, et al. 1990. Mechanisms of cell injury by activated oxygen species. *Lab Invest* 62:670.

Golstein P. 1997. Controlling cell death. *Science* 275:1081.

Good PF, et al. 1996. Evidence for neuronal oxidative damage in Alzheimer's disease. *Am J Pathol* 149:21.

Green DR, Reed JC. 1998. Mitochondria and apoptosis. *Science* 281:1309.

Guillemin K, Krasnow M. 1997. The hypoxic response. *Cell* 89:9.

Hack CE, et al. 1997. A role for secretory phospholipase A_2 and C-reactive protein in the removal of injured cells. *Immunol Today* 18:111.

Kroemer G. 1997. The proto-oncogene *Bcl-2* and its role in regulating apoptosis. *Nat Med* 3:614.

Moore RM, et al. 1995. Mechanisms of gastrointestinal ischemia-reperfusion injury and potential therapeutic interventions. *J Vet Intern Med* 9:115–132.

Moslen MT. 1994. *Free radicals in diagnostic medicine.* D. Armstrong, ed., Plenum Press, New York.

Nieminen A-L, et al. 1997. Mitochondrial permeability transition in hepatocytes induced by *t*-BuOOH: NAD(P)H and reactive oxygen species. *Am J Physiol* 272:C1286.

Ojcius DM, et al. 1998. Pore-forming proteins. *Sci Med* (Jan–Feb):44.

Trump BF, Berezesky IK. 1995. Calcium-mediated cell injury and cell death. *J FASEB* 9:219.

Cell protection and recovery

Adams JM, Cory S. 1998. The Bcl-2 protein family: arbiters of cell survival. *Science* 281:1322.

Jortner BS, et al. 1996. Ubiquitin expression in degenerating axons of equine cervical compressive myelopathy. *Vet Pathol* 33:356.

Wu MX, et al. 1998. IEX-1L, an apoptosis inhibitor involved in NF-κB–mediated cell survival. *Science* 281:998.

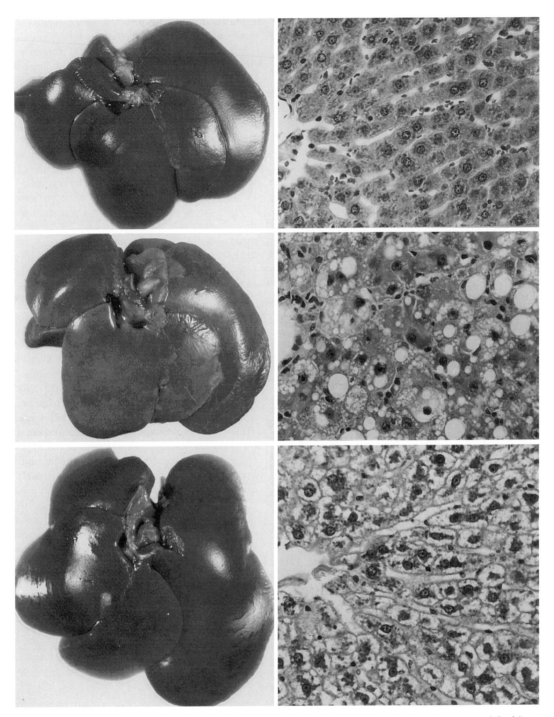

FIGURE 2.1. Cellular degeneration in the liver, rat: *left,* gross appearance; *right,* histologic changes. *Top,* normal liver with normal hepatocytes, central vein, and parallel sinusoids. *Middle,* fatty degeneration, sublethal carbon tetrachloride toxicity. *Bottom,* glycogen degeneration, treatment with large dose of cortisol (glycogen has been removed during tissue processing, leaving empty spaces).

▦ CHAPTER 2

Cell and Tissue Responses to Sublethal Injury

In sublethal injury, cells degenerate more slowly than when the cell is lethally injured. Cellular degeneration (L. *degeneration,* deterioration) is characterized by accumulation of catabolic products and abnormal protein complexes. The manifestations of injury are not swelling and lysis or cellular collapse and death, but more slowly developing shifts in metabolic pathways, causing molecules of lipids, proteins, or glycogen to accumulate and distort the cell (Fig. 2.1).

The type of pathologic change that develops in response to injury depends on (1) **duration of the etiologic agent's effect** and its **concentration** in tissue; (2) **tissue vascular supply and blood flow** to the injured cell, including oxygen availability, pH, and temperature; and (3) **metabolic characteristics of the cell**. Metabolically active cells are, in general, most susceptible to injury, and that is why patterns of degeneration are so meaningful in liver, kidney, and muscle.

METABOLITE OVERLOAD

The production and accumulation of small amounts of lipids, glycogen, and proteins in the cytoplasm occur as part of the normal physiologic processes in liver, kidney, muscle, and other organs with high rates of metabolism. Sublethal injury shifts metabolic pathways, so that these substances accumulate in large amounts, a condition that, if severe, alters cellular structure and function.

Fatty degeneration

Fatty degeneration (fatty change, lipidosis) is the accumulation of neutral lipids in the cytoplasm. Fat is a normal product, and fatty degeneration is an exaggeration of triglyceride production in which fats accumulate as large cytoplasmic globules of triglycerides. In theory, fatty degeneration can oc-cur in any tissue. However, the swollen, yellow, greasy appearance of fatty degeneration is characteristic of liver and, less commonly, of kidney and heart. Nearly all tissues develop cytoplasmic lipids upon injury, but few others produce lipid globules sufficient to alter the gross appearance so strikingly.

In fatty degeneration, triglyceride production exceeds the slower, more elaborate events in the production of lipoproteins or in the shunting of fatty acids into mitochondria for energy production. Normally, the amount of triglycerides awaiting processing is small, and few lipid globules are in hepatocytes. When injury destroys any part of the lipid metabolic pathway, substrate molecules begin to accumulate (e.g., cholesterol, phospholipids, or fatty acids). It is the massive backlog of triglycerides, however, that dominates the changes of fatty degeneration (Fig. 2.2).

Fatty degeneration is a diagnostic clue for liver injury. Excess lipids in hepatocytes indicate that sublethal injury has occurred. Clinical diseases associated with hepatic fatty degeneration include the following:

- Acute toxic injury that affects pathways of lipid metabolism
- Chronic metabolic diseases, with loss of enzymes or receptors (diabetes)
- Chronic hypoxia, which suppresses lipid-metabolizing enzymes
- Long-standing elevation of blood lipids

Microscopically, lipid accumulation causes cells to be enlarged, pale, and lacy. Solvents used in routine histologic processing dissolve out fats, leaving clear spaces. To distinguish lipids from the clear spaces of hydropic degeneration, tissue sections are specifically stained for fats using lipid-soluble dyes such as Sudan III or oil red O. In hepatocytes with fatty degeneration, the distribution and size of lipid

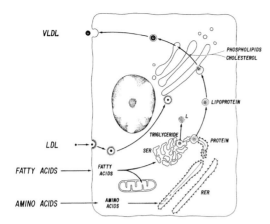

FIGURE 2.2. Hepatocyte lipid metabolism. Triglycerides are formed from fatty acids and shunted from the site of their production in the smooth endoplasmic reticulum (SER) to lipid globules (L) in the cytoplasm. Low-density lipoproteins (LDLs), which carry cholesterol, bind (via apoprotein) to LDL receptors on hepatocyte surfaces and stimulate formation of coated vesicles for endocytosis. LDLs are delivered to vacuoles where their proteins and cholesterol are hydrolyzed. Lipoproteins are assembled by combination of triglycerides from smooth endoplasmic reticulum and apoprotein from rough endoplasmic reticulum (RER). After further processing, the final product—very low density lipoproteins (VLDLs)—is released at the hepatocyte surface.

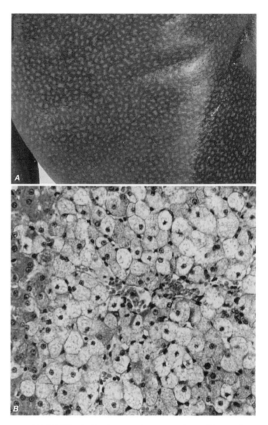

FIGURE 2.3. Fatty degeneration, liver, dog with diabetes mellitus. A. Centrolobular distribution of pale areas of necrosis. B. Foamy, lipid-laden hepatocytes around a central vein.

globules are a crude indication of the type of injury. Small-droplet degeneration is typical of acute metabolic disease and is always coincident with ionic imbalance and some degree of acute cell swelling (Fig. 2.3). Large-droplet fatty degeneration is characteristic of more slowly developing toxic or viral injury.

Toxic injury and fatty liver

Toxins that cause imbalance among supply, utilization, synthesis, and release of lipids typically cause fat to accumulate. Toxins may shunt fatty acids into triglycerides by preventing fatty acid activation by CoA or by blocking the passage across the mitochondrial membrane for entry into mitochondrial matrix energy pathways in the citric acid cycle. Toxins also may form lipids by blocking protein synthesis, lipoprotein granule assembly, or release of lipoprotein granules at the cell surface. Lipid production is also altered by interference with enzymes bound to membranes of the smooth endoplasmic reticulum (such as the triacylglycerol synthetase complex) that transfer fatty acids to glycerol to form triglycerides. The kidney is also apt

to be involved in acute injury or metabolic disease.

Sublethal doses of some toxins produce fatty degeneration in the liver by depressing protein synthesis. Toxins as diverse in mechanism as carbon tetrachloride and aflatoxin ultimately affect ribosomes and their ability to produce peptide chains. If cells are not killed outright by acute cell swelling, they survive to develop massive triglyceride accumulation. Deprived of newly emerging peptide chains, the hepatocyte cannot conjugate triglycerides and is deprived of proteins that serve as enzymes in lipid metabolism. Because apoproteins are not formed, lipoproteins cannot be synthesized and the continuing production of triglycerides results in a progressive accumulation in the cytoplasm.

Excess fatty acids: starvation and diabetes

The abnormal carbohydrate metabolism that occurs in starvation and diabetes mellitus is accompanied by defects in lipid metabolism and fatty de-

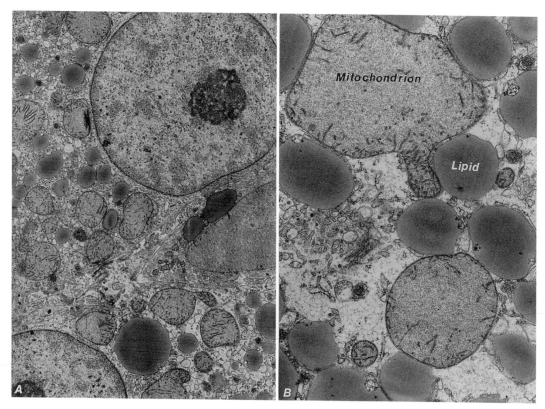

FIGURE 2.4. Fatty degeneration, liver, dog with diabetes mellitus. Lipid globules have a close relationship with mitochondria. A. Hepatocytes. B. High magnification of *A*.

generation in the liver. Accumulation of fat begins around central veins, and the expanding lesion precisely outlining individual liver lobules is called **centrolobular fatty degeneration**. Large lipid globules composed of triglycerides accumulate in the cytoplasm of the hepatocytes (Fig. 2.4).

Carbohydrate stores in liver and muscle are depleted in starvation and diabetes mellitus (through continual loss of glucose via urine). In both diseases, this leads to breakdown of fat and protein (gluconeogenesis, the formation of glucose and glycogen from noncarbohydrate sources). Lipolysis in adipose tissue accelerates, and free fatty acids increase in the blood. In the liver, acetyl CoA fails to enter the citric acid cycle and is diverted to acetoacetate and hydroxybutyrate, which diffuse out of the cell to circulate.

Suppression of fatty acid oxidation: hypoxia

Although hypoxic cells attempt to accommodate to oxygen deficit, they undergo several changes. Mitochondria enlarge as the respiratory chain becomes inhibited. In the smooth endoplasmic reticulum, enzymes that catalyze fatty acid oxidation are inhibited, and this promotes synthesis and accumulation of triglycerides. For example, the hypoxic liver of chronic congestive heart failure develops fatty degeneration in centrolobular zones—areas where hepatocytes are most susceptible to oxygen deficiency.

Excessive lipid metabolism: the fatty liver syndromes

Insufficient sources of energy in the diet often lead to fatty degeneration, especially in lactating dairy cows or in hens during peak egg production. Fat accumulates in the liver of cows around the time of parturition, because of excessive mobilization of fatty acids from adipose tissue in response to the negative energy balance of early lactation. Any metabolic defect that interferes with intracellular transport and exocytosis in the liver will cause fatty degeneration. Syndromes of abnormal lipid metabolism with accumulation of large amounts of fat are also seen in adult cats.

Glycogen inspissation

Glycogen, a branched polymer of glucose molecules, is the storage form of glucose. It is a normal component in the cytoplasm of most cells, but it accumulates when excessive amounts of glucose enter the cell. Major deposits occur in liver, muscle, and kidney during normal physiologic variation in blood glucose. The shift to massive **glycogen inspissation** arises in some metabolic disorders and is an important diagnostic clue in these tissues. The term **glycogen degeneration** is used when cells are so distended with glycogen that degenerative phenomena occur in other organelles.

In the liver, glycogen inspissation is found in hepatocytes in the following conditions: (1) hyperglycemia of any cause (commonly that of diabetes mellitus); (2) drug-induced metabolic disease with disturbed carbohydrate metabolism (e.g., hepatocytes of animals treated with corticosteroids); (3) enzymatic deficiencies associated with rare hereditary glycogen storage diseases; and (4) glycogen-storing "clear cell" hepatocellular tumors.

The most common instance of hepatic glycogen inspissation occurs after the injection of large doses of corticosteroids. The liver in treated animals becomes markedly enlarged and pale. Microscopically, all hepatocytes are affected and consist of massively enlarged cells with remnants of normal cytoplasm pushed to the periphery of the cell, along with large, clear structureless areas containing glycogen particles.

In the cytoplasm of the hepatocyte, glycogen granules are located at sites containing the enzymes that carry out glycogen synthesis and degradation (Fig. 2.5). In **glycogenesis** (synthesis), glycogen synthetase and a branching enzyme link glucose molecules into a large polymer, a process that is enhanced by natural (cortisol) and synthetic (dexamethasone) glucocorticoids. **Glycogenolysis** (degradation) requires a different set of enzymes. Glycogen breakdown in liver and skeletal muscle is markedly affected by epinephrine and glucagon. Both hormones are transported to the liver in the bloodstream and attach to hepatocyte surfaces to activate signals that initiate the cytoplasmic process for degradation. Intranucleolar glycogen is sometimes seen in hepatocytes of aged ruminants and of dogs with diabetes mellitus.

Protein inclusion bodies

Cells with large aggregates of proteins are commonly an important clue in making an etiologic diagnosis. These inclusions may be nuclear or cytoplasmic,

FOCUS

Diabetes Mellitus

AN 11-YEAR-OLD INTACT CHIHUAHUA-TERRIER mongrel had been treated symptomatically for 1 year for cardiac failure. It was brought to a clinic because of a severe, seeping, ulcerating dermatitis; excessive thirst and urination; and abdominal pain. The dog had a serous nasal discharge and foul-smelling fluid feces. Hematology and clinical chemistry data from blood were as follows (normal values in parentheses):

Hemoglobin	17.9 g	(12–8 g)
Hematocrit (PCV)	44%	(37–55%)
WBCs, total	42,200/μl	(6,000–17,000/μl)
Glucose	371 mg/100 ml	(65–115 mg/100 ml)
Blood urea nitrogen (BUN)	38 mg/dl	(10–25 mg/dl)

The clinical pathology findings indicate that this dog had both acute pancreatitis and diabetes mellitus. At necropsy, there was chronic, diffuse fibrinopurulent pancreatitis with destruction of acinar tissue and vacuolar degeneration of the pancreatic islet β cells.

Diabetes mellitus is **pathologic hyperglycemia** (the persistence of excessive blood glucose during fasting). As a result of insulin deficiency, carbohydrate and lipid metabolism are abnormal, which leads to ketosis, fatty degeneration of the liver, and progressive emaciation.

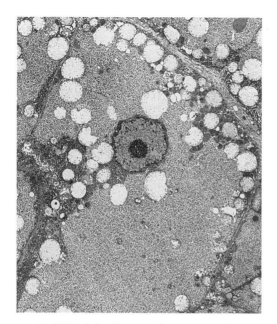

FIGURE 2.5. Glycogen degeneration, hepatocyte, dog treated with cortisol. Cell is enlarged and contains masses of glycogen particles. Mitochondria are swollen. Dense remnants of degenerate rough endoplasmic reticulum are around nuclear and plasma membranes.

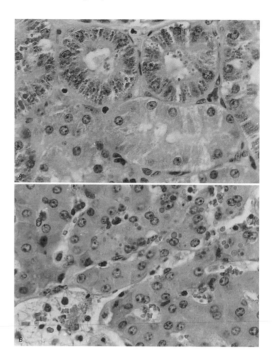

FIGURE 2.6. Protein droplet (hyalin) degeneration. A. Hyalin droplets in proximal renal tubules, dog with chronic renal failure. Droplets represent inspissated proteins acquired by the tubule cell from the glomerular filtrates. B. Hyalin droplets formed by excessive protein secretory product in the cytoplasm, hepatocytes, pig.

spherical or globular, homogeneous or complex, and eosinophilic or basophilic. Inclusions arise in diverse and unrelated conditions, and differences in structure and staining affinities provide evidence for a diagnosis. Origins of inclusion formation include the following:

- Absorption inclusions
- Secretory inclusions
- Inclusions of toxic injury
- Viral inclusions
- Inclusions of protein aggregation disorders

Absorption inclusions

Absorption inclusions, or "absorption droplets," are common in renal tubules and in other organs that reabsorb proteins from lumens. As proteins attach to renal tubular epithelial cells lining lumens of the nephron, they are taken into the cell. Cytoplasmic inclusions develop as proteins are sequestered into large phagolysosomes. In renal disease, where plasma albumin passes into the glomerular filtrate and into urine (albuminuria), proximal tubule cells reabsorb albumin that passes the renal glomerulus, and albumin-bearing phagosomes accumulate in the cytoplasm as hyalin droplets (Fig. 2.6). Proteins of some neoplasms (e.g., Bence Jones proteins of the plasmacytoma) are secreted into urine and taken up into lysosomes of renal tubules; they can be found as cytoplasmic crystals.

Secretory inclusions

Secretory inclusions are giant secretory granules that accumulate in the cytoplasm because protein synthesis exceeds the capacity for release of the protein from the cell. Once newly synthesized proteins reach a critical concentration, they begin to polymerize and to appear as inclusion bodies. For example, hepatocytes producing large amounts of **albumin** will develop inclusions if the secretory pathway is blocked. Another form of secretory inclusion occurs in plasma cells. These cells produce **globulins** (antibodies) and accumulate in healing inflammatory lesions. The inclusions, called Russell's bodies, are formed from globular condensations of globulins in the cytoplasm.

Large cytoplasmic inclusions are common in the liver and develop by accumulation of tiny granular precipitates of protein that expand into large vacuoles of the protein-synthesizing organelle, the rough endoplasmic reticulum. The specific protein that has accumulated can be identified by immunocytochemistry using a bank of reagents for individual proteins that are produced by the hepatocyte. The most common proteins found in these inclusions are albumin, fibrinogen, and α_1-antitrypsin.

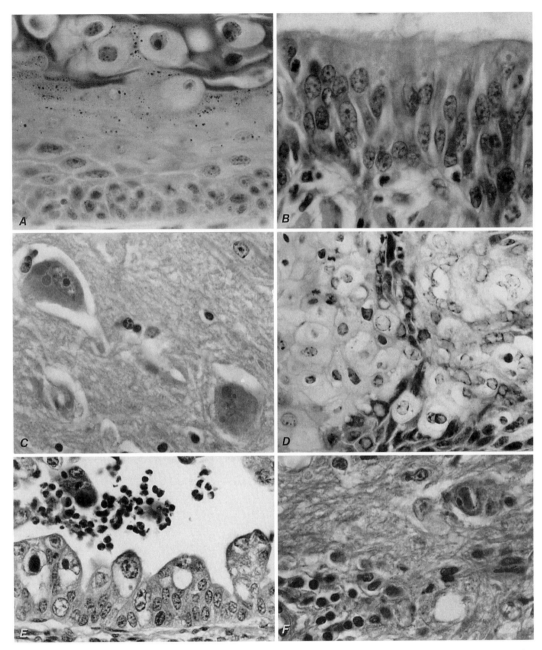

FIGURE 2.7. Viral inclusion bodies are used in diagnosis. A. Pleomorphic, irregular nuclear inclusions, oral epithelium, canine oral papilloma. B. Spherical, homogeneous (eosinophilic) cytoplasmic inclusions in respiratory epithelium, canine distemper. C. Large, irregular cytoplasmic inclusions in neurons, bovine rabies. D. Diffuse "ground-glass" nuclear inclusions, infectious bovine rhinotracheitis. E. Large nuclear inclusions in enlarged bronchiolar epithelial cells, ovine adenovirus. F. Large nuclear inclusions in enlarged nuclei of neurons, chronic canine distemper.

Inclusions of toxic injury

Cytoplasmic inclusions consisting of aggregated filamentous material occur in several chronic toxicologic liver diseases. Large spherical cytoplasmic inclusions of acute toxicity develop from movement of proteins into cytoplasmic vacuoles that arise from cellular injury. Nuclear inclusions of protein-heavy metal aggregates are diagnostic in prolonged toxicity with mercury, bismuth, and some other metals.

Filaments of abnormal aggregates of **prekeratin** polypeptides develop in some toxicities. The insoluble material results from liver cytokeratins that have been cross-linked by a transglutaminase enzyme in the hepatocyte. Ethanol and other agents that damage the cytoskeleton of the hepatocyte will ultimately diminish the excretory capacity through bile canaliculi, and this effect underlies the accumulation of precursors of cytokeratin filaments. **Ubiquitin**, the protein that binds to denatured proteins, is involved in processing of abnormal intermediate filaments.

Viral inclusion bodies

Viruses kill cells by shutting off normal protein synthesis. During viral replication, cell metabolism is disrupted as protein synthesis is shut down. Viral nucleic acid templates are liberated into the host cell cytoplasm and are used as codes to create new viral genetic material, viral enzymes, and structural proteins that will become part of the external coat of the new virion. Although some of the viral peptides are directly toxic to the cell, most cellular injury arises from failure of the infected cell to produce critical enzymes and energy for its own metabolism. Production of proteins for new virions is unbalanced, and aggregates of the various peptides and other excess components accumulate as inclusion bodies (Fig. 2.7).

Specific identification of viral inclusions using immunologic reagents applied to tissue sections is routine in diagnostic laboratories. Most viral inclusions are remnants of viral factories and are composed of excess viral structural proteins and lipoprotein membranes with viral particles of varying maturity distributed in the periphery. In some cases, viral inclusions are composed of mature viral particles (virions) arranged in lattice formations.

Inclusions of protein aggregation disorders
Inclusions of abnormally folded proteins.
Insoluble aggregates of normally well-behaved proteins form a group of abnormal protein inclusions. Improperly folded intermediate stages of protein molecules are the building blocks of many of these abnormal proteins; that is, formation of an aggregate occurs through the abnormal folding intermediate. Aggregation and polymerization of these abnormal proteins can lead to their massive accumulation in the cytoplasm.

A syndrome of deficiency of the acute phase protein α_1-antitrypsin occurs because the protein is not folded properly in the endoplasmic reticulum of the hepatocyte. The mechanism is a single amino acid substitution that causes the protein not to be secreted but to be retained. The chronic accumulation of α_1-antitrypsin in the hepatocyte leads eventually to chronic liver disease, a disorder seen most often in Cocker spaniels.

Blocks anywhere in the pathway of protein synthesis are associated with accumulation of protein and with the subsequent formation of aberrant fibrillar and tubular forms in the cell. The location and character of a protein inclusion are determined by the site in the synthetic pathway that is damaged. Injury to transcription in the nucleolus leads to nuclear inclusions. When a block occurs in pathways of protein synthesis, aggregates of incomplete proteins polymerize in cisternae of the endoplasmic reticulum and Golgi saccules.

Aging inclusions in the brain. In aging cells, particularly in neurons, proteins polymerize and aggregate into cytoplasmic inclusions. Generally not associated with specific diseases, they are found incidentally at autopsy or biopsy of tissue. In some cases, proteins polymerize into rigid, highly insoluble filaments in which specific amino acids are cross-linked by unusual covalent bonding of glutamyl-lysine side chains. Some data suggest that the enzyme transglutaminase is activated by the rising Ca^{2+} concentrations in degenerating cells and promotes polymerization of normal peptide chains.

In the brain, filamentous cytoplasmic inclusions develop in neurons and glia. These inclusions are composed of various filaments whose component proteins have been **ubiquitinated** during the process of denaturation; that is, the stress protein ubiquitin has bound to the abnormal protein to facilitate its sequestration in the cytoplasm. **Neurofibrillary tangles** are large inclusions that develop as perikaryonal masses in neurons of human patients with Alzheimer's disease and in some animals with Alzheimer-like lesions, e.g., sheep and wolverines. The major component of neurofibrillary tangles are **paired helical filaments**, insoluble fibers composed of two helically wound filaments containing microtubule-associated proteins (tau).

ACCUMULATION OF NONDEGRADABLE PRODUCTS

The end result of persistent abnormal metabolism is often an accumulation of amorphous, irregular inclusions in the cytoplasm. **Inclusions** of undegraded cytoplasmic components such as membranes, protein filaments, and lipid complexes are common in tissues with high metabolic rates. Proteins and glycoproteins are degraded in highly regulated processes, and those molecules that fail to fold or assemble correctly are not released from the endoplasmic reticulum for export. Instead, the defective molecules are retained in the cisternae and removed by proteolytic degradation. Normally, the proteolytic system for removal is rapid and highly selective. However, when overwhelmed, cytoplasmic aggregates and crystals of these defective proteins accumulate in otherwise normal cells and appear as dense masses that can be seen by light microscopy. Uncontrolled production of certain proteins is associated with giant autophagosomes that sequester cellular proteins, debris, and membrane fragments.

Lipofuscin

Lipofuscin is a golden brown pigment formed in lysosomes of cells undergoing progressive and prolonged autoxidation of unsaturated lipids. It tends to develop in cells with high rates of metabolism such as liver, heart, and muscle. Lipofuscin increases with advancing age—hence the term aging pigment, or wear-and-tear pigment. Microscopically, lipofuscin is found in the cytoplasm of parenchymal cells of the heart, brain, thyroid, adrenal cortex, and gonads of aged animals. In these cells, lipofuscin develops in large autophagolysosomes from nondegradable materials that result from the continual recycling of membranes and other cellular components.

Lipofuscins accrue as older cells must degrade more lipids and membranes at a time when their antioxidation mechanisms wane. After peroxidation of double bonds of lipids, oxidized forms are condensed into solid polymers that give the color and reactivity of lipofuscin. Deposits fluoresce brown in ultraviolet light and stain with fat-soluble dyes, acid-fast stains, and the periodic acid-Schiff (PAS) reaction.

Lipofuscins are a group of complex lipopigments. As oxidation proceeds in lipofuscin-bearing lysosomes, there are changes in the nature and histochemical reactivity of the pigment. Early forms with many lipid globules and strong acid-fastness give way to dominance of membranogranular debris and weak acid-fast staining. Ceroid, an early form of lipofuscin, consists of partially oxidized and polymerized unsaturated fatty acids. Ceroid is produced by macrophages, hepatocytes, and other cells. It is associated with vitamin E deficiency in several species. Hepatic ceroidosis is common in salmonids and catfish fed rancid diets. Livers of the fish are brown orange, with autofluorescent, acid-fast pigments that distort the hepatocyte. Some lipofuscins stain for iron because this metal is incorporated into the lysosome during the autophagocytic process.

The ceroid lipofuscinosis diseases are a group of neurodegenerative diseases characterized by accumulation of fluorescent lipopigments in neurons and many other cells of the body. They have been reported in sheep, cattle, goats, dogs, and cats. In humans, at least 10 phenotypes have been described, associated with four or more gene loci.

Neuronal ceroid lipofuscinosis is an autosomal recessive disease in English setter dogs, characterized by intracellular accumulation of lipopigments in neurons and associated with progressive loss of neurons and cerebral function. Autofluorescent pigments are about 50% acidic lipid polymers. There is a defect in detoxification of peroxides, based on markedly decreased tissue levels of p-phenyldiamine-linked peroxidase. Neuronal ceroid lipofuscinosis has also been reported in Beefmaster cattle, cats, and South Hampshire sheep.

In dogs, lipofuscin deposits are found in smooth muscle of the intestine in chronic diarrheal disease, steatorrhea, and pancreatic acinar deficiency (Fig. 2.8). Peculiar deposits of lipofuscin in specific organs, for which the cause is unknown, occur in various species; e.g., "black kidneys" of cattle with renal lipofuscin.

Phospholipid inclusions

In normal cells, membranes are continually recycled. Tiny portions of the membrane are sequestered by autophagosomes as part of normal cellular reconstruction. This material is then shunted to enzyme-bearing lysosomes, where it is degraded and either stored or released from the cell. Specific enzymes catalyze this normal breakdown of membrane phospholipids. When membrane repair is driven to excess, or when enzymes involved in the process are missing or damaged, phospholipid fragments accumulate in lysosomes, giving rise to the foam cells of phospholipid degeneration.

Some tranquilizers and plant poisons produce phospholipid degeneration in neurons that leads to central nervous system clinical signs. The familial, systemic lipid storage diseases, which are due to the absence or diminution of enzymes that degrade glycolipid cerebrosides and gangliosides, also produce phospholipid degeneration. In affected brains, the degradation of myelin gradually overwhelms the capacity of brain to recycle this important molecule.

Membranes, which are composed of dense arrays of phospholipids, are fragmented, and fragments are taken into lysosomes to be degraded. Aggregates of these granules engorged with cellular membranes and other fragments give the cell its characteristic foamy, granular appearance, and the condition is referred to as granulovacuolar de-

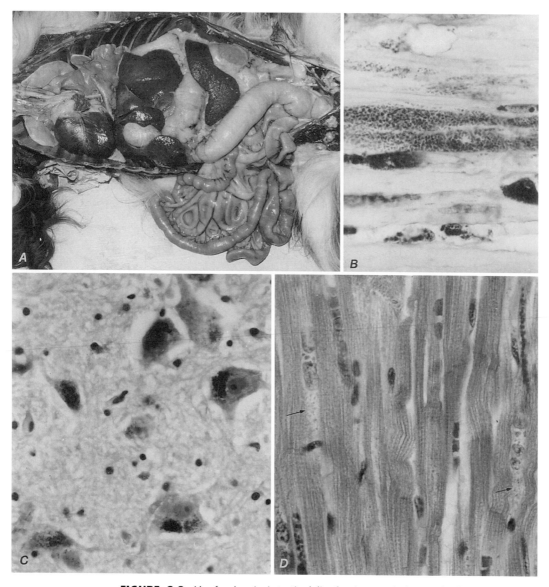

FIGURE 2.8. Lipofuscin. A. Intestinal lipofuscin, aged dog with chronic relapsing pancreatitis (note difference in pigment of colon and jejunum). B. Histology: accumulation of granules in smooth muscle cells in the intestine. C. Neuronal lipofuscinosis, dog. D. Lipofuscin in cardiac myocytes, dog with dirofilariasis. Small granules around nuclei *(arrows)* are lipofuscin.

generation. Histologically, foam cells resemble cells with severe vacuolar degeneration and small-droplet fatty degeneration, so that the phospholipid nature of the cytoplasmic material must be demonstrated with special stains.

Intracellular calcification

Calcium deposits develop in cells that undergo marked ionic imbalance. The abnormal aggregates of calcium phosphate salts appear as dense, deep blue or purple spicules or granules in the cytoplasm. Proof that these structures contain calcium is established by histochemical staining with the von Kossa procedure. Ca^{2+} is critical for many cell activities. Even though intracellular and extracellular amounts of calcium may be similar, free Ca^{2+} is more than 100 times that in the cytoplasm. The two major homeostatic mechanisms that maintain

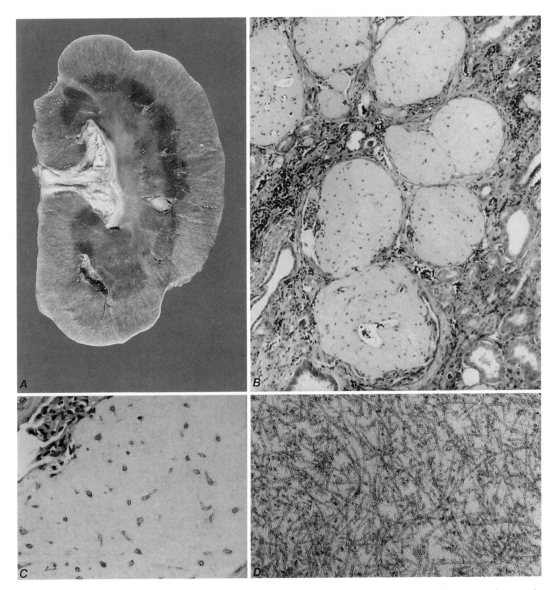

FIGURE 2.9. Amyloidosis, 19-year-old collie with chronic enteritis treated recently with corticosteroids. A. Kidney, pallor of cortex. Cortex is pale and irregular with white stripes between areas of nephrons. B. Massive deposition of amyloid in glomeruli. C. Enlargement of *B:* amyloid-producing stellate cells among delicate amyloid deposits. D. Ultrastructure of amyloid fibrils.

cellular calcium use mechanisms that move Ca^{2+} back and forth between free cytosol and cytoplasmic organelles: (1) **passive influx** into the cytosol from extracellular spaces, mitochondria, and endoplasmic reticulum, and (2) **active extrusion** of Ca^{2+} from the cytosol back into these zones by Ca^{2+} pumps in their membranes.

Amyloid

Amyloid (Gr. *amylon,* starch) is a homogeneous, fibrillar protein. It is most common in spleen, liver,

and kidney and causes these organs to be large, pale, and waxy. A discrete cellular defect in protein processing underlies amyloidosis. The new abnormal protein is not processed normally, and peptide units are assembled into fibrils. Although fibrils are uniform physically, they may be composed of abnormal peptide segments of such diverse proteins as albumin, growth hormone, immunoglobulin, insulin-like proteins, and serum amyloid A, an acute phase protein of inflammation.

Amyloid can be detected in biopsy tissue or at

necropsy by applying aqueous solutions of iodine to tissue surfaces, because iodine stains amyloid brown. Histologically, amyloid is stained by Congo red, and a characteristic green birefringence is induced under polarized light because of the peculiar alignment of the dye on parallel amyloid fibrils. Crystal violet and the fluorochrome thioflavin T are also useful, but staining is variable and nonspecific.

Electron microscopic examination of amyloid reveals characteristic amyloid fibrils, 7.5–10 nm in diameter (Fig. 2.9). Fibrils are rigid, nonbranching, hollow-cored tubules whose length is indeterminate because they crisscross into and out of the plane of section. When examined by X-ray diffraction, the peptides that form the fibrils have a characteristic β-pleated sheet configuration. This macromolecular helix of 100-nm periodicity formed from two twisted β-pleated sheet micelles is responsible for the resistance of amyloid fibrils to proteolytic digestion. The implacable deposition of these inert fibrils leads to pressure atrophy and interference with tissue function. In addition, some types of amyloid have been reported to induce programmed cell death.

Amyloid fibrils form a matrix onto which glycosaminoglycans are secreted and which absorbs some of the proteins of connective tissue fluids. Variations in density and staining of amyloid result from differences in amounts of nonamyloid components that have attached to the fibrillar scaffold. Fibrin, collagen, complement, and globulin can all be found to be present in amyloid. Depending on its stage of deposition, amyloid is contaminated with varying amounts of these substances.

Glycosaminoglycans give amyloid its carbohydrate character. Amyloid-secreting cells alter the connective tissue stroma and facilitate amyloid deposition by releasing glycosaminoglycans, which enhance the polymerization of amyloid fibrils. The **P component**, a tiny 8-nm-diameter, pentagonal, doughnut-like body, is also a component of amyloid. Chemically unrelated to the amyloid fibril, this glycoprotein is identical to an α_1-glycoprotein of normal serum (which is related to complement component C1t and to C-reactive protein). The iodine-staining characteristics of amyloid are imparted by the glycosaminoglycans.

Sources of amyloid

The common denominator of all amyloids is that they are aggregates of proteinaceous, twisted, β-pleated sheet fibrils. Despite their physical homogeneity, the chemical nature of each fibrillar protein is distinct. That is, the fibril is composed of repeated units of specific peptides that are identical (or highly similar) to a normally occurring protein. The differing chemical structure and source of these peptides provides the basis for classifying different types of amyloid.

Amyloid fibrils can be formed by the abnormal processing of such diverse proteins as acute phase proteins, immunoglobulins, endocrine secretions, and many other cellular proteins (Table 2.1). Many of these amyloids arise from a soluble precursor protein that has an amyloidogenic primary structure and, after proteolytic cleavage, assembles into a β-pleated sheet configuration. This form is resistant to further enzymatic digestion and accumulates in tissue; for example, the fibril composed of amyloid A that develops in chronic infection and sepsis.

Serum protein AA (apoSAA)–derived amyloid: AA amyloid

AA amyloidosis is the dominant form of systemic amyloidosis in animals. It is most common in dogs, cattle, and horses but is reported throughout the animal kingdom. AA amyloidosis is pathogenetically linked to chronic inflammatory, immunologic, and neoplastic diseases and is referred to as secondary amyloidosis.

AA amyloid is a low-molecular-weight, single-chain protein and is the major component of fibrils that have been purified from the amyloid of chronic inflammation. Amyloid A is **formed in macrophages** by proteolysis of antigenically related but larger molecules that circulate in the blood, serum amyloid A.

Serum amyloid A (SAA) is an acute phase reactant of plasma that is present in normal animals. It increases during the early phases of acute inflammation, although its function is not understood. Plasma concentrations of SAA rise within a few hours after fever or infection and decline rapidly to normal values after recovery. SAA, which is markedly elevated in animals with amyloidosis, is synthesized in hepatocytes and transported in the bloodstream, associated with high-density lipoproteins.

TABLE 2.1. Types of amyloid

Type of amyloid	Precursor	Occurs in . . .
AA	Serum amyloid A (SAA)	Chronic disease, sepsis
AL	Immunoglobulin light chains	Plasmacytoma
AI	Apolipoprotein AI	Pulmonary arteries
IAPP	Islet amyloid polypeptide	Pancreatic islets
Senile	β-protein	Brain of aged animals

SAA amyloid develops in long-standing, progressive infections or tissue-destructive processes. It is common in tuberculosis, malaria, leishmaniasis, and bacterial osteomyelitis. In these diseases, the clinical sequelae of amyloid deposits are often masked by the severity of the causal septic disease.

Immunoglobulin-derived amyloid: AL amyloid

AL amyloidosis is rarely seen in animals and is largely a disease of humans. AL amyloid is produced by immunoglobulin-secreting cells, the prototype being the neoplastic plasmacyte found in patients with plasmacytoma. In dogs, AL amyloidosis is associated with localized forms of plasmacytoma. Local nodular deposits of AL amyloid associated with the nasopharyngeal mucosa or subcutis occur in horses and are formed from light chains of the immunoglobulin molecule.

AL protein is the precursor of amyloid in this plasmacytoma-associated amyloid. Analysis of concentrated amyloid fibrils produced by purification of tissue amyloid reveals that amino acid sequences of the amyloid proteins are similar, if not identical, to immunoglobulin light chains and to the light chains excreted in the urine of plasmacytoma patients. Furthermore, fibrils can be synthesized in vitro from urinary immunoglobulin fragments (Bence Jones proteins) from human patients with plasmacytoma and amyloidosis. Studies suggest that reticular cells produce amyloid by intralysosomal proteolytic digestion of circulating light-chain fragments.

Apolipoprotein AI (apoAI)–derived amyloid

A unique form of apoAI-derived amyloidosis occurs in intimal and medial regions of pulmonary arteries of dogs. ApoAI is a major component of high-density lipoprotein molecules and is the major activator for the enzyme lecithin:cholesterol acyltransferase, a critical participant in reverse cholesterol transport. There is no evidence to date that this form of age-associated apoAI-derived amyloidosis in dogs is associated with point mutations. Pulmonary vascular amyloid deposits of this type occur in 12–22% of dogs (no extrapulmonary deposits have been reported).

Islet amyloid polypeptide (IAPP)–derived amyloid

Amyloid can be formed during the processing of normal peptides such as insulin, calcitonin, growth hormone, and other hormones. Islet amyloid polypeptide (IAPP) is a normal component of pancreatic islet β-cell secretory granules and is co-secreted with insulin. IAPP amyloid occurs in the pancreatic islet and is especially common in old cats and nonhuman primates. In cats, islet amyloid may be associated with β cells. There is an association of pancreatic islet amyloid and diabetes mellitus in cats. IAPP-induced amyloid occurs in more than 90% of humans with type 2 diabetes and in more than 80% of cats with a similar form of age-associated diabetes.

β-protein-derived cerebral amyloidosis

The cerebral cortex of aged mammals develops tiny foci of degenerate axons and neurites that surround a core of amyloid fibrils. Called neuritic plaques (or senile plaques), these foci develop in aged dogs and cats and, in humans, are the hallmark of Alzheimer's disease. The amyloid filaments found in senile plaques of dogs, bears, monkeys, and humans are similar biochemically. A survey of dogs showed that diffuse plaques occurred in 36% of dogs 11.1–12.9 years of age and in 73% of dogs 15.1–17.8 years of age. There appears to be an increase in plaque density with increasing age.

Amyloid in neuritic plaques is composed of a unique protein, amyloid protein (βAP). βAP appears to be toxic to neurons, and the accumulation of amyloid fragments within the neuron may lead to cell death and the formation of neuritic plaques. βAP is synthesized in neurons as a component of a larger protein, β-amyloid precursor protein (βAPP). βAPP is an integral membrane glycoprotein that is synthesized in the neuron body and is shunted to the surface of the neuron by rapid anterograde transport to maintain adhesion of nerve cells at nerve termini. When there is a mutation in βAPP, the abnormal fragments are moved into lysosomes, where they can re-form as amyloid. βAPP develops after cytoskeletal damage to the neuron and has been used as a marker for brain injury.

Systemic amyloidosis (AA or AL types)

Amyloidosis is the disease resulting from deposition of amyloid in tissue. Amyloidosis is complicated in the terminal stages by two major events: (1) overload of the monocyte-macrophage system by circulating amyloid precursors, and (2) the progressive destruction of parenchymal cells and capillaries by masses of amyloid. Although amyloid interferes with the function in any organ, the fatal effects occur in the kidney.

Spleen is a common site of amyloid deposition

Spleen is the primary site of SAA amyloid deposition. First appearing in atrophic lymphoid tissue at the periphery of periarterial lymphoid sheaths, this

Amyloidosis in Cyclic Hematopoiesis of Collies

Plasma protein abnormalities occur early in amyloidosis

As amyloidosis develops, marked abnormalities are found in plasma proteins, especially in globulins. Synthesis of α_2-, β-, and γ-globulins is increased, and degradation of α_2-globulin is accelerated. Studies of gray collies with cyclic hematopoiesis illustrate that plasma changes occur long before amyloid is deposited in tissue. Neutrophils in these dogs disappear from their bloodstream for 24 hours every 11 days. Affected puppies suffer recurring bacterial infections that correlate with neutropenic episodes. Gradual elevations in α_2-globulin occur early, and progressive increases in all plasma globulins characterize late disease.

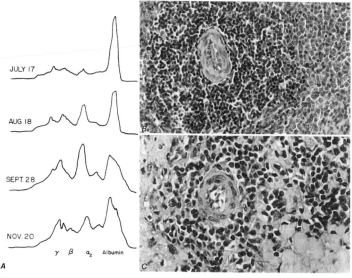

Plasma protein changes and lesions in spleen biopsies, dog with progressive amyloidosis. A. Plasma proteins. B. Splenic histology on Sept. 28 is normal. C. Splenic histology on Nov. 20 shows loss of lymphoid cells and infiltrates of amyloid.

Amyloid deposition occurs in two phases

Secondary amyloidosis begins with a long, clinically silent period. This **preamyloid (initial) phase** is characterized by an accumulation of reticular cells and macrophages in spleen and other lymphoid tissues and a rise in serum amyloid A (SAA) and globulins in plasma. SAA synthesis in the liver is stimulated by a macrophage cytokine, possibly interleukin-1. The **amyloid (second) phase** is characterized by development of PAS-staining cells (filled with abnormal glycoproteins), amyloid deposition, and a decrease in peak SAA levels. Transition from the initial phase to the amyloid phase is dependent on suppression of proliferating reticuloendothelial cells, either by exhaustion of the immune mechanism following protracted antigenic stimulation or by immunosuppressive drugs. Corticosteroid therapy markedly hastens the transition from preamyloid to amyloid phases.

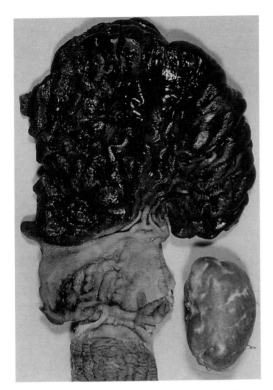

FIGURE 2.10. Necrosis (infarction) of the stomach, dog with uremia due to renal amyloidosis. Body and fundus are affected with diffuse necrosis and hemorrhage, but antrum is spared. *Bottom right,* kidney with amyloid.

perifollicular amyloid causes splenic corpuscles to be large, gray, and translucent. Perifollicular amyloid bulges from the cut surface to resemble grains of tapioca; even though rare, this "sago spleen" is a classic lesion of SAA amyloid. Histologically, splenic amyloid can also be seen between adventitial and smooth muscle cells of the central artery and arterioles and as discrete clumps in the red pulp.

Renal glomerular amyloid leads to uremia

Animals with progressive renal amyloidosis die with renal failure and uremia (Fig. 2.10). Kidneys of these animals are enlarged, pale, and yellow to orange brown. Gray, translucent areas of amyloid occur as spots in the cortex and as streaks in the medulla. Histologically, amyloid is deposited in the renal glomerulus, in and below basement membranes of the renal tubules, and in small arteries. Within the glomerulus, amyloid is produced by mesangial cells and accumulates in the mesangium and along the basement membranes of capillaries. Deposition of amyloid in glomeruli interferes with function of the renal filtration apparatus and re-

sults in marked loss of protein, especially albumin, into the glomerular filtrate.

Amyloidosis is progressive

Amyloid is inefficiently removed by macrophages and other phagocytes. Amyloid fibrils are resistant to phagocytosis and proteolysis. They are not remarkably immunogenic, because of the large size of the amyloid molecule. The persistence of the underlying defect in amyloidosis usually causes production to dominate resorption. However, if the underlying cause of amyloidosis is removed, amyloid fibrils may gradually disappear. Neutrophils take up degraded amyloid, and further hydrolytic destruction occurs in neutrophil lysosomes.

CALCIFICATION

When tissue encountered in postmortem dissection feels gritty and scrapes against the knife, it is probable that calcium deposits are present. They appear in histologic sections as granular, amorphous, blue black deposits. The von Kossa stain, which detects phosphates associated with calcium, is used to establish that the substance is calcium (Fig. 2.11). Two forms of pathologic tissue calcification occur: **dystrophic calcification**, in which calcium salts are deposited in degenerating tissues and cells, and **metastatic calcification**, in which calcium is deposited in normal tissues in the presence of hypercalcemia. This dichotomy is not entirely satisfactory, because hypercalcemia can rarely be directly correlated with tissue calcification. Hypercalcemia also enhances dystrophic calcification. The role of cellular injury is difficult to assess, and nearly all forms of calcium deposition involve some previous cellular defect.

Dystrophic calcification

Dystrophic calcification is seen at sites of tissue damage, especially at sites of scarring, hemorrhage, and necrosis. Lesions of chronic diseases such as tuberculosis, trichinosis, histoplasmosis, and caseous lymphadenitis are frequently mineralized.

Calcium salts develop within foci of damaged interstitial ground substance that contain altered glycosaminoglycans. One of the more serious sites of dystrophic calcification is the degenerating smooth muscle layer of arteries. Calcium is deposited on altered microfibrillar portions of the elastic tissue, and calcification spreads to involve large parts of the artery.

Tumorous calcinosis is a variant of dystrophic calcification in which tissues are converted into masses of calcium salts surrounded by foreign body giant cells. These hard, circumscribed deposits, also

FOCUS

Uremia

UREMIA IS THE COMPLEX SYSTEMIC DISEASE brought about by decreased renal glomerular filtration and by failure of tubular reabsorption and secretion. Alterations in uremia include failure to conserve water, electrolyte imbalance, acid-base imbalance, and failure in the excretion of urea and other nonprotein nitrogenous wastes.

As renal tubules fail to reabsorb water, urine volumes may remain large until shortly before death. The ornithine-urea cycle is shifted markedly, and failure of the kidney to secrete ammonia and to absorb Na^+ leads to progressive metabolic acidosis.

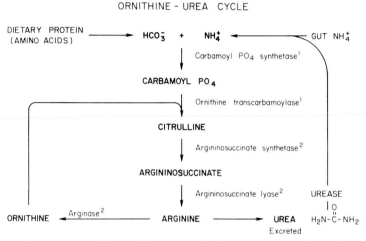

Metabolic pathways of the ornithine-urea cycle. Enzymes are located in mitochondria (1) or in the cytoplasm (2).

Vomiting, weakness, congestion of mucous membranes, and paleness and coolness of the skin are seen in animals with uremia. Neurologic signs range from drowsiness to coma. The abnormal electroencephalographic changes in dogs are related to increased Ca^{2+} in the brain. An ammonia odor of the breath is common. In dogs, ulceration and inflammation of the tongue, oral mucosa, and stomach are nearly always present in severe uremia. Mechanisms of disease include depression of glomerular filtration, tubular secretion and reabsorption, and tubular detoxification.

Gastrointestinal lesions
Uremic gastropathy with edema and ulceration is common in dogs. There is striking diffuse arteriopathy with marked calcification of arterial walls throughout the stomach; edema and hemorrhage correlate with the degree of vascular injury. Ulceration occurs via a mucosal energy deficiency due to vascular lesions superimposed over both local and systemic hypoxia. These are compounded by bile reflux and back diffusion of H^+ from the gastric lumen. Gastric surface mucus, which acts as a diffusion barrier and inhibits the proteolytic action of pepsin, is diminished in uremia, and this contributes to ulcer formation. Mast cell histamine promotes gastrointestinal lesions via its functions in vascular permeability, calcification, and parietal cell chemostimulation.

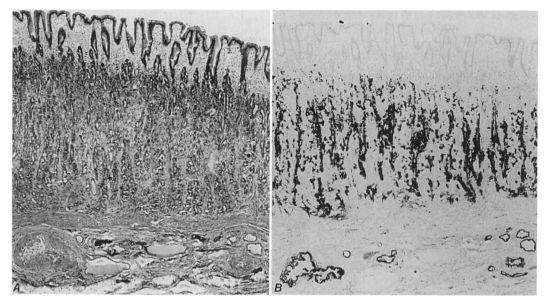

FIGURE 2.11. Calcification in the stomach, dog with uremic gastropathy. A. Fundic mucosa: edema in foveolar (surface) regions, calcified pale areas in glandular regions, arterial lesions and dilated lymphatics in submucosa. B. Section adjacent to that in *A*, stained by the von Kossa technique for calcium salts, which are deposited in the mucosa and submucosal arteries.

called calcinosis circumscripta, occur in the skin over bony prominences and in the tongue of dogs.

Metastatic calcification

Persistent hypercalcemia leads to deposition of calcium salts in tissue. The most common causes of metastatic calcification are

- Vitamin D toxicity
- Parathyroid hormone hypersecretion
- Renal failure (uremia)
- Bone destruction

Kidneys calcified by **hypervitaminosis D** have been used as models to study metastatic calcification. Vitamin D causes a progressive uncoupling of oxidative phosphorylation in mitochondria, which are the organelles first involved in the pathogenesis of this calcifying disorder. Widespread soft tissue calcification occurs in a variety of diseases for which the mechanisms of calcification are not known.

Some plant toxins are calcinogenic

Livestock grazing plants of the genera *Solanum, Cestrum,* and *Trisetum* develop hypercalcemia, hyperphosphatemia, and widespread tissue calcification. Soft tissue mineralization and progressive debilitation are due to the vitamin D–like action of toxins in the plant. Leaves contain steroid-glycoside conjugates similar to 1,25-dihydroxycholecalciferol (the active metabolite of vitamin D), which stimulates calcium-binding protein synthesis and enhances intestinal calcium absorption.

Neoplasms can cause hypercalcemia

Persistent hypercalcemia that accompanies disseminated neoplastic disease is often due to ectopic secretion of parathyroid hormonelike peptides by the tumor cells. Calcification is not common in these syndromes, and the hypercalcemia does not play a major role in mortality (see Neoplasia, Chapter 12).

Bacteria can be calcinogenic

Calcium-sequestering bacteria produce deposits of calcium salts in tissue, especially in late stages of inflammation. The extreme example of bacteria-induced calcification is the calcified microbial plaque on teeth. Dental calculi of dogs contain the calcite form of $CaCO_2$ mixed with small amounts of apatite, $Ca_5(PO_4)_3OH$. Bacteria secrete unique acidic phospholipids that complex with soluble electrolytes in saliva to initiate precipitation of calcium carbonate and apatite in the calculus overlying the tooth surface.

Calcified bodies

Calculi are abnormal masses, usually of calcium and other mineral salts, that develop in organs as a

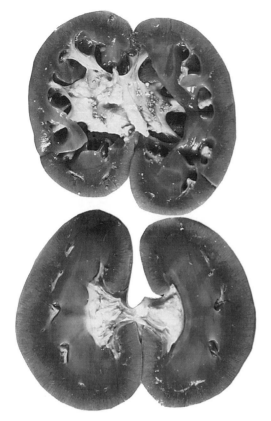

FIGURE 2.12. Renal calculi, goat. Kidney with hydronephrosis due to calculi in the renal pelvis and ureter *(top)* and normal kidney *(bottom).*

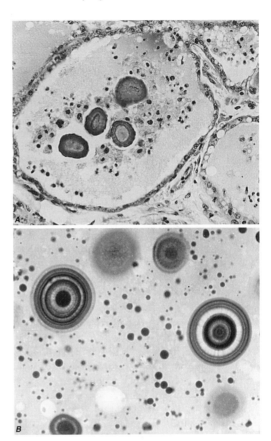

FIGURE 2.13. Corpora amylacea. These calcified spherical bodies form from progressive layering of glycosaminoglycans. They sequester calcium salts. A. Mammary acinus, cow. B. Yolk sac, 2-day-old turkey.

result of accretion or inspissation (thickening) of luminal contents (Fig. 2.12). The combined effects of stasis, bacterial infection, and high mineral content of tissue fluids are usually associated with their presence. Calculi are classified by anatomic location. The following are some of the more common calculi:

- Salivary gland (calculus)
- Intestinal (enterolith)
- Dental (plaque)
- Biliary (gallstone)
- Renal (urolith)
- Bladder (cystolith)

Corpora amylacea are large, laminar, round bodies of diverse origin and are associated with secretory processes in brain, pineal, pituitary, thyroid, and mammary gland (Fig. 2.13). In the bovine mammae, they occur within glandular acini. In primate brains, corpora amylacea develop in the cytoplasm of astrocytes and other glia. They are derived by polymerization of acidic glycosaminoglycans of interstitial ground substance and appear to originate from degenerating neurons. Giant laminated calcified bodies called psammoma bodies, or "sand bodies," are important diagnostic features of some tumors and chronic inflammatory lesions. In tumors they may form from calcification of thrombi or from foci of dead tumor cells.

PIGMENTS

The **endogenous pigments** are produced within the body. In mammals, four major endogenous pigments accumulate in tissue: melanin, lipofuscin, hemosiderin, and bilirubin. Melanin is a normal pigment that is involved in defective pigmentation disorders and in neoplasms. Lipofuscin, the "wear-and-tear" pigment of aged animals, is a complex of nondegradable lipoproteins that accumulate in cells with inadequate intracellular digestion. The last two pigments are derived from erythrocyte breakdown.

Melanin

Melanin is the brown pigment of skin, hair, leptomeninges, and choroid of the eye. It is a large biochrome molecule bound to protein. Formed in melanocytes, it resides in characteristic granules called **melanosomes**. In skin, melanin is also transferred from melanocytes to phagocytic storage cells called **melanophages**. The only known function of melanin in mammals is protection against solar ultraviolet radiation. It is thought to capture injurious free radicals generated in the skin during injury. In lower animals, melanin has a protective effect in inflammation.

Melanin synthesis

Many of the different coat color mutations of animals are attributed to different genetic loci, which determine the expression of genes for melanin synthesis. The **agouti** locus controls synthesis of two different melanin molecules, eumelanin and pheomelanin. In most vertebrates, genes direct the production of the more common black-brown insoluble **eumelanin**. In some avian and mammalian epidermal melanosomes (including those in human red hair), the light-colored, sulfur-bearing melanin **pheomelanin** is formed.

During dermal pigmentation, melanosomes are transferred from the dendrites of melanocytes into keratinocytes. Increased transfer causes increased pigmentation. Tanning of human skin by ultraviolet radiation involves an increase in the length of dendrites and increases in melanosomes and tyrosinase activity but not in the numbers of melanocytes.

Tyrosinase, a copper-protein enzyme, facilitates oxidation of tyrosine to dihydroxyphenylalanine (dopa), and dopa to dopaquinone. Detection of tyrosinase (the **dopa reaction**) is the basis of the histochemical identification of melanocytes and melanoblasts in tissue. In melanocytes, tyrosinase accumulates in small, membrane-bound Golgi vesicles called premelanosomes. During maturation of the melanosome, melanin develops into oriented protein strands, and melanin polymers are deposited on the protein framework.

Abnormal melanin pigmentation can result from changes anywhere in the pathway of melanin production (Table 2.2). In chronic dermatitis, for example, the skin may show pigmented defects caused by failure of transfer to hyperplastic keratinocytes. **Contact depigmentation** of skin is caused by some chemicals, notably phenol. **Melanosis**, the aberrant accumulation of melanin foci, occurs in young animals of several species. In ruminants, melanosis of the brains is common (melanin arises from astrocytes), but these foci are not known to proliferate or cause disease. Melanotic lesions of the skin, in contrast, carry the potential for malignant transformation (see Neoplasia, Chapter 12).

Chromatophore pigments other than melanin

Chromatophores (contractile pigment cells) of cold-blooded vertebrates produce rapid color changes of skin by intracellular aggregation and dispersion of pigment granules. Dermal color changes are under hormonal control and are used for camouflage, sexual attraction, and protection. In addition to melanophores, chromatophores of fish and amphibians include red **xanthophores** and refractile **iridophores**. Chromatophore movements are important in responses to injury. In inflammation, chromatophores protect subcutis from ultraviolet rays of sun, allowing recovery to occur. In fish, massive aggregates of chromatophores are characteristic of chronic inflammation.

TABLE 2.2. Pathologic changes in melanization

Defect in . . .	Occurs in . . .	Pathologic change
Melanoblast differentiation	Focal hypomelanosis (merle dogs, piebald mice, white spotting) Diffuse hypomelanosis (white tiger, gray collie syndrome) Vitiligo	Melanocytes absent because of inadequate differentiation or migration of melanoblasts from neural crest
Tyrosine synthesis	Albinism	Melanocytes do not synthesize tyrosine and melanin; any melanosomes present are normal and transferred normally to keratinocytes
Melanosome formation	Chédiak-Higashi syndrome	Abnormal aggregation of melanin molecules with bizarre shapes
Transfer to keratinocyte	Chronic dermatitis	Melanocyte normal, but keratinocytes lack melanosomes; melanin not transferred to abnormal keratinocyte
Autoimmune destruction of melanosomes	DAM chickens	Lymphocytes destroy melanocytes

Pigments derived from hemoglobin

Hemoglobin, the oxygen-carrying pigment of erythrocytes, is a combination of **globin** and the pigment complex **heme**. Hemoglobin occurs in tissue as reddish brown casts—it is common in renal tubules after intravascular hemolysis of erythrocytes. During normal and pathologic breakdown, different types of pigment complexes are formed. Most of these are heterogeneous and, except for ferritin, are not chemically defined. Ferritin and hemosiderin are the principal **iron storage compounds** in animal tissue. Both contain trivalent iron in the form of hydrous ferric oxides $(FeOOH)_x$, and both are detected histochemically by the Prussian blue reaction.

Ferritin is a tiny (10-nm), iron-laden aggregate of the protein apoferritin. It has a hydrous iron oxide core surrounded by several protein subunits and is water soluble. In diseases that involve lysis of erythrocytes, iron is sequestered by macrophages. Particles of ferritin are formed as iron is added to apoferritin. Ferritin accumulates in lattice arrays free in the cytoplasm and moves to the lysosome, where it is converted to hemosiderin. Cell iron overload may result either from massive accumulation of iron pigments or from a deficiency of lysosomal excretion of hemosiderin.

Hemosiderin

Hemosiderin, a brown, granular, iron-containing pigment, is found in macrophages at sites of erythrocyte lysis or breakdown. It is common in liver, spleen, lymph nodes, and bone marrow and at any site of hemorrhage. Hemosiderin consists of densely packed micelles of hydrous iron oxide derived from degenerating ferritin. Biochemical analysis is hampered because hemosiderin is always contaminated by other cell proteins.

Microscopically, hemosiderins develop as aggregates of ferritin and erythrocyte debris, most of which is in lysosomes. Confirmation of **hemosiderosis** in tissue is by the Prussian blue stain for ferric iron. Lung alveoli often contain "heart failure cells" (hemosiderin-laden alveolar macrophages). **Systemic hemosiderosis** results from excessive iron uptake and iron overload and affects macrophages throughout the body, especially in the liver.

Bilirubin

Bilirubin is a yellow or yellow brown pigment in macrophages of the spleen, liver, bone marrow, and sites of hemorrhage that is derived from degradation of heme, a component of hemoglobin. Bruises are colored by the yellow of bilirubin and its precursor, **biliverdin**, which is green.

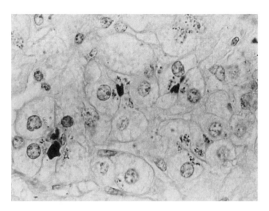

FIGURE 2.14. Bile stasis (dark structures) in biliary canaliculi and secretory granules of bilirubin in hepatocytes, liver, aflatoxicosis.

Bilirubin stains tissue yellow. Because of excessive production or failure of removal by damaged hepatocytes, bilirubin accumulates. Bilirubin appears in cells only when there is some derangement in its secretion by the liver or by obstruction of the biliary tract. When deposited in tissues, it is responsible for their yellow color in **icterus** (also known as **jaundice**). Histologically, bilirubin appears in cells as amorphous, globular cytoplasmic deposits. Commonly limited to hepatocytes (Fig. 2.14), it also can be found in renal tubules and other tissues when icterus is severe.

Bilirubin is produced by macrophages. Bilirubin develops from breakdown of hemoglobin as macrophages process senescent erythrocytes. Porphyrin, the heme pigment, is cleaved, iron is released, and bilirubin is produced after a series of oxidation-reduction reactions within lysosomes. Although the hemoglobin-bilirubin conversions can occur in macrophages elsewhere, the principal organ of production is the spleen. Bilirubin enters the bloodstream, is bound to albumin, and is transported to the liver. Being insoluble in water, it is not passed through the renal glomerulus and either is processed in the liver or, if the liver is abnormal, accumulates in the bloodstream.

Bilirubin is conjugated in the liver and excreted into bile. The albumin-bilirubin complex dissociates at the plasma membrane of the hepatocyte, and bilirubin enters this cell to be conjugated, largely to glucuronide. Conjugated bilirubin, which is water soluble, is secreted into biliary canaliculi (it can also be excreted in urine). As bile reaches the duodenum, the diglucuronide is cleaved and bilirubin is converted by bacteria to urobilinogen. Most urobilinogen is reabsorbed in the distal small intestine and transported to the liver (the **enterohepatic circulation**). Some is excreted by the kidneys. The unabsorbed urobilinogen is transformed in the gut to urobilin and excreted in the feces. The bilirubin pathway may be summarized as follows:

- **Macrophage:** heme is converted to biliverdin, and biliverdin to bilirubin
- **Bloodstream:** bilirubin + albumin → albumin-bilirubin complex
- **Hepatocyte:** carrier-mediated uptake → glucuronidation in endoplasmic reticulum
- **Bile:** excretion of water-soluble, nontoxic bilirubin diglucuronides
- **Intestine:** deconjugation of bilirubin by bacterial glucuronidases + reabsorption

Hyperbilirubinemia can be caused by conjugated or unconjugated bilirubin. The two major forms of bilirubin, conjugated and unconjugated, have important diagnostic and prognostic implications, and they can be distinguished by a specific test of serum. The **van den Bergh test** shows a direct reaction with conjugated bilirubin and an indirect reaction with unconjugated bilirubin.

Any derangement in excretion of conjugated bilirubin into the gut causes urinary urobilinogen to decrease and conjugated bilirubin to appear in urine; that is, **conjugated hyperbilirubinemia**. Conversely, defective conjugated bilirubin in the hepatocytes (the liver secretes the increased amounts of unconjugated bilirubin delivered to it) leads to **unconjugated hyperbilirubinemia**, in which no bilirubin appears in urine, but since more urobilinogen is formed in the gut, urinary urobilinogen increases.

Porphyrin

The **porphyrias** are a group of rare diseases of heme synthesis in which excessive amounts and abnormal types of porphyrins accumulate in tissue, blood, and feces. Porphyria may be hereditary or acquired and occurs in two forms (based on the tissue in which the metabolic defect is expressed): **erythropoietic** and **hepatic**. Porphyrins are small, soluble molecules and cannot be easily detected in histologic sections of tissue.

Copper-containing pigments

Copper-bearing pigment granules accumulate in hepatocytes in a genetic disease caused by the inability to excrete copper into bile, the main route of disposal by mammals. Copper accumulates in lysosomes in the cytoplasm. **Inherited copper toxicosis** occurs in Bedlington terriers. Affected dogs begin to accumulate copper as pups, and as hepatic copper exceeds 2,000 µg/g dry liver, signs of liver failure appear. Copper localizes in centrolobular areas in the liver and also appears in kidney, cornea,

and brain. Focal and periportal hepatitis develops and leads to cirrhosis.

EXOGENOUS PIGMENTS

Exogenous pigments enter via the skin, lung, and intestinal tract. They are most common and most serious in the **lung**, where the diseases are known collectively as **pneumoconioses**. Some of these diseases, such as **anthracosis** (caused by coal dust pigment), cause little tissue reaction. Others, including **silicosis** (caused by silicon dioxide), may produce severe inflammation with extensive fibrosis. In dogs, accumulation of carbon dust in lungs is an indication of environmental contamination. Carbon pigments in macrophages of alveoli and lining the lymphatic vessels of alveolar septae blacken the lungs; pigments are also trapped in draining lymph nodes in the hilar region of the lungs.

Pigments entering the **intestine** are generally of less import to health than are those in lungs. Metallic poisons such as lead (which causes **plumbism**) and silver (which causes **argyria**) may cause pigmentation following ingestion and absorption. Poisoning by these metals can produce a lethal disease in which intestinal pigmentation plays little role.

Tetracyclines, used widely as broad-spectrum antibiotics in antimicrobial therapy, are known to be incorporated into **bone**, where they form a fluorescent compound and stain the tissue yellow in visible light. This characteristic, which is unrelated to antibacterial effects, is used by experimental pathologists as a specific label for calcifying tissues.

Only a few pigments enter through the **skin**. The best examples are Prussian blue, India ink, and mercuric sulfide (vermilion), which are used in tattooing and reside both in macrophages and free in the dermis.

Several **parasites** excrete pigmented compounds into tissue. *Pneumonyssus simicola*, the lung mite of monkeys, is surrounded by dense deposits of excreta. Brownish **malarial pigment** is formed by excretion of catabolized hemoglobin from certain species of plasmodia. In infected animals, massive deposits develop in macrophages of spleen and liver. Malarial pigment arises from degradation of hemoglobin, usually within lysosomes.

CRYSTALS

Oxalosis

Crystals of calcium oxalate are deposited in tissue in toxic diseases, causing increased oxalic acid in blood (**oxalemia**) and urine (**hyperoxaluria**). Causal agents are most often poisons of plants that contain large amounts of oxalic acid (e.g., rhubarb, greasewood, halogeton) or the antifreeze component ethylene glycol (Table 2.3).

Sheep are commonly poisoned by ingestion of oxalate-containing plants; dogs and cats, by drinking ethylene glycol. In the latter case, oxalate is derived by a series of reactions that begin with conversion of ethylene glycol to a toxic glycoaldehyde by the action of the enzyme alcohol dehydrogenase. The subsequent pathway is glycoaldehyde → glycolic acid → glyoxylic acid → oxalic acid. Cattle are resistant to oxalate poisoning because of oxalate-utilizing bacteria in the rumen and oxalate-metabolizing enzymes in the liver.

Dietary ingestion of oxalates causes three disease patterns

Different patterns of disease depend on the species of animal and the amount of oxalate ingested. **Peracute toxicity**, due to corrosive action of oxalate on gastrointestinal mucosa, is associated with gastroenteritis, hemorrhage, and ulceration. This syndrome occurs in horses, which are resistant to oxalate nephropathy. **Acute toxicity** is due to hypocalcemia, the initial systemic effect of oxalates. Hypocalcemia and metabolic acidosis caused by formation of acidic products of oxalate metabolism combine to produce ataxia, convulsions, tetany, and abnormalities of cardiopulmonary function. If animals survive the above episodes, they are prone to develop a third manifestation, **oxalate nephropathy**.

Renal oxalate deposits cause tubular necrosis

Deposits of doubly refractile, translucent, yellowish oxalate crystals occur in tubular lumens, interstitium, and tubular epithelium (Fig. 2.15). Tubular necrosis is particularly prominent, but cortical necrosis may also occur, caused by a secondary ischemic phenomenon. Anuria results from obstruction of tubule lumens by crystals, and uremia kills the animal.

Silicosis

Desert atmospheres are rich in silicate dusts, and animals that roam these areas commonly have crystal-laden macrophages in peribronchiolar tissues in their lungs. The deposits are complex silicates and aluminum-potassium silicate. These lesions are especially common in animals that root about in the ground. In clinical disease resulting from silicates, animals usually have multiple granulomas in the lungs, composed of large, foamy macrophages. The granulomas often have necrotic centers, some with multinucleate giant cells.

Histologically, macrophages contain refractile, crystalline particles, usually smaller than 1 μm, both free in the cytoplasm and within lysosomes. Backscattered electron scanning electron microscopy shows that these crystals are silicon dioxide and aluminum silicate; other silicates also present contain iron and other metals.

Silica exists in dust in amorphous and crystalline forms. The latter is particularly important in induction of fibrosing alveolitis in the lung. Following phagocytosis by alveolar macrophages, necrosis occurs because of damage by crystals of 0.5 μm or less to lysosomal membranes. Hydrolytic enzymes leak into the interstitium of alveolar septa and produce lysis. Cycling of the silica that cannot be broken down results in prolonged destruction of macrophages. Silica and necrotic debris are finally walled off by a granulomatous reaction. Collagen production is stimulated, and there may be diffuse pulmonary fibrosis.

Sulfonamide crystals

Nephrosis and uremia may result from ingestion of large doses of sulfonamides, particularly if associated with deficient fluid intake. These disorders are apt to occur in animals that are febrile and dehydrated. Sulfonamide crystals are often visible grossly in the pelvis and as pale, yellowish, radial lines in the medulla. Tubular degeneration and plugging of the nephron, especially of the collecting ducts, cause anuria. Sulfonamides also produce renal disease by an allergic mechanism.

Urates and uric acid

Deposits of uric acid crystals and urates characterize **gout**, a disease of purine metabolism. Seen most commonly in birds, snakes, and humans, it is due to excessive production or insufficient excretion of uric acid. Chalky white masses of uric acid (referred to as *tophi*) develop in tissue and cause local inflammatory reactions.

Avian gout. Birds normally excrete much uric acid, which predisposes them to gout. Avian gout occurs in two forms. **Visceral gout** is common; plasma uric acid is increased, and urates are deposited in kidney, liver, joints, and pericardium. It is a common sequela to dehydration. **Articular gout** is limited to synovia and tendon sheaths of joints, especially of the foot and hock. The diagnosis can be established by identification of urate crystals via

TABLE 2.3. Classification of oxalosis

Primary	Defect in oxalate metabolism	Inborn metabolic error
		Thiamine deficiency
Secondary	Ingestion of oxalates	Ethylene glycol
		Poisonous plant oxalates
		Fungal oxalates

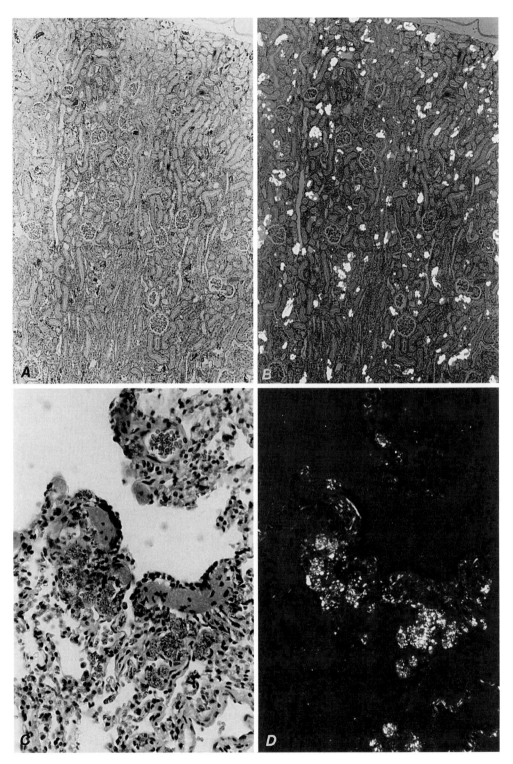

FIGURE 2.15. Crystals in tissue. A. Oxalate nephropathy, cat with ethylene glycol toxicity, hematoxylin and eosin (H&E) section (crystals not apparent). B. Same section as *A* but using polarizing optics (crystals show clearly). C. Peribronchiolar silica crystals, dog lung, section stained with H&E. D. Same section as C in polarized light.

polarizing microscopy of synovial fluid or renal tissues (Fig. 2.16).

Both forms of avian gout are initiated by renal failure in uric acid secretion and are promoted by dehydration and diets high in protein. Occurrence depends on hereditary variations; strains susceptible to gout have defective renal uric acid secretion. Experimentally, avian gout can be produced by administration of nephrotoxic agents and diets deficient in vitamin A and high in calcium.

Gout in other species. Urate nephrolithiasis has been reported in mink and is probably due to an inherited defect in uric acid metabolism. In snakes, the nephrotoxic antibiotic gentamicin is associated with a high incidence of gout. In the dog, uric acid is converted to allantoin in the liver by uricase. Dalmatian dogs differ in that hepatic metabolism lacks this conversion. They excrete uric acid in urine and tend to develop urate or uric acid uroliths.

CONNECTIVE TISSUE SUBSTANCES

Interstitial ground substance is the extracellular gel of proteoglycans, glycosaminoglycans, and fluids in which connective tissue fibers are embedded. Its viscosity and gel nature are due to proteoglycans, both free and attached to collagen, and to elastic fibers. Ground substance contains mixtures of **glycosaminoglycans** (GAGs), which are polysaccharides that contain amino sugars (glucosamine, galactosamine) on their chains. Dermatan sulfate is the most common molecule in skin, tendon, and gastric mucus. Hyaluronic acid is prevalent in synovial fluid, umbilical cord, and vascular walls, whereas chondroitin sulfate dominates in cornea and cartilage. Enhanced synthesis or reduced degradation may produce excesses of GAGs in tissue, and this occurs in metabolic, inflammatory, and neoplastic disease.

Glycosaminoglycans

Striking accumulation of glycosaminoglycans in ground substances is associated with stimulation by sex hormones. Growth of the cock's comb under the influence of testosterone, and swelling of the vulva due to progesterone, are two examples. In some female monkeys, a striking "sex skin" develops that is an attractant to males. The edematous, red, moist character of the skin is caused by subepidermal capillary dilation, accumulation of fluid, and massive deposition of glycosaminoglycans (Fig. 2.17).

Adrenal corticosteroids also have a promoting ef-

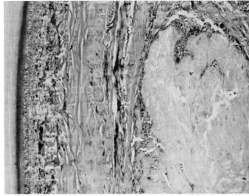
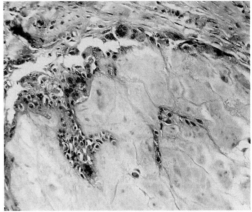

FIGURE 2.16. Avian gout. Deposits of pale, homogenous gout crystals in a tendon sheath of the hock joint, chicken. *Bottom,* enlargement of top photo.

fect on glycosaminoglycans in ground substances. In massive doses they act on capillaries to decrease permeability and edema, thereby playing a significant role in suppressing acute inflammation.

Myxedema

The influence of thyroid hormones on ground substance is clearly seen in **myxedema**, the accumulation of glycosaminoglycans, albumin, water, and mast cells in subcutis that accompanies hypothyroidism. Primarily a disease of adult humans, myxedema has also been reported in the dog. Glycosaminoglycans accumulate around capillaries and veins. Accumulation of fluid is due partly to the great capacity of hyaluronic acid to bind to water and to the subsequent suppression of lymphatic drainage. Changes similar to those in skin occur throughout the body, including skeletal and cardiac muscle, and the net clinical effect is weakness and cardiac failure. Affected renal glomeruli alter plasma filtration and enhance fluid and electrolyte problems.

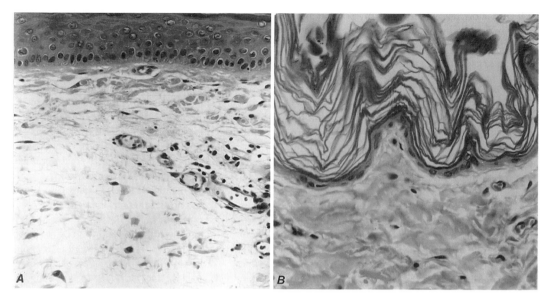

FIGURE 2.17. Mucosubstances. A. Epidermal hyperplasia and dermal swelling with edema fluid and proteoglycans; perineal skin (sex skin), female rhesus monkey during estrus. B. Epidermal atrophy, decreased mucosubstances, inactive collagen; skin, dog with chronic treatment of adrenocorticosteroid hormones.

Basement membranes

Basement membranes (syn: basal lamina) are extracellular, homogenous sheets of dense granular material interposed between epithelium, endothelium, and other cellular layers. Basement membranes are composed of type IV collagen, which is complexed with the noncollagenous glycoproteins laminin and fibronectin and to glycosaminoglycans.

Type IV collagen is synthesized by endothelium, epithelium, and myoepithelial cells, which also produce laminin, the substance that forms the other major network in basement membranes. Heparin sulfate, which predominates in most basement membranes, imparts a filter function because it is a strong polyanion. **Laminin** is a specific attachment factor for epithelial cells to type IV collagen. **Fibronectin** is associated with fibroblast surfaces, where it promotes attachment of fibroblasts to collagen; fibronectin plays important roles in migrating and adhesion, particularly of platelets to collagen during inflammation. **Chondronectin** promotes attachment of cartilage cells to collagen.

Excessive production of basement membranes

Starvation. Tissue atrophy of starvation is characterized by increased thickness of basement membranes in several organs, as well as by excessive deposits of collagen and proteoglycans. The mecha-

nism is continued synthesis in the face of an inhibition of degradation and removal of basement membrane materials.

Diabetes mellitus. Systemic thickening of capillary endothelial basement membranes underlies the chronic complications of diabetic microangiopathy. This lesion may be responsible for severe renal membranous glomerulopathy, a common cause of death. Hyperglycemia-induced glycosylation is the major pathogenetic factor in basement membrane expansion. Hyperglycemia also produces nonenzymatic glycolysis of basement membranes and affects hemoglobin and lens crystallin.

ADDITIONAL READING

Metabolic overload

Daryl-Hart B, et al. 1991. Hepatotoxicity of phenobarbital in dogs: 18 cases (1985–1989). *J Am Vet Med Assoc* 199:1060.

Helman RB, et al. 1995. The lesions of hepatic fatty cirrhosis in sheep. *Vet Pathol* 32:635.

Sevelius E, et al. 1994. Hepatic accumulation of alpha-1-antitrypsin in chronic liver disease in the dog. *J Comp Pathol* 111:401.

Shirota K, Nomura Y. 1994. Ultrastructural appearance of hyalin droplet-laden cells in the glomerular mesangium of pigs. *Vet Pathol* 31:705.

Accumulation of nondegradable products

Birdfell R, et al. 1995. Neuronal ceroid-lipofuscinosis in a cat. *Vet Pathol* 32:4–85.

DiBartola SP, et al. 1990. Familial renal amyloidosis in Chinese Shar Pei dogs. *J Am Vet Med Assoc* 197:4–83.

Edwards JF, et al. 1994. Juvenile-onset neuronal ceroid-lipofuscinosis in Rambouillet sheep. *Vet Pathol* 31:48.

Hall DG, et al. 1998. Lafora bodies associated with neurologic signs in a cat. *Vet Pathol* 35:218.

Johnson KH, et al. 1992. Islet amyloid polypeptide: mechanisms of amyloidogenesis in the pancreatic islets and potential roles in diabetes mellitus. *Lab Invest* 66:522.

Johnson KH, et al. 1996. Amyloid proteins and amyloidosis in domestic animals. *Int J Exp Clin Invest* 3:270.

Linke RP, Trautwein G. 1989. Immunoglobulin lambda-light-chain derived amyloid (A2) in two horses. *Blut* 58:129.

Newsholme SJ, et al. 1985. A suspected lipofuscin storage disease of sheep associated with ingestion of the plant *Trachyandra divaricata* (Jacq.) Kunth. *Onderstepoort J Vet Res* 52:87.

O'Brien TD, et al. 1993. Islet amyloid protein. *Vet Pathol* 30:317.

O'Brien TD, et al. 1995. Human islet amyloid polypeptide expression in COS-1 cells. *Am J Pathol* 147:609.

O'Brien TD, et al. 1996. Islet amyloid and islet amyloid polypeptide in cynomolgus macaques *(Macaca fascicularis):* an animal model of human noninsulin-dependent diabetes mellitus. *Vet Pathol* 33:479.

Roertgen KE, et al. 1995. Apolipoprotein AI–derived pulmonary vascular amyloid in aged dogs. *Am J Pathol* 147:1311.

Tani Y, et al. 1997. Amyloid deposits in the gastrointestinal tract of aging dogs. *Vet Pathol* 34:415.

Westermark P. 1998. The pathogenesis of amyloidosis. *Am J Pathol* 152:1125.

Wetzel R. 1996. For protein misassembly, it's the "I" decade. *Cell* 86:699.

Yoshino T, et al. 1996. A retrospective study of canine senile plaques and cerebral amyloid angiopathy. *Vet Pathol* 33:230.

Calcification

Gilka F, Sugden EA. 1984. Ectopic mineralization and nutritional hyperparathyroidism in boars. *Can J Comp Med* 48:102.

Hansen DE, et al. 1994. Photosensitization associated with exposure to *Pithomyces chartarum* in lambs. *J Am Vet Med Assoc* 204:1668.

Yanai T, et al. 1994. Vascular mineralization in the monkey brain. *Vet Pathol* 31:546.

Pigments

Haynes JS, Wade PR. 1995. Hepatopathy associated with excessive hepatic copper in a Siamese cat. *Vet Pathol* 32:427.

Kucera J, et al. 1997. Bilateral xanthine nephrolithiasis in a dog. *J Small Anim Pract* 38:302.

Owen CA, Ludwig J. 1982. Inherited copper toxicosis in Bedlington terriers. *Am J Pathol* 106:432.

Pawelek JM, Korner AM. 1982. The biosynthesis of mammalian melanin. *Am Sci* 70:136.

Crystals

Rhyan JC, et al. 1992. Severe renal oxalosis in five young Beefmaster calves. *J Am Vet Med Assoc* 201:1907.

Sorensen JL, Ling GV. 1993. Metabolic and genetic aspects of urate urolithiasis in Dalmatians. *J Am Vet Med Assoc* 203:857.

Woodard JC, et al. 1982. Calcium phosphate deposition disease in Great Danes. *Vet Pathol* 19:464.

Connective tissue substances

Atkins ME, et al. 1988. Morphologic and immunocytochemical study of young dogs with diabetes mellitus associated with pancreatic islet hypoplasia. *Am J Vet Res* 49:1577.

Doliger S, et al. 1995. Histochemical study of cutaneous mucins in hypothyroid dogs. *Vet Pathol* 32:628.

Hardy MH, et al. 1988. An inherited connective tissue disease in the horse. *Lab Invest* 59:253.

Haskins ME, et al. 1980. The pathology of the feline model of mucopolysaccharidosis. *Am J Pathol* 101:657.

Miner JH, Sanes JR. 1996. Molecular and functional defects in kidneys of mice lacking collagen α3(IV): implications for Alport syndrome. *J Cell Biol* 135:1403.

Potter KA, Besser TE. 1994. Cardiovascular lesions in bovine Marfan syndrome. *Vet Pathol* 31:501.

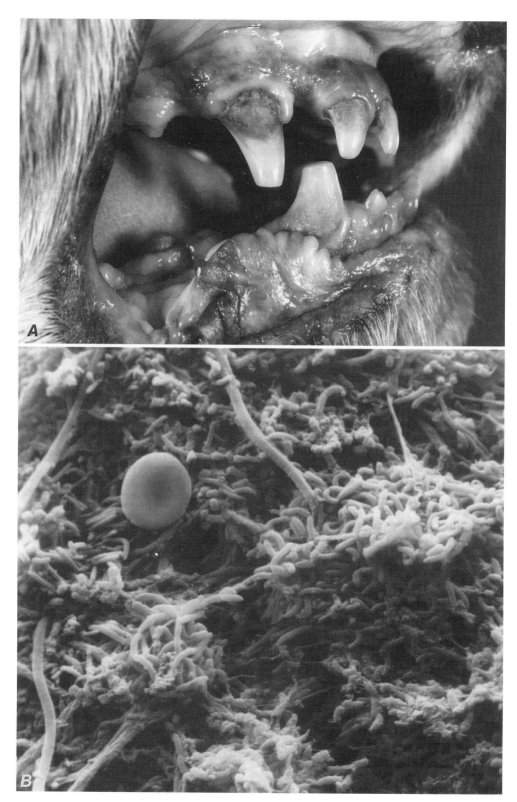

FIGURE 3.1. Microbial plaque, tooth, dog. A. Supragingival calculi with fibrotic gingivae. B. Bacilli and cocci attached to large filamentous bacterium, probably *Actinomyces* sp.

■ CHAPTER 3

Etiology

Etiology is the study of the causes of disease (Fig. 3.1). The word *etiology* is also used synonymously with **etiologic agent**, the actual causal agent of disease (Table 3.1). Some etiologic agents directly and consistently cause a pathologic tissue reaction and a predictable set of clinical signs of disease. Cyanide stops mitochondrial function in the cell and will kill an animal regardless of nutritional and immune status. Rabies virus, once established as an infection, replicates in neurons and invariably produces neuronal degeneration, inflammation of the brain, and death. The only determinants of disease for these dangerous agents are the total dose received by the host and the portal of entry.

It is rarely sufficient, however, to explain disease in terms of single causes and unremitting, step-by-step progress. With most etiologic agents, production of disease is not uniform. Bacteria of the genus *Mycobacterium* cause tuberculosis, yet only a small fraction of infected animals develop clinical disease. Feline leukemia virus infects large numbers of kittens but induces leukemia in only a few. In these

TABLE 3.1. Etiologic agents of tissue injury and disease

External agents	
Physical	
Mechanical trauma	Cutting objects, blows, compression
Electrical trauma	Lightning, high-frequency currents
Heat	Heatstroke, sunstroke, fever, burns
Cold	Local tissue freezing, cold shock
Radiant energy	Ultraviolet light, x-irradiation
Pressure	Increased, decreased
Chemical	
Biologic toxins	Bacterial and fungal toxins, venoms
Pesticides	Organophosphates (parathion)
Herbicides	Paraquat, 2,4-D, dinitrophenols
Environmental toxins	Metals, nitrates, PCBs
Dietary excess	Vitamins A and D
Biologic	
Acellular agents	Viruses, prions
Prokaryotes	Bacteria
Eukaryotes	Fungi, protozoa, algae
Metazoan parasites	Cestodes, nematodes, trematodes, insects
External deficiencies	
Nutritional deficiency	Protein, vitamins, calories
Environmental deficit	Water, oxygen, sunlight
Internal defects	
Aging	Natural, premature
Immunologic defects	Autoimmune disease
Genetic defects	Single mutant gene to chromosomal breaks

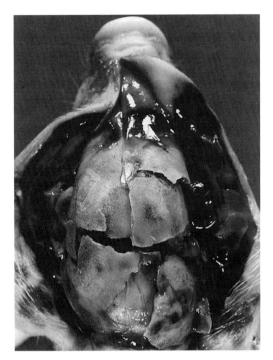

FIGURE 3.2. Fracture of skull, newborn piglet crushed by the sow.

diseases, pathogenesis involves a balance of agent viability and host defense. Genetic, nutritional, immunologic, and environmental characters of the host animal determine, in large part, the development and extent of disease. Thus the pathologist must seek multiple factors as causes of disease, searching for patterns and groups of lesions, and multiple etiologic agents that have combined to produce the clinical manifestations of disease.

Clinical disease is often caused by two or more etiologic agents. In the liver, one drug may inhibit detoxifying enzymes that predispose the liver to hepatotoxicity by another drug; for example, a single dose of ethanol produces a markedly enhanced susceptibility to barbiturate anesthetics. Two or more infectious agents may act together to cause tissue injury. Viruses may induce respiratory disease of little importance, yet in so doing, predispose the lung to severe secondary bacterial infection, such as when swine influenza (caused by a virus) becomes complicated with bacterial pneumonia, or canine distemper suppresses host immunity to enhance growth of *Toxoplasma gondii*.

PHYSICAL INJURY

Trauma

Traumatic lesions arise from any force or energy that is applied to the body. In large animals, trauma is especially common during confinement and shipping. Factors that determine the severity of wounding by mechanical trauma include amount of force, rate of application of the force, surface area involved, and type of tissue that is wounded. Viscera are more friable than skin and muscle. Abnormal tissues are usually more susceptible to mechanical injury than are normal tissues; that is, wounding to fatty livers and congested spleens will be more extensive.

Direct trauma to the heart may lead to contusions, rupture of a chamber, injury to valves or septum, or sudden death from electrical disturbance. Abrupt change in hydraulic pressure—that of compression of the column of blood in the aorta—may cause heart valve injury. A lacerated valve may be the nidus for bacterial infection.

Trauma that does not wound the external surfaces of the body may still cause internal injury and is sometimes referred to as "nonpenetrating trauma." Splenic rupture is a frequent intra-abdominal complication of trauma and may be coincident with rib fracture and injury to the left kidney. Hemorrhage may be immediate or, if the hematoma is subcapsular, may be delayed.

Types of wounds

Contusions (bruises) arise from blood vessel rupture with disintegration of extravasated blood. **Abrasions** are circumscribed areas where epithelium has been removed; they may or may not penetrate to the dermis. The displacement of epithelium in an abrasion may indicate the direction of the force applied. On mucous membranes, the term **erosion** is used to indicate partial loss of surface epithelium. **Incised wounds**, or cuts, are produced by sharp-edged instruments and are longer than they are deep. **Stab wounds** are deeper than long. **Lacerations**, or tear wounds, involve severance of tissue by excessive stretching and are common over bony prominences and on the skull; they occur with dull instruments that macerate and tear tissue with much blood loss.

Compression injuries result from the force of slowly applied pressure. These are common during parturition or in the neonatal period (Fig. 3.2). **Blast** injury arises from explosive force transmitted (in air or water) to body surfaces. In air blast injury, a force of compression waves is exerted unidirectionally against surfaces, followed by a wave of diminished pressure. This can rupture muscles and viscera to cause extensive hemorrhage. Gas emboli may arise and lead to infarction of lung and other viscera. In water blasts, pressure is applied more uniformly to body surfaces, usually propelling the animal to the surface. In fish, rupture of the swim bladder is often lethal.

Bullet wounding

As a spinning bullet produces an entry wound in the skin, it indents, stretches, and scrapes out epidermis. Research done in the 1940s on dogs and goats showed that bullets hitting the skin at a right angle produce uniform margins of abrasion; those that hit at less than 90° produce asymmetric margins in which the widest margin indicates the direction from which the bullet came. In exit wounds, bullets are traveling at slower speeds and are deformed, so they tend to produce irregular, lacerated wounds with everted edges. Contamination of bullet wounds with bacteria occurs directly from bullet surfaces and indirectly by suction induced by violent cavity formation and collapse of tissue.

Lead bullets are rapidly encapsulated in fibrous connective tissue and seldom cause clinical problems, except for rare cases of lead toxicosis. Lead bullets retained in joints are exposed to synovial fluid that serves as a solvent and promotes entry of lead into the systemic circulation. New steel shot (used since 1991), when embedded in tissue, undergoes surface corrosion that may cause a more severe inflammatory response, leading to foreign body reaction and fistulae.

Fragmentation of the bullet greatly increases the severity of injury. Pure lead tends to fragment after hitting the target, especially if the tip has been scored (a dumb-dumb bullet) or if the bullet has a hollow point. Jacketed bullets are usually scored by a metal harder than lead, such as copper or nickel—required for military use by the Geneva Convention; they resist fragmentation upon hitting the target.

The wounding capacity of bullets can be determined by weight (W) and velocity (V)—that is, force + $WV^2/2g$, where g is the acceleration of gravity. The kinetic energy of a bullet increases arithmetically in relation to weight and geometrically in relation to velocity. When two bullets weigh the same, but one travels twice as fast as the other, the energy is 4 times as great in the fast bullet. A bullet fired from a rifle (2,000–3,000 ft/s) has a muzzle velocity 3–4 times greater than that fired from a pistol (500–1,000 ft/s), and such high-velocity bullets have kinetic energies 9–16 times greater than at low velocity. Rotation of the bullet also enhances its energy and thus the injury production of flying metal.

Electrical injury

Electrical injury depends on the kind (direct or alternating), amount (amperage), and electromotive force (voltage) of an electrical current. The path, duration, and area of current flow are also important. A 60-cycle alternating current as small as 100 mA is sufficient to cause ventricular fibrillation in a dog if it passes through the heart.

Electricity causes injury both directly (electric flow through the cardiac conduction system or respiratory centers of brain) and indirectly (heat produced in tissue and fractures on falling during tetany). High voltage produces severe flash burns that are serious if the animal survives. Death from low-voltage current is usually due to ventricular fibrillation. High-voltage currents induce tetanic spasm of respiratory muscles and directly inhibit respiratory centers in the brain. High voltage also produces severe flash burns that are serious if the animal survives.

Lightning

The diagnosis of death by lightning is based on history of a severe thunderstorm, absence of any other disease, and presence of lesions (which are not pathognomonic): singed haircoat (occurs in about half the cases), and tiny hemorrhages in lungs, endocardium, and superficial lymph nodes. Cyanosis, postmortem bloat, and congestion of viscera are common in animals killed by lightning. In pregnant cows, lightning may kill the fetus but not the cow. Postlightning sequelae in surviving cattle include ocular degeneration and myoglobinuria, often with renal tubular necrosis. Because of legal considerations, it is important to remember that lightning can kill without leaving any of these signs of injury.

Ground fault voltage

The term *stray voltage* is used to describe electricity on metals and other conducting materials, especially on feeders and waterers on dairy farms. In a recent survey in Michigan, 32 of 59 dairy farms had sources of stray voltage. Animals in contact with stray voltage may show excitability and abnormal behavior of other types. Water consumption is reduced when waterers are charged with as little as 3.7 volts, so dehydration may be important. Affected piglets are excitable and are prone to tail biting. Cows exposed to voltage that exceeds 1 volt alternating current may show increases in abnormal behavior: poor milk production, reduced feed or water intake, and abnormal behavior at milking time. An increase in clinical mastitis also has been seen on affected farms.

Power lines

Despite the lack of evidence on effects of power lines on animal health, especially cattle, veterinarians are questioned on this matter. Recent studies in Oregon have shown no effect on beef cattle that were grazing under high-voltage, direct-current power lines. There were no differences in nervousness, weight gain, or number of calves born between exposed and control cattle.

Temperature injury

Thermal burns

The clinical significance of thermal burns depends on the proportion of the body surface involved and the depth of the burn. Burns are classified as follows:

- **First degree**—partial thickness injury; superficial burns with erythema and/or vesicles
- **Second degree**—partial thickness injury; epidermis is destroyed but skin appendages remain
- **Third degree**—full thickness injury, with necrosis through entire dermis

Only hyperemia and injury to the superficial layers of epidermis are involved in first-degree burns (e.g., sunburn of hairless, white-skinned animals). In second-degree burns, the epidermis is destroyed, although hair follicles remain and provide a nidus for the epithelization of healing. In third-degree burns, the dermis is destroyed. Regeneration of the skin to cover burned surfaces can occur from skin appendages in both first- and second-degree burns. An infection can convert a second-degree burn to a third-degree burn, so that regeneration will not occur.

The effects of burns are **local tissue destruction, fluid loss,** and secondary **bacterial infection.** Increased vascular permeability with extensive fluid loss may lead to shock and death. These effects arise from blistering, serous exudation, and surface evaporation from large, denuded wounds. Late complications of severe thermal burns include **laryngeal and pulmonary edema** from inhalation of smoke and toxic gases, **renal failure** that accompanies shock-induced necrosis of renal tubules, and **sepsis** arising from secondary bacterial infection. Immediately after burning, the wound is sterile for about 20 hours. Thereafter, bacterial contamination is progressive, and by 72 hours there may be millions of bacteria per gram of burned tissue. Bacteria invade the deep layers of skin, reaching inflammatory zones that demarcate healthy tissue. Although staphylococci and streptococci are major problems, the bacterium *Pseudomonas aeruginosa* has a predilection for skin, where it invades vascular tissues and produces septicemia.

Thermal injury to skin results in transient neutropenia, sequestration of neutrophils in lung capillaries, and activation of the **complement system** in serum (C5-related chemotactic activity). Oxygen-derived free radicals released by activated neutrophils play a crucial role in lung injury in severe burns. Immunosuppression occurs in severe burns and is related to impaired phagocytosis by neutrophils.

Sunburn

The cellular response of skin to prolonged sunlight exposure is keratinocyte swelling within the basal epidermis, blistering of the epidermis, and an associated inflammatory response in the dermis. Sunburn of the skin occurs in hairless, white-skinned animals. Dogs raised in temperate zones are apt to develop sunburn of the tongue because of prolonged panting when transferred to hot, tropical climates. Fish held in shallow waters in uncovered concrete ponds (especially at high altitude) develop focal necrosis of the skin with blistering and ulceration.

Hyperthermia

Hyperthermia due to high environmental temperature in mammals leads directly to water loss, and this in turn causes increases in blood pH, hemoglobin concentration, and erythrocyte counts. In **heatstroke,** there may be degenerative changes in the myocardium, renal tubules, and brain that lead to permanent damage. Heatstroke frequently occurs in small pets confined in a hot environment without water. The early signs are hyperpnea (abnormal increase in rate and depth of respiration), tachycardia (rapid heart action), and vomiting, and these may be related to brain injury caused by elevated body temperature. Several days after heatstroke occurs, there is often evidence of renal failure caused by degeneration and necrosis of renal tubules.

Hypothermia

Hypothermia, a low body temperature, is due in clinical settings to exposure to cold weather. It is especially important in poorly nourished animals. Cold injury in animals relates to the requirement for increased caloric intake in cold environments. Range cattle can withstand very cold temperatures if the food supply is adequate, but their susceptibility to cold increases markedly if they are poorly nourished.

Hibernation is a precisely regulated lowering of the central thermostat in the hypothalamus designed to conserve energy. Regulated by the effects of day-length cycles on the pineal, hibernation is mediated by a protein called thermogenin and by stimulation of heat production in brown fat cells in which mitochondrial oxidative phosphorylation and respiration are uncoupled.

Freezing

Freeze-induced necrosis of extremities occurs in prolonged severe cold environments. Frozen tissue undergoes necrosis because water crystallizes, leaving high salt concentrations in the cytoplasmic matrix. Necrotic tissue is swollen, blotchy, and discolored. Freeze damage is enhanced by injury to blood vessels. As frozen tissue thaws, vasodilation, increased vascular permeability, and thrombosis occur and increase parenchymal cell damage. There may also be significant damage to peripheral nerves.

Laser injury

Lasers emit light in the near infrared spectrum that passes unimpeded through tissues to induce injury at a point of focus. As the laser beam is focused, it creates ionized atoms and free electrons that cause capillary damage with edema, hemorrhage, and coagulation. Absorption of energy is most intense in pigmented tissues. If the beam is delivered continuously, the effects are chiefly thermal, with damage being governed mainly by wavelength of light.

Radiation injury

Radiation includes **electromagnetic radiation** (UV, X-rays, gamma rays) and **particle radiation**, which usually needs to be ingested to cause injury, because particles may not travel far through tissue. These particles are of two types: **uncharged particles** (neutrons) and **charged particles**, which include alpha particles (protons), beta particles (electrons), and positrons (antimatter positively charged electron equivalents). The initial tissue damage in radiation is instantaneous, but the clinical effects may not be apparent for days.

Radiation-induced cell damage

Radiation injury is caused when energy in radiation is transferred to the cell. Atoms can be ionized, or electrons can be excited. Both states are unstable and likely to cause secondary reactions. Radiation injury can be either nuclear (DNA, genetic) or somatic (cytoplasmic), but both are involved in any exposure. Disruption of linkages and bonds of DNA is the most serious event, although enzymes, membranes, and other macromolecules are typically broken.

Cells acutely injured by radiation develop cell swelling, usually with vacuolation of the endoplasmic reticulum and swelling of mitochondria. Chromosomal damage may include breakage, deletion, and translocation. Radiation injury to vascular and connective tissue enhances parenchymal cell damage. Erythema is one of the early tissue changes seen in acute radiation sickness. At high doses, blood vessels may rupture or develop thrombosis.

We are constantly being exposed to both cosmic radiation and radioactive elements in the earth's crust. Because radiation is ubiquitous and animals have evolved in a radiation environment, nature has given animals the enzyme systems that allow the capacity to withstand certain amounts of radiation. These enzyme systems reverse radiation-induced injury to DNA and cytoplasm.

Radiation-induced disease occurs in patients that

FOCUS

Mechanisms of Heat Loss and Conservation

ON A HOT DAY A WHIPPET can keep a rabbit running until the rabbit dies of heat exhaustion. Although running raises the temperature of both animals, and both are cooled by airflow over oronasal mucosae, the dog's brain has a cooling system that the rabbit lacks. A network of blood vessels branching from the carotid artery, the carotid rete mirabile, passes through a venous sinus that draws cooled blood directly from the nasal cavity. In the rete mirabile, the warm arterial blood loses heat to the cooler venous blood, thereby cooling the blood supply to the brain. These countercurrent heat-exchange networks occur in the brain of carnivores and artiodactyls (cattle and other even-numbered-hoofed mammals) but are lacking in horses, primates, rodents, and lagomorphs.

receive large doses of therapeutic, antineoplastic radiation. Tissue injury generally results from vascular lesions. In the **heart**, early changes of endothelial cell swelling and altered capillary permeability are followed by basement membrane reduplication, platelet aggregation, and phagocytosis. Late phases of injury lead to myocardial fibrosis. In the **brain**, ultrastructural evidence of radiation injury is seen in the neuropil and in vascular tissues. In rodents, changes are seen as early as 1.5 hours after large doses of radiation.

Radiation injury is generally a property of radiosensitivity of a particular tissue. However, radiation injury to vascular components makes all organs susceptible. Salivary glands, which are unavoidably irradiated during treatment of pharyngeal and oral tumors, may develop sialoadenitis. Salivary glands are generally viewed as radioresistant; damage occurs largely in the capillary endothelium and secondarily to the acinar cells.

Radiation sensitivity is in direct proportion to a tissue's mitotic activity and inversely proportional to its degree of differentiation. Germinal cells of the ovary are the most sensitive, followed by sperm, lymphocytes, erythropoietic and myeloid cells of bone marrow, and intestinal epithelium. Neuron and muscle cells are relatively insensitive to radiation. Radiation injury is diminished in the absence of oxygen, and hypoxia is a protective factor. This is important in cancer therapy, because the centers of tumor nodules are often hypoxic.

Generally, the higher the animal species is phylogenetically, the more sensitive it is to radiation. The X-ray dose that is lethal for 50% of a group of animals (LD_{50}) is 100,000 R for amoebae, 700 R for frogs, 400–650 R for mice and humans, 315 R for dogs, and 275 R for pigs. These differences are partly due to variation in activity of cell replication. Frogs can be given a dose of radiation that will kill

in 6 weeks. If irradiated frogs are kept at 5°C, they remain alive for several months, but on being warmed, they will die within 6 weeks, like the control animals kept at normal temperature.

Total body radiation

Acute radiation sickness from large doses of radiation given by a point source arises from killing of cells in the bloodstream, bone marrow, and intestine (Table 3.2). Anorexia and vomiting develop within 2 hours of radiation and may arise from brain injury. These signs decline, but at 24–48 hours they recur, accompanied by severe diarrhea due largely to necrosis of gastrointestinal epithelium and to dehydration, hemoconcentration, and shock.

In the 1960s, radioactive fallout from military bomb tests resulted in massive liberation of neutrons and gamma radiation. Effects of this type of radiation are complicated by cloud movement and deposition of radioactive particles on plants. Acute radiation sickness in exposed animals results not so much from external radiation but from internal radiation from ingestion of contaminated plants.

INFECTIOUS DISEASES

Prion disease

The transmissible agents that cause the slowly progressive spongiform encephalopathies have been designated as **prions** (for "proteinaceous infectious particle"). Diseases associated with prions are characterized by vacuolation of nervous tissue and reactive astrocytosis. Human prion diseases include kuru, Creutzfeldt-Jakob disease, and Gerstmann-Straussler syndrome. Animal prion diseases are as follows:

- Scrapie
- Bovine spongiform encephalopathy
- Transmissible mink encephalopathy
- Wasting disease of deer/elk

Scrapie, the prototype prion disease, is a progressive, degenerative neurologic disease of sheep and goats. It begins insidiously with the animal scraping its fleece against fixed objects and progresses to tremor, ataxia, and death. Neuropathologic changes in natural scrapie of sheep include diffuse vacuolation (status spongiosis), loss of neurons, and astrogliosis of the gray matter. Vacuoles are chiefly in neurons, although some glia may be affected. Extracellular spaces are not enlarged. Typically, nerve cells degenerate, but astrocytes proliferate in response to infection.

A critical role is played by both agent strain and host genotype in the transmissible spongiform en-

TABLE 3.2. Clinical signs of acute radiation injury

Signs	Pathology
Leukopenia	Immediate onset, especially lymphopenia
Vomiting	Early (neurologic) and late (intestinal) onset
Thrombocytopenia	Bone marrow destruction
Hemorrhage	Especially in heart, intestine, urogenital tract
Bone marrow aplasia	Diminished blood cell production
Anemia	Predisposes to cardiovascular injury
Epithelial necrosis	Intestine affected: diarrhea, ulceration, tarry stools
Lymphoid necrosis	Widespread infection, necrosis

cephalopathies. The major host factor that controls the incubation period in scrapie is a gene called *Sinc*, or *Prn-i*, which is closely related to the gene encoding PrP^{Sc}.

Prions contain a single major protein that is required for infectivity (they appear to lack nucleic acids) and are highly resistant to most disinfectants. In scrapie the prion protein is called PrP^{Sc} and is a modified, protease-resistant form of a normal tissue protein called PrP^{C}. PrP^{C} is a normal host protein encoded in a single exon of a single-copy gene. It is located on neuron surfaces anchored to the plasma membrane by glycoinositol phospholipid moieties. PrP^{Sc} differs from PrP^{C} in its resistance to proteolysis, sedimentation properties, ability to aggregate into β-pleated sheets of amyloid, and association with infectivity. In scrapie, there is a direct correlation between PrP^{Sc} concentration and pathologic changes in the brain. PrP^{Sc} does not anchor to the plasma membrane but accumulates in the cytoplasm.

FOCUS

Failure to Conduct Necropsies: The Utah Radiation Incident

DURING MAY 1953, two atomic bomb blasts at a test site in Nevada rained fallout on herds of sheep grazing nearby. The U.S. Atomic Energy Commission had tested "Nancy" and "Harry," two high-yield bombs. As clouds of dust and radiation rolled down Utah valleys, ranchers reported radiation burns on sheep grazing downwind of detonation sites. Wool sloughed off in clumps. Within a short period, 2,000 ewes and 2,200 lambs died, roughly one-eighth of the ewes and one-fourth of the lambs.

Complaints were made, and a team of veterinarians was dispatched to collect tissues and bone samples from surviving sheep for radiologic analysis at the radiation lab in Oak Ridge. Later, sheep were experimentally exposed to intense radiation at Los Alamos in an attempt to duplicate the lesions. Scientists at a Hanford, Washington, lab who studied effects of radioiodine on ewes suggested that the sheep did not die from irradiation, because "doses were too low," and they did not die from doses to thyroid, because "that is a slower cause of death." However, two veterinarians concluded that the lesions on surviving sheep were similar or identical to those produced at Los Alamos and that "radiation was at least a contributing factor to the loss of these animals."

The sheep probably died from effects of contaminated grass in their stomachs. Sheep exposed to only 4 rad of external gamma radiation might have gotten a dose of 1,500–1,600 rad in the gastrointestinal tracts, and fetal lambs may have received a thyroid dose of 20,000–40,000 rad (*Science* 218:545, 1982).

Thirty years after this incident, previously classified documents were released that stimulated lawsuits against the government in relation to human leukemia. Utah ranchers initiated a lawsuit, also alleging suppression of information after atomic testing. The courts found that the U.S. government had suppressed scientific data and pressured veterinarians to revise their conclusions. Motivated by a desire to prevent general alarm, the Atomic Energy Commission had extensively investigated these events but had not revealed potentially compromising field observations and critical data from laboratory experiments.

TABLE 3.3. Patterns of viral disease

1. Acute cytolytic disease—viral replication leads to cell death
    a. Direct—herpes
    b. Preliminary proliferation (stimulation of growth factors)—pox
    c. Massive proliferation (presence of growth genes)—papilloma
2. Immunopathic reactions—interaction with antibodies/lymphocytes
    a. Immunosuppression—feline immunosuppressive virus
    b. Hypersensitivity—lymphocytic choriomeningitis
3. Asymptomatic infection—no clinical disease
4. Neoplasia—virus inserts into host cell genomes—retroviruses

Viral disease

Viruses produce disease by replicating inside cells to cause degeneration and cell death. The mature infectious viral particles, which are called virions, do not have ribosomes to synthesize protein and must use cellular organelles to reproduce. As viral replication proceeds, cellular organelles disappear and are replaced by viral proteins and other structures that are used to form new virions (Table 3.3).

Acute cytolytic viral infection

Replication of highly pathogenic, cytolytic viruses results in cell death, often with marked lesions of necrosis in tissue (Fig. 3.3) and severe signs of systemic disease. Clinical signs of systemic disease are provoked when infected cells are lysed, with release of potent cytokines and cellular debris into lymphatic and blood-vascular systems. These **biologically active peptides**, membrane fragments, and viral protein remnants act on the vascular and nervous systems as pyrogens and chemoattractants for inflammatory cells, and are responsible for many of the clinical signs. For example, infection of monocytes by influenza virus causes those cells to release several peptide cytokines that send signals to other tissue systems—pyrogens act on the hypothalamus to produce fever, interleukins act on lymphocytes to induce immune reactions, and a metabolism modulating factor induces gluconeogenesis in skeletal muscle (and the amino acid drain that leads to myalgia, or muscle pain).

Tissue may also be injured by severe inflammatory responses provoked by the virus. Many viruses, especially those producing systemic disease, tend to replicate within leukocytes and endothelium; these cells release **cellular signal** molecules (e.g., cytokines, prostaglandins, and leukotrienes) that induce fever, anorexia, and myalgia). The disintegra-

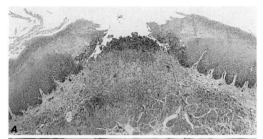

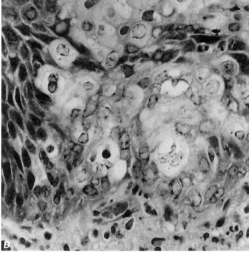

FIGURE 3.3. Epithelial necrosis and ulceration, herpesvirus-infected esophageal epithelial cell, infectious bovine rhinotracheitis. A. Severe focal necrosis with ulceration of epithelium. B. Acute cell swelling and lysis of herpesvirus-infected cells at the periphery of the necrotic area, at the interface of epithelium and dermis.

tion of neutrophilic leukocytes and macrophages releases tissue-destructive enzymes that enhance the primary viral injury.

Proliferative response to viruses

Many viruses produce a proliferative response in cells as part of the infectious process. The most extreme examples are papilloma viruses, which cause marked proliferation of epithelial cells. This response, although controlled by the host, leads to large proliferative lesions called **infectious papillomas** (see Fig. 2.7A). Most acute cytolytic viruses incite proliferative responses in tissues (note the increased epithelial layer even in the highly cytolytic herpesvirus infection in Fig. 3.3). Epithelial lesions caused by poxviruses typically have strong proliferative and cytolytic responses (see Fig. 1.9).

Proliferative responses to viral infections in skin

and mucous membranes leave characteristic gross lesions that often lead to the diagnosis. Cutaneous lesions commonly seen in viral disease include the following:

- **Macule**—discolored spot on skin that is not elevated
- **Papule**—small, circumscribed, solid elevation of the skin
- **Vesicle**—small (<1 cm) circumscribed epidermal space with serous fluid
- **Pustule**—pus within the epidermis or its glands

Lesions of poxviruses move progressively through these four stages. Acute cytolytic herpesviruses and many other viruses develop one or more of these lesions, and many are pathognomonic for the disease they produce.

Some viruses infect without producing disease

Viral infection may occur without signs of disease. These infections are subclinical, or **asymptomatic**. Asymptomatic infection may occur because viral replication is very slow (without inducing cell degeneration) or because a virus does not replicate at all. Viral genetic material may hide at some location in the cell until later provoked to replicate and thus produce an acute lytic infection. Herpesviruses often act in this way; they remain latent until some stressful event occurs (often associated with adrenal corticosteroid release) that stimulates viral replication.

Viruses that induce tumors act in this way, except that their association with the nucleus eventually leads to the uncontrolled cell replication of **neoplasia**. Neoplastic disease occurs long after infection and usually involves the integration of viral genetic material into the chromosomes of the host cell.

Viruses must bind to cell surfaces to infect

To be pathogenic, viruses must be capable of specifically attaching to the surfaces of target cells. Attachment must alter the cell membrane so that a specific signal for uptake of virions occurs. After entering the cell, viruses must contain enzymes (or genomic codes to produce enzymes) that alter cell metabolism in favor of viral replication. Viruses shut down host cell synthesis and subvert it toward replication of new virus-induced nucleic acids and proteins. This causes the acute lytic infection of cells that, if uncontrolled, leads directly to tissue destruction and systemic signs of illness.

Viruses kill cells by shutting off protein synthesis

In the process of viral replication, normal cell metabolism is disrupted as protein synthesis is shut down. Viruses contain either DNA or RNA as their genetic material. These nucleic acid templates are liberated into the host cell cytoplasm and are used as codes to create new viral genetic material, viral enzymes, and structural proteins that will become part of the external coat of the virion. Although some of the viral peptides are directly toxic to the cell, most cellular injury arises from failure of the infected cell to produce critical enzymes and energy for its own metabolism.

As viral replication proceeds, production of the various proteins used to assemble new virions becomes unbalanced. Masses of virus-induced proteins and other excess components of virions accumulate as **inclusion bodies** that distort the cell. Energy sources are depleted, electrolyte pumps on the cell surface decline, and intracellular pH drops. The result may be a shrunken necrotic cell or a lysed cell that has liberated its cytoplasmic debris into tissue spaces (Fig. 3.4).

Viruses are released by cell lysis or budding from cell surfaces

Viruses vary considerably in size and complexity and thus in how they replicate within cells. Most virions are released from cells when the cell dies and disintegrates. In acute herpesviral infections, cells are quickly killed and virions are released into tissue. Some viruses do not kill the host cell but allow it to survive in order to shed new virions over a longer period. For example, influenza virus is shed into the lumen of the airways to be coughed up in respiratory exudates. In influenza-infected cells, the surface membrane is altered at sites where virions are to emerge. Immature viral particles migrate to the cell surface, are stitched into the plasma membrane by special viral proteins, and are drawn into the membrane and surrounded. After total envelopment, the virion is pinched off from the cell and released into the respiratory tract.

Laboratory diagnosis of viral infections

Analysis of the cellular changes and the character of the inflammatory response leads to the proper diagnosis. The presence of **inclusion bodies** is a major factor in pinpointing the virus group involved (see Fig. 2.7). **Immunolabeling** of viral proteins present in tissue sections will establish a specific diagnosis. In these techniques, specific

Influenza

INFLUENZA VIRUSES OCCUR in birds and in four species of mammals: swine, horses, seals, and humans. All of these viruses produce disease by destroying epithelial cells of the respiratory tract. Soon after the initial foci of infection begin in epithelia of the nasal turbinates, virus spreads to involve the entire upper respiratory tract. An acute, intense inflammatory response (rhinitis, tracheitis, and pneumonitis) is accompanied by coughing, fever, and myalgia. In the lung, epithelium of the terminal bronchioles is especially vulnerable to infection. Affected epithelial cells swell and develop cytoplasmic basophilia, but definite inclusion bodies are not present.

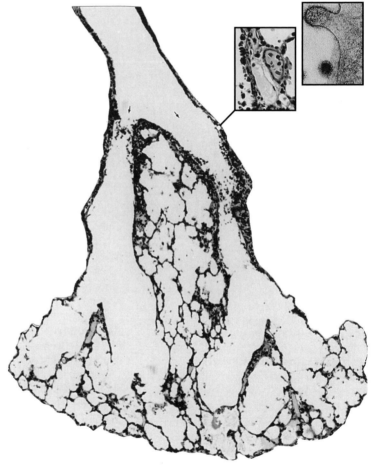

Swine influenza. Virus first replicates in respiratory epithelium as it terminates in the ends of the bronchioles *(arrows)*. As epithelial cells are destroyed *(left inset),* virions bud from cell surfaces *(right inset)* and are released into exudates in the airway.

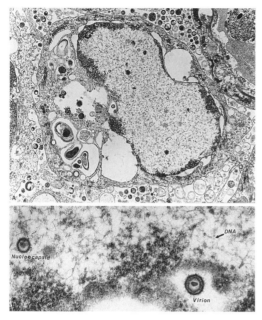

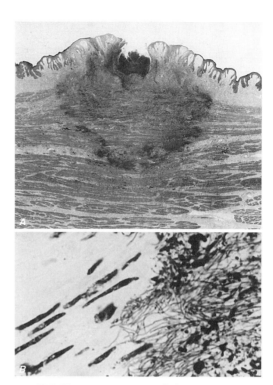

FIGURE 3.4. Epithelial cell infected with herpesvirus (from Fig. 3.3). A. Viral DNA and viral structural proteins are combined in the nucleus to form immature viral particles called *nucleocapsids*. B. Nucleocapsids bud through the nuclear membrane to acquire an exterior coat and become complete viral particles called *virions*. Virions accumulate in vacuoles in the cytoplasm and are shed from the cell to the extracellular spaces.

FIGURE 3.5. Necrosis of the rumen caused by *Fusobacterium necrophorum*, cow. A. Histology: central area of epithelial necrosis with ulcer; necrosis extends deep into the muscle layers. B. Bacteria are located at the margin of healthy and necrotic muscle tissue.

antiviral antibody molecules are conjugated with a dye or other signal molecules. Smears or frozen sections of tissue are fixed, stained with the antibody-signal conjugate, and examined. Detection of the signal stain indicates sites of viral proteins.

Bacterial disease

Pathogenic bacteria produce disease in several different ways. The nature of the cellular response in infected tissue provides clues to the identity of bacteria. Bacteria are grouped according to the predominant tissue reaction that occurs, as follows:

- **Pyogenic**—producing pus by attracting leukocytes
- **Toxigenic**—secreting toxins that cause disease
- **Intracellular**—replicating inside macrophages and other host cells

Pyogenic bacteria such as streptococci and staphylococci produce pus by releasing factors that increase permeability of blood vessels and that are chemotactic for neutrophils. Toxigenic bacteria in-

cite little pus but cause great tissue destruction by releasing toxins that directly kill specific cells (Fig. 3.5). Intracellular bacteria do neither of these but replicate inside macrophages or parenchymal cells to produce subacute or chronic disease. All bacteria, after being taken up by phagocytosis, release substances called **virulence factors**, which suppress the host cell's bacteriocidal mechanisms and allow the bacterium to survive.

Pyogenic bacteria colonize skin and body orifices

Bacteria associated with acute inflammation are typically pyogenic—that is, they attract neutrophils to sites of infection. *Streptococcus* spp. cause inflammatory lesions in the skin, lymph nodes, heart valves, and meninges. These are important agents of mastitis in cattle, strangles and other respiratory diseases of horses, and many diseases of pigs, including septicemia, meningitis, arthritis, endocarditis, and lymphadenitis. Streptococci can colonize normal skin for long periods and then, after some minor trauma, cause **pyoderma**. The initial lesion is a microabscess or small pustule that expands into adjacent areas.

Staphylococcus spp. are residents of normal skin, nasal passages, and lower gut, depending on individual species. They are frequent causes of infection of skin and body orifices. Some strains of staphylococci produce toxins that cause vacuolar changes and microvesicles in epithelium. Dogs with diabetes mellitus commonly develop severe staphylococcal infections because their neutrophils are inhibited by persistent hyperglycemia.

Granulomatous lesions of chronic infections by pyogenic bacteria, such as staphylococci and *Pseudomonas aeruginosa,* and by *Actinomyces* spp. and *Actinobacillus* spp. often contain peculiar but diagnostically useful granules that are formed by aggregation of bacteria, debris, and proteins of plasma. They are called **sulfur granules** because of their yellow, granular appearance. Histologically, sulfur granules stain bright red with eosin and have a central mass of amorphous debris from which club-shaped processes radiate outward. Reactions of antibodies with antigens in these masses produce aggregates of hyalin material.

Bacterial toxins

Toxins produced by bacteria fall into two major categories: **structural components** of the bacterium, which are released after bacterial destruction, and **soluble peptides**, which are released by the living bacterium. The dominant structural toxins are the **endotoxins**, lipopolysaccharides present in the cell

---

FOCUS

Rabies

RABIES ENCEPHALITIS has been a fearsome scourge of dogs, humans, and other animals since the beginning of recorded history. Rabies persists in nature because of the unique duality of host infection. First, the encephalitis induces a change from the normal fearful attitude of the host to one of aggressive behavior in which, in carnivores at least, the host will attack other potential host animals. Second, virus replicates to high titer in the salivary glands of carnivores and is excreted in the saliva.

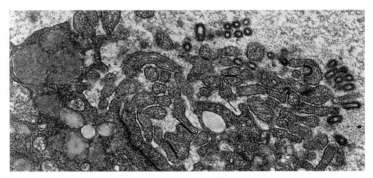

Virions at the surface of a ductal epithelial cell in the parotid gland of a fox. (Photograph: Richard Dierks, *Am J Pathol*)

In superficial bites, virus replicates in the stratum germinativum of skin and is transmitted to unmyelinated nerves. In deep bites, it first replicates in striated muscle cells, with release of virus to neuromuscular spindles and motor endplates. Rabies virus ascends to the central nervous system by axonal flow through nerves and by transneuronal transfer. To enter nervous tissue, it uses the normal **acetylcholine receptor** located at the synapse as the receptor for viral attachment.

wall of gram-negative bacteria. Endotoxins produce profound effects on the blood-vascular system and are important in septicemia, in which they cause "endotoxic" shock.

Exotoxins may be potent lysins that **damage cellular membranes** (clostridial phospholipases, hemolysins, and other lysins), they may act by entering the cell to **suppress metabolism**, or they may be **pore-forming toxins**—toxins that embed in the cell surface to form a channel for ions that leads to lysis of the cell. In the first group, the toxins destroy phospholipids in the lipid bilayer of the cell surface. Small holes are produced in the membrane, the cell gains unwanted electrolytes and water, and cell swelling progresses to cell lysis. The highly lethal α-toxin produced by clostridia in

Once signs of rabies develop, viral antigens are found to be disseminated throughout the body. Infected corneal epithelial cells provide the basis of a corneal smear immunofluorescent diagnostic test. Smears from snout epithelium are used to detect rabies infection in living dogs.

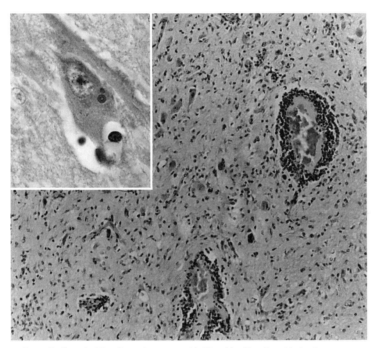

Perivascular lymphoid cuffs and neuron with Negri bodies *(inset)* in brain.

In the brain, virus has a predilection for the brain stem, where it produces an **acute, lymphocytic leukoencephalomyelitis** and **polioencephalomyelitis**. Neuronal degeneration is accompanied by perivascular lymphoid infiltrates and gliosis, often with glial nodules. The medulla, cerebellum, basal ganglia, spinal cord, and dorsal root ganglia may be severely affected, reflecting the clinical picture of ascending paralysis. Infected neurons undergo **cell swelling** and **chromatolysis**. Large aggregates of dense granular viral proteins develop in the cytoplasm. Called **Negri bodies**, these multiple, eosinophilic, cytoplasmic inclusion bodies are used histologically for the diagnosis of rabies.

FOCUS

Colibacillosis

ESCHERICHIA COLI, a major pathogen in mammals and birds, causes **diarrhea** in young animals, **mastitis**, and **purulent infections** of the umbilicus and genitourinary tract. Because some strains of *E. coli* enter the bloodstream, they not only cause **septicemia** but also lodge in organs and produce organ infections such as meningoencephalitis, osteomyelitis, and pyelitis. In the intestine, two distinct mechanisms of disease are caused by *E. coli:* **diarrhea** results from **enterotoxin** production, and **dysentery** from direct invasion of the gut wall.

Acute **enterotoxic colibacillosis** occurs in pigs, calves, lambs, and humans as profuse watery diarrhea that can lead to fatal dehydration and acidosis. Bacteria adhere tightly to the surface of intestine and are not washed out of the gut by peristalsis. Even though bacteria are confined to the gut, they secrete **enterotoxins** that produce little or no structural damage. They do cause absorptive cells of the small intestine to secrete increased water and electrolytes, and when secretion exceeds the capacity of the colon to absorb water, diarrhea occurs.

Enteroinvasive colibacillosis is rare relative to enterotoxin disease. It occurs when *E. coli* attach to and actually invade absorptive cells of the gut to cause dysentery. The lesions involve severe inflammation of the mucosa, often with microulceration. Enteropathogenic *E. coli* closely attaches to apical surfaces of epithelial cells of dome epithelium of Peyer's patches in the ileum, and later to enterocytes of the distal small intestine, cecum, and colon.

Poorly characterized toxins of *E. coli* are associated with **angiopathy** and **edema disease** of baby pigs. Degenerative angiopathy of arterioles and small arteries in several tissues develops as necrosis of smooth muscle cells of the media is followed by exudation of albumen and other plasma proteins into the necrotic media. Vascular degeneration in the brain can cause ischemia, focal necrosis (malacia), and hemorrhage.

---

blackleg of cattle and gas gangrene of humans, for example, is a **lecithinase** that destroys membrane lecithins. The enterotoxins of staphylococci, shigellae, and some of the other clostridia damage intestinal absorptive cells in the same way.

Toxins that suppress metabolism are typically large glycoproteins with two-unit construction: an A chain produces cell injury, and a B chain binds to cell surfaces. After the B chain binds to surface receptors, the exotoxin enters the cell by receptor-mediated endocytosis (into coated vesicles). The subsequent cleavage of the molecule allows fragment A to exert its toxic effect. Some bacterial exotoxins act by ADP ribosylation; that is, the toxin catalyzes cleavage of endogenous NAD with covalent attachment of the adenosine diphosphoribose moiety to a cell substrate. In some cases this process inactivates a critical component of protein synthesis, whereas in others it increases cell activity.

Pore-forming toxins aggregate to form ion-permeable channels on cell surfaces—pores that cause cells to become leaky and undergo lysis. The staphylococcal α-toxin is composed of protein components that aggregate on the cell surface and insert through the membrane, causing the cell to become leaky to ions and water (see Fig. 1.12). Some bacterial toxins that act by creating pores on the surfaces of cells include the following:

α-Toxin	*Staphylococcus aureus*
Perfringolysin	*Clostridium perfringens*
Pneumolysin	*Streptococcus pneumoniae*
Streptolysin O	*S. pyogenes*
Listerolysin O	*Listeria monocytogenes*

α-Hemolysin	*Escherichia coli*
Enterohemolysin	*E. coli*
Cytotoxin	*Pseudomonas aeruginosa*

Intracellular bacteria

Pathogenic bacteria that replicate inside living cells for at least part of their life cycle are called **facultative intracellular bacteria**. Mycobacteria, brucellae, and salmonellae all replicate within cells of the host to cause disease. Like other bacteria, they are taken up by macrophages as they enter tissue, but they are able to survive within the cytoplasm of macrophages and replicate to produce disease (Figs. 3.6 and 3.7). Although macrophages kill most of these intracellular bacteria within a few hours, a small residual population survives and begins to multiply intracellularly to slowly incite a granulomatous or pyogranulomatous lesion.

Bacteria colonize normal mucosal surfaces

Surfaces of the upper respiratory tract, urogenital tract, oropharynx, stomach, and intestine have normal bacterial populations. The microflora of the tongue, orifices of salivary glands, and teeth are similar among different individuals. Tiny microbial plaques occur at the gingival margins of teeth when streptococci cling to tooth surfaces (see Fig. 3.1).

FOCUS

Tetanus

MARCH 30, 1819. I was requested to attend a chestnut colt, four years old, that had been taken up to be broken, the property of Mr. Bamford Bradely, near Bilstone, Staffordshire. I was immediately convinced that it was Tetanus, from the following symptoms: Jaw completely closed, saliva flowing from the mouth; rigidity of the principle muscles of the body, pulse slow and irregular, and tail elevated. (From *The Veterinarian*, vol. 2)

Severe spasms of striated muscle spread progressively from muscle to muscle from a site of wound infection with *Clostridium tetani*. The bacterial toxin suppresses, as does strychnine, all synaptic inhibition. The cause of death is usually asphyxia following paralysis of respiratory muscles. The toxin causes disruption of spinal inhibitory pathways; the resulting unopposed stimulation of motor nerves is the primary cause of unremitting rigidity of skeletal muscle. Muscle rigidity leads to locomotor disturbances; stiffness of limbs, ears, and tail; and curious facial expressions.

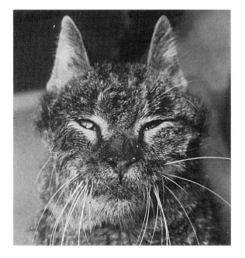

▶

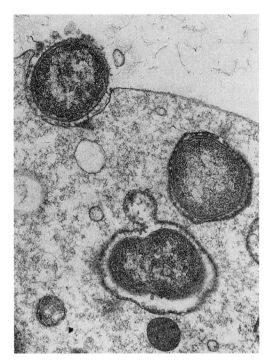

FIGURE 3.6. Phagocytosis of bacteria *(Salmonella choleraesuis)*. Bacteria occur at the surface of the cell, within a phagosome, and within a phagolysosome (which results from phagosome-lysosome fusion).

They secrete enzymes that cleave sucrose (into glucose and fructose), and enzymes called glycosyltransferases in the bacteria polymerize the glucose into long chains called glucans. Glucans adhere to enamel and trap other bacterial species. Each animal species has its characteristic plaque population.

Some parts of the alimentary canal are important fermentation areas whose microflora is of great diversity (e.g., the rumen in many species and the colon in the pig and horse). These normal microflora are changed markedly in disease. This microbial shift probably plays an important secondary role in the diarrhea of dysentery. Staphylococci and streptococci are the most commonly isolated aerobic bacteria obtained from the vagina, prepuce, and urethral orifice of dogs; during genital disease of the female, *E. coli*, which is normally present in low numbers, replicates to much larger numbers.

Identification of bacteria in tissue

Bacteria in tissue can be detected by the Gram stain (a dark blue crystal violet–iodine complex). This stain separates bacteria into two major groups: in **gram-positive** bacteria, dye is fixed in the cell wall and cannot be removed by alcohol because of the presence of mucocomplexes containing muramic acid; **gram-negative** bacteria, which stain pink, have thin cell walls that permit removal of the dye

C. tetani produces several toxins. The most important is the neurotoxin **tetanospasmin** (generally referred to as *tetanus toxin*), which is highly toxic for horses and man. Tetanospasmin binds selectively to ganglioside receptors at peripheral nerve endings, is taken into the nerve, and passes via retrograde transport to nerve cell bodies in the spinal cord, where it diffuses back to exert its action presynaptically. Its major effect is to suppress neuroinhibitory Renshaw cells. Within these neurons, toxin localizes on membranes of endoplasmic reticulum and suppresses the production of neurosecretory substances.

Tetanus toxin also produces central effects in the brain—for example, reflex motor convulsion. In rare cases, these effects may dominate in a syndrome of "cephalic tetanus." Toxin may also bind to cells of the sympathetic nervous system in later stages of disease, producing hypertension, tachycardia, and peripheral vasoconstriction.

A second toxin, **tetanolysin**, is a hemolysin that destroys cells by acting on plasma membranes. Experimentally, it causes hematologic alterations and cardiovascular alterations, and some of the signs seen in terminal tetanus are due to this toxin—for example, pulmonary edema and azotemia. There is a direct lytic effect on skeletal muscles late in the disease, and this effect may be due to tetanolysin, possibly by its inhibition of ion flux in sarcoplasmic reticulum.

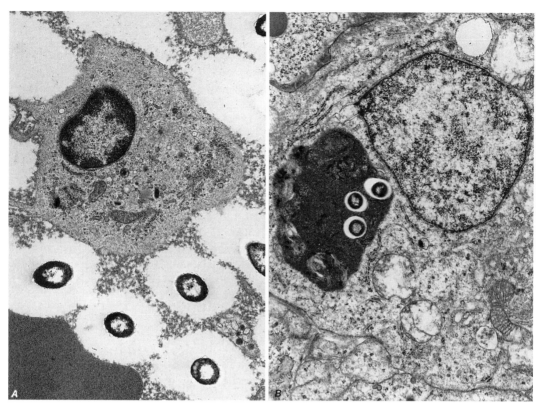

FIGURE 3.7. Bacteria suppress macrophage function by different mechanisms. A. Anthrax. *Bacillus anthracis* produces a thick capsule that is antiphagocytic and prevents uptake by the monocyte or macrophage. B. Tuberculosis. *Mycobacterium* spp. are taken into macrophage phagosomes but produce cell wall lipids that prevent fusion of bacteria-containing phagosomes with lysosomes, which contain the enzymes needed for bacterial killing.

by alcohol treatment. Special stains are useful in diagnosis of some pathogenic bacteria (e.g., silver impregnation techniques for spirochetes, the Giemsa stain for rickettsiae, and the acid-fast stain, which uses basic fuchsin and phenol, for mycobacteria).

Colonies of bacteria may be present in tissues, especially if a terminal or comatose state existed prior to death (Fig. 3.8). When they are found in the renal glomerulus, lung capillaries, and other vascular tissue, they may indicate an origin from septic emboli. Bacterial replication also continues after death, particularly the large saprophytic rods that are found in foci of postmortem autolysis in visceral organs.

Microbial agents may be destroyed by host defenses between the times of infection and death of the animal. Clinical treatment commonly obliterates the cause of death. Bacteria may be killed by antibiotics and cannot be cultured from even severe inflammatory foci in treated animals. In rare infections, antibiotic treatment may even promote

death; in anthrax, for example, treatment kills the circulating bacteria, but the host may die from the ensuing massive liberation of bacterial toxins.

Bacterial structures important in the capacity to cause disease include cell walls, capsules, fimbriae, and flagella. In tissue sections, bacteria are found in interstitial tissue, within cells (especially phagocytic cells), and on epithelial surfaces. Although especially common on lumens of intestine and respiratory tract, they are usually washed away during routine tissue processing.

Bacterial virulence factors

Surfaces of bacteria contain structures that are important **virulence factors** (e.g., fimbriae, capsules, cell walls). Virulence factors enhance bacterial attachment and colonization in tissue, inhibit phagocytosis, or depress host immunity. When produced in sufficient concentrations, these substances cause the organism to resist the opsonic and lytic effects of antibody and complement. Although true viru-

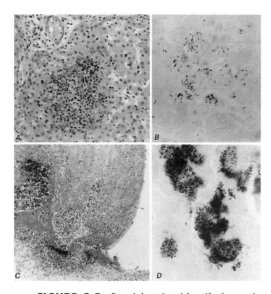

FIGURE 3.8. Special stains identify bacteria in tissue sections. A and B. Necrosis of liver with neutrophil infiltrates and microabscess. A. H&E. B. Gram stain for bacteria identified bacilli in the microabscess. C and D. Vegetative valvular endocarditis, pig. C. Valve at bottom with fibrinous endocarditis extending upward. D. Gram stain identified cocci in the lesion.

lence of bacteria is detectable only in living animals, microbiologists use those components that develop in cultures as markers of virulence (Table 3.4).

Bacterial secretions (exotoxins, coagulase, hyaluronidase) are also important virulence characteristics. They suppress the natural antimicrobial effects of glucosaminoglycans and enable bacteria to move through connective tissue.

Fimbriae are small filamentous appendages that project from the surface; they are important in adhesion of bacteria to the gut lumen and in colonization of tissue surfaces. In several species of bacteria, virulent isolates are fimbriated, whereas nonvirulent isolates lack fimbriae. Fimbriae may be composed of different proteins that function in adhesion. Fimbriae on enteropathogenic *E. coli* of swine contain a protein called K88 that promotes attachment to intestinal epithelium. Vaccines made of purified K88-containing fimbriae have been effective in preventing colibacillosis of pigs and calves.

Several bacteria possess a slimy amorphous **capsule** of complex polysaccharides that inhibits phagocytosis. The capsule of *Bacillus anthracis* effectively prevents phagocytosis by neutrophils and macrophages so that septicemia can develop. Other pathogenic bacteria elaborate soluble factors that suppress the host's cellular defense mechanisms. *Mycobacterium* spp. contain complex lipids that in some way inhibit the fusion of phagocytes and

TABLE 3.4. Bacterial virulence factors

Factor	Mechanism
Structural components	
Capsules	Inhibit phagocytosis (streptococci, anthrax bacilli)
Peptidoglycans	Degranulate platelets (streptococci, staphylococci)
Lipopolysaccharides (endotoxin)	Bind to and destroy cell surface membranes; pyrogen release; prostaglandin release
Lipoteichoic acid	Adhere to epithelium
Cytoplasmic lipids	Inhibit phagosome-lysosome fusion (tuberculosis)
Fimbrial proteins (pili)	Adhere to epithelium
Soluble factors	
Protein synthesis inhibitor	Splits NAD to suppress elongation factors that catalyze translocation of peptide chains
Phospholipase D	Membrane lysis (*Listeria* spp., *Corynebacterium ovis*, *Clostridium* spp.)
Sphingomyelinase	Sphingomyelin lysis (staph β-toxin)
Cholesterol lysin	Cholesterol lysis (streptolysin O)
Hyaluronidase	Proteoglycan disintegration (staphylococci)
Coagulase	Activates fibrinogen; coats bacteria with fibrin; inhibits phagocytosis; promotes intravascular coagulation (staphylococcal coagulase)
Streptokinase	Activates plasma; initiates fibrinolysis
IgA protease	Neutralizes antibodies (streptococci, *Haemophilus* spp., *Neisseria* spp.)
Protease	Degrades fibronectin; inhibits phagocytosis *(Pseudomonas aeruginosa)*
Adenyl cyclase stimulator	Stimulates adenyl cyclase in membranes to produce cyclic AMP and enhance electrolyte secretion (*Vibrio cholera, E. coli*)

Anthrax

ANTHRAX IN ANIMALS and humans is caused by *Bacillus anthracis,* a gram-positive, spore-forming bacterium. Discovered by Koch, *B. anthracis* was used by Metchnikoff in his classic studies on phagocytosis. The bacterium infects most mammals and can cause a rapidly fatal septicemia. Goats, sheep, cattle, horses, pigs, and dogs are susceptible (in that order).

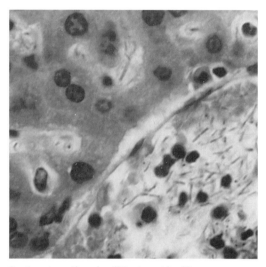

Septicemia, anthrax bacilli in sinusoids of liver.

The bloodstream of septicemic animals swarms with chains of capsulated, square-ended bacilli. The host is killed by a combination of the lethal peptide toxins and massive amounts of antiphagocytic capsular material, which prevents opsonization and killing of *B. anthracis.* When the host animal dies, vegetative bacilli from the carcass are rapidly killed by putrefaction. However, bacilli contaminate the soil and form highly resistant spores that survive for decades.

Grazing mammals ingest spores, which enter through mucous membranes, aided by local lesions. Cutaneous infection (common in humans) is rare in animals. **Pulmonary anthrax**, a particularly lethal form, results from inhalation of spore-laden grasses and dust. Infection can also be transmitted by insects; this mode, however, has not been clearly established.

The absence of anthrax in an area for several years followed by an explosive outbreak with large death losses may lead to popular misconceptions regarding the origin of the disease. *B. anthracis* has been widely studied in the United States, Great Britain, and the former Soviet Union in relation to biological warfare. In theory, airborne dissemination of spores could devastate livestock populations. In April 1979 an outbreak of human anthrax occurred in Sverdlovsk, a city of more than 1 million people. It was believed to have arisen from an accident at a Russian military base. The outbreak was perceived as a threat to Western countries, and fears promoted in the press added to the generally popular fear of anthrax.

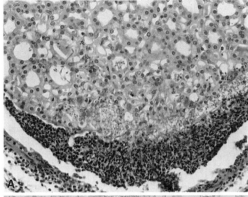

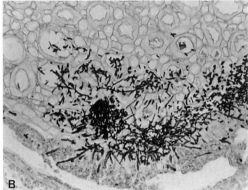

FIGURE 3.9. Special stains identify fungi in tissue sections. A. Necrosis of renal papilla with neutrophil infiltrates. B. Adjacent tissue section stained for fungi, methenamine silver stain to show *Candida* sp.

lysosomes. Intracellular killing and digestion are suppressed, and bacteria can replicate to produce disease.

Gram-negative bacteria contain lipopolysaccharides in the cell walls, known as **endotoxin,** that greatly modify the host's inflammatory responses. Cell degeneration and death may be caused by **exotoxins** (toxic components of the bacterium) or by soluble toxins released during bacterial replication. The ultimate pathogenicity of a bacterium is largely determined by how effectively it produces these toxic factors.

Fungal disease

Fungi are single-celled, nucleated plant organisms that include not only a wide variety of pathogenic species but also yeasts, molds, mushrooms, and mildews. The simplest form is the single-celled budding yeast. In culture, most fungi consist of networks of hyphae called mycelia. Individual hyphae form by elongation of the fungal cells without separation into new cells. Fungi grow by producing new hyphae at the edge of the mycelium (vegeta-

tive growth). Many fungi form specialized reproductive bodies, or **spores.** Asexual spores arise by differentiation of cells of spore-bearing hyphae without fusion; sexual spores are produced by fusion of two cells.

With few exceptions, fungi pathogenic for vertebrates are classed as Fungi Imperfecti; the two important groups are the pathogenic yeasts and the dermatophytes. Most of the important pathogens are **dimorphic;** that is, their typical growth forms are different in tissue and in saprophytic stages in culture. For example, in histoplasmosis, the causal organism, *Histoplasma capsulatum,* is found as small, budding yeast cells within macrophages. In culture, this organism grows as septate mycelia with microconidia and tuberculate chlamydospores.

Fungi cause three types of disease in animals:

- **Mycosis**—direct invasion of tissue by fungal cells
- **Allergic disease**—development of hypersensitivity to fungal antigens
- **Mycotoxicosis**—ingestion of toxic fungal metabolites

It is not unusual for mycosis and allergic disease to occur together, especially when infection of the lung is involved.

Imperfect immune responses lead to fungal infections

Most fungi are omnipresent in the environment, so host resistance is a dominant factor in disease. Opportunistic fungal infections result when animals are immunosuppressed, when mechanisms of inflammation are inhibited, when host protective bacterial microflora is altered, or when stress is placed on their systems over long periods. Newborn and very old animals are most often affected by these factors. In immunosuppression produced by drugs, *Aspergillus* spp. and *Candida* spp. commonly produce complicating systemic infections. Whereas aspergillosis usually occurs in the lungs, candidiasis commonly involves the urogenital tract. Localization in renal tissue involves attachment by specialized glycoproteins on the surface of the fungal spore. Tissue invasion occurs by specialized germ tubules that penetrate between and directly through surface epithelium of the renal cortex (Fig. 3.9).

Aerosol exposure is especially dangerous

Inhalation is the most significant factor in enabling fungal pulmonary infections to become established. The size of the fungal cell inhaled is important. In the mammalian lung, nothing larger than 10 μm that penetrates the nose reaches the lungs, whereas almost everything under 2 μm reaches the alveoli and is retained. The gastrointestinal tract, despite the ingestion of large numbers of spores, is seldom the site of primary fungal infection. This is due, in part, to the protective effect of the normal bacterial microflora. One notable exception involves fungi associated with bovine mycotic placentitis and abortion, in which the disease appears to follow ingestion of spores. The urogenital tract is rarely affected, because fungi are swept away by mucous secretions. The bovine teat is an important orifice for infection, and mycotic mastitis results from several species of fungi.

Protozoa

Only a few of the thousands of protozoal species are pathogenic for animals, and most pathogenic species are associated with diseases of the blood, reticuloendothelial system, or intestinal tract. The major classes of pathogenic protozoa include flagellates, amoebas, telosporeans, toxoplasmas, and piroplasmas (plasmodia, babesia, and other blood cell parasites). Most protozoal life cycles involve a specific host and a specific vector. Many protozoa stop the replicative cycle during adverse environmental conditions in order to survive. For example, the trophozoites of amoebae, which replicate in the gut lumen, can transform into cysts that survive outside the gut.

As the parasite moves from vector to host and back again, its surface is often altered to reflect the requirements for attachment and uptake by the host involved. For example, the malarial protozoa in the genus *Plasmodium* infect hepatocytes and emerge again in new form with new surface antigens. New progeny are unaffected by host immune responses that are incited by the parental organisms during initial infection.

Some protozoa are pathogenic only under certain conditions. *Entamoeba* spp., *Giardia* spp., and many other protozoa can colonize the intestinal tract without causing disease or tissue invasion. With certain immune deficits of the host or with very virulent strains of protozoa, disease can result. The replication cycle and its effect on the host caused by **intracellular protozoa** have many similarities to those of viruses and intracellular bacteria. Parasite metabolism differs from that of the host; for example, many intracellular protozoa, such as *Trypanosoma cruzi* and *Leishmania donovani,* lack purine synthesis capacity and depend on salvage of purines to form purine nucleotides.

Protozoa kill host cells by a wide spectrum of virulence factors, including pore-forming proteins se-

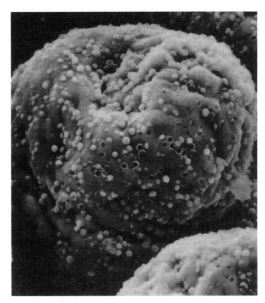

FIGURE 3.10. Cryptosporidia. Scanning electron micrograph of atrophic villi to which cryptosporidia adhere. (Micrograph: Joachim Pohlenz, *Vet Pathol* 15:417, 1978)

creted onto membranes of the host cells, toxin secretion, and intracellular replication that blocks metabolic activity to the point of lysis. *Cryptosporidium* spp. attach to epithelial cells of the intestine in large numbers, leading to cellular damage, malabsorption, and diarrhea (Fig. 3.10). *Leishmania* spp. and *Trypanosoma* spp. produce pore-forming toxins that insert into membranes of the host cell and cause cytolysis.

Protozoa are major causes of red blood cell damage. *Babesia* spp. are small (1–5 μm) tick-transmitted intraerythrocytic parasites that cannot survive outside the host. Feeding, development, and reproduction require factors provided by erythrocytes. During infection, erythrocyte destruction occurs by direct action of the parasite. However, anemia is out of proportion to the number of parasitized red cells, and it is believed that a late destructive immunologic reaction occurs. In some other parasitisms, cell-mediated immune responses of the host play a major role in tissue damage. Immune complex glomerulonephritis is a common lethal end result of malaria.

Algae

Algae are aquatic, nonvascular plants. The most serious pathogenic group is *Prototheca* spp., colorless algae that replicate freely in stagnant water and decaying organic matter. They are associated with focal and disseminated granulomatous lesions of animals and humans, generally as a rare, isolated

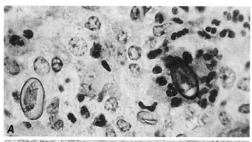

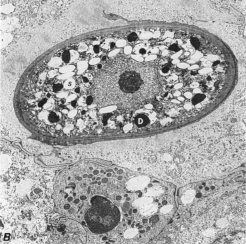

FIGURE 3.11. *Prototheca zopfii,* cow with chronic granulomatous mastitis. A. Algae are killed by neutrophilic leukocytes when they are extracellular *(right).* When phagocytized by macrophages *(left),* algae are protected from neutrophil activity. B. Within the macrophage, the thick outer wall of glycoproteins prevents fusion with lysosomes and permits replication. Starch granules *(S)* and dense bodies *(D).* Note vacuolated, granular neutrophil *(bottom),* which has cell membrane interdigitated with that of the macrophage.

disease in an immunosuppressed host. In tissue, algae occur as single endospores or as large sporangia containing multiple sporangiospores (daughter cells); both occur in macrophages. Protothecal cells have thick cell walls, large nuclei, and large numbers of starch granules. *Prototheca* spp. are an important cause of **mastitis** in cattle (Fig. 3.11) and occur incidentally in most other species. Occasionally, enteric prototheocosis will occur in dogs, resulting in severe enterocolitis. This may progress to systemic prototheocosis with involvement of the eyes and brain.

In ruminants, ingestion of large amounts of **blue-green algae** can cause enteric infection, liver necrosis, and death. Young sheep inoculated intrarumenally with an algal bloom of *Microcystis aeruginosa* developed elevations in serum enzymes and reduced blood glucose. They died 18–24 hours later, with widespread hemorrhages and acute cell swelling and necrosis of hepatocytes.

Invertebrate parasites

Metazoan parasites of vertebrate animals fall into five major groups: arthropods, pentastomids, platyhelminths (flatworms), acanthocephalids, and nematodes (roundworms). The last group, which deserves special emphasis because it causes the most serious economic losses, is the largest and most diverse. Each group of parasites has gross characteristics and produces typical eggs or young that parasitologists use for identification.

In tissue sections, parasites are identified by comparing their integuments, musculatures, body cavities, digestive tracts, and reproductive systems. **Eggs** are commonly present in tissue sections and are an important aid in diagnosis; for example, eggs of *Trichuris* spp. have a single polar cap. **Larvae,** which are also used for identification, may be present surrounding the parasite or in cross sections of the ovary or uterus of the female. In viviparous nematodes, ova embryonate and hatch in the uterus. Ovoviviparous nematodes produce ova that develop to embryos, but with larvae remaining within the eggshell as the eggs are deposited.

Invertebrate parasites produce disease by a wide variety of mechanisms (Table 3.5). Most parasites damage the host by mechanically obstructing ducts or vascular channels. Obstruction may result from masses of parasites or from the granulomas produced by the parasites' presence. Parasites nearly always are themselves infected with bacteria. After creating wounds in epithelium, they carry pathogenic bacteria into tissue (Fig. 3.12).

Parasites that suck blood produce chronic anemia

Chronic anemia caused by bloodsucking nematodes or insects may be lethal, especially in young animals. Some bloodsucking nematodes release an anticlotting substance that promotes blood flow. Adult hookworms, using a buccal cavity and hooklike teeth, attach to villi of the small intestine. The hookworm secretes a protease that inhibits fibrin clot formation and even promotes dissolution of clots as they form. Each worm can extract 0.2 ml blood per day, and in heavy infestations, this eventually leads to both hypoalbuminemia and chronic iron deficiency anemia.

Parasites can alter the host's immune response

Parasite surfaces are especially important in recovery stages because they contain substances that make the parasite refractory to an immune response. Large amounts of proteins shaved off the

Trichinosis

JAMES PAGET, a first-year medical student at St. Bartholomew's Hospital in London in 1835, discovered larvae of the roundworm *Trichinella spiralis*. Dissecting a human cadaver, he noted that small white specks in muscle were cysts with tiny worms inside. It was not until 1859 that clinical trichinosis was diagnosed. A German girl, preparing meat for Christmas, developed fever and myalgia. Brought to a Dresden hospital, she died after 15 days of excruciating muscle pain. When the pathologist Zenker removed a sliver of muscle from her arm, crushed it, and examined it microscopically, he saw dozens of tiny worms wriggling about. Once trichinosis was established as a disease, several severe outbreaks were recorded, and the life cycle of the parasite was determined.

The adult life of *T. spiralis* is spent in the small intestine of many species of carnivores. Adult worms lie within the cytoplasm of absorptive and goblet cells. Threaded through rows of enterocytes, they often cannot be seen on the mucosal surface. The viviparous female burrows into the lamina propria of the intestinal villi and deposits her larvae directly into the intestinal lymphatics. Larvae exit in lymph, pass through the mesenteric lymphatics and thoracic duct, and enter the bloodstream. During circulation through the skeletal muscles, they enter myocytes and encyst.

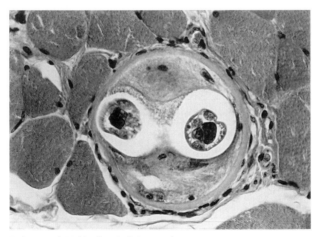

Early cyst of *Trichinella spiralis* in muscle.

The cyst both nourishes and protects the larvae from host defense mechanisms. Eosinophilic and neutrophilic leukocytes and plasmacytes (which contain antitrichina antibody) develop around the cysts, but their effect on encysted larvae is negligible. When the host is killed and its muscle eaten by a new potential carnivore host, intestinal enzymes digest the capsule, and the liberated larvae burrow into the intestine to begin their life cycle anew.

parasite surface may inhibit responses of inflammatory cells. On the other hand, some parasites release fragments of surface proteins or secrete toxins that act as potent antigens to induce **hypersensitivity reactions**. For example, ascaris surface antigens cause the host to become hypersensitive. Smashing ox warbles in the skin of cattle releases enough surface antigens to cause **anaphylaxis**.

TOXICOLOGIC DISEASE

Biologic toxins

Arthropod toxins and venoms

Spiders are uniformly venomous, but most attack only other arthropods, using venom to paralyze their prey. Venom of the black widow spider causes paralysis of the mammalian nervous system by affecting release of neurotransmitters. The result is severe inflammation at the site of the bite and ascending motor paralysis with destruction of peripheral nerve endings. Envenomation into blood vessels may lead to cardiovascular collapse and respiratory paralysis. The brown recluse spider produces a hemolytic and necrotizing venom that incites a chronic ulcerating wound.

Hymenopterous insect bites (from bees, wasps, hornets, and yellow jackets) may cause death due to systemic anaphylactic shock, in which respiratory distress is followed by vascular collapse. Bee venom contains histamine, phospholipase A_2, hyaluronidase, and several toxic peptides. The latter include melittin (which is hemolyzing), apamin (which is neurotoxic), and a mast cell–degranulating peptide. Melittin, 50% of the dry weight of bee venom, acts on plasma membranes of vascular endothelial cells to increase capillary permeability and incite necrosis and inflammation.

Blister beetles, when ingested in hay, produce necrotic lesions in the alimentary canal. This is a recurring problem in horses in the southwestern United States. Hemorrhage and necrosis with ulceration in the gastrointestinal tract and urinary bladder occur in equine blister beetle toxicity. Focal necrosis of the myocardium and swelling of renal tubule cells contribute to the lethal effect of the toxin. Cantharidin ("Spanish fly") is the toxic principle responsible for the tissue necrosis.

Snake venoms

Snake venoms are mixtures of up to 30 different peptides, most of which are toxic, either directly or via activity as enzymes (Table 3.6). All snake venoms contain **phosphodiesterase, peptidases, hyaluronidase** ("spreading factor"), and **phospholipase A_2**, which has a direct lytic action on

TABLE 3.5. Mechanisms of tissue injury by metazoan parasites

Mechanism	Parasite	Animal
Obstruction of lumina	*Dirofilaria immitis*	Dog (heart)
	Ascaris spp.	Pig (intestine)
	Metastrongylus spp.	Pig (lung)
	Liver fluke	Several (bile duct)
Irritation	Fleas	Many (skin)
Epithelial destruction	*Trichostrongylus* spp.	Sheep (stomach)
	Hookworms	Dog (intestine)
	Strongylus spp.	Horse (large intestine)
Anemia	Hookworms	Dog (intestine)
	Strongyles	Horse (intestine)
	Stomach worms	Sheep
Carry pathogenic viruses: Bluetongue African horse sickness Bovine ephemeral fever Viral encephalitides	*Culicoides* spp.	Many (skin)
Carry pathogenic protozoa: *Haemoproteus* *Leukocytozoon* *Hepatocystis*	Several spp.	Mammals, birds, etc.
Carry pathogenic nematodes: *Dirofilaria immitis* *Wuchereria bancrofti* *Onchocerca cervicalis*	*Culicoides* spp.	Dog, humans

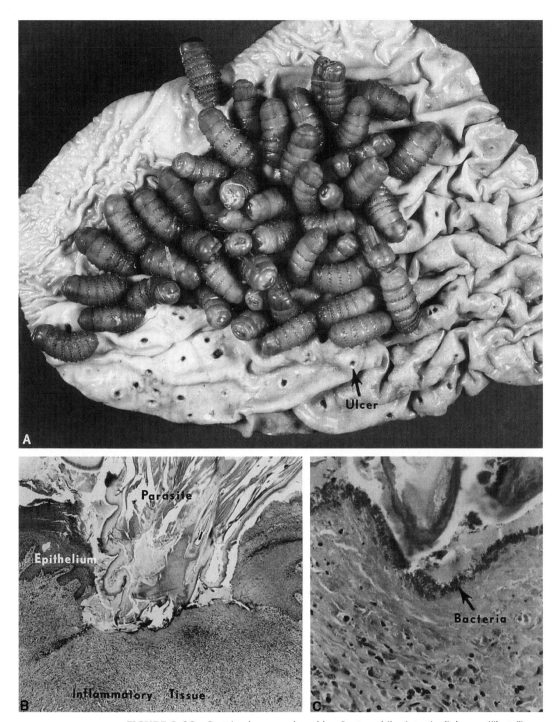

FIGURE 3.12. Gastric ulcers produced by *Gasterophilus intestinalis* larvae ("bots") are walled off by chronic inflammation. A. Detachment of larvae reveals ulcers on the gastric surface. B. Chitinous oral hooks of the parasite produce erosions and ulcers surrounded by hyperplastic squamous epithelium and chronic focal fibrosing gastritis. C. Surfaces of pits contain many aerobic and anaerobic bacterial species. Lymphoid cells infiltrate the chronic fibrous tissue underlying the ulcer.

membranes of erythrocytes, platelets, and other cells. Hyaluronidase cleaves internal glycoside bonds of acidic mucopolysaccharides to facilitate diffusion of toxin into tissue. Superimposed on these enzymes are different toxins in individual venoms that act specifically on nerve tissue, coagulation systems, and other organs.

Rattlesnakes and other pit vipers have fangs that reach deeply into muscle. They produce large puncture marks that rapidly develop severe edema and erythema. In animals in which curiosity leads to probing the snake, bites are apt to occur on the nose. These bites lead to swelling of facial and pharyngeal tissues and to respiratory distress. Hemolytic anemia (with hemoglobinemia) and kidney damage reflect the necrotizing toxins in venom. When much venom is involved, cardiac irregularities, a fall in blood pressure, and shock may occur.

Neurotoxins of snake venoms kill by blocking neuromuscular transmission at motor endplates of skeletal muscle, by blocking the cardiac conduction system, and by producing central effects that suppress both respiratory and cardiac action. The most prominent of these is motor endplate dysfunction and paralysis of the respiratory muscles of the diaphragm and rib cage. Neurotoxin action on neuromuscular transmission may be presynaptic, via inhibition of acetylcholine release; synaptic, by cholinesterase acting within the synaptic cleft; or postsynaptic, by binding to acetylcholine receptors to prevent the depolarizing action of acetylcholine.

Cobra and krait have postsynaptic toxins that bind tightly and irreversibly to acetylcholine receptors and act as antagonists, like curare. Cobra venom in mammals produces a flaccid muscle paralysis, and death occurs by respiratory failure. Neurotoxic peptides bind specifically to nicotinic acetylcholine receptors, producing a nondepolarizing block. In addition to postjunctional neurotoxins, cobra venoms contain large amounts of similar peptides that act directly on cell membranes. They cause depolarization and contracture of cardiac (and skeletal) myocytes.

Fish and amphibian toxins

All toads contain skin glands that secrete repulsive chemicals. The more poisonous amphibians are the Colorado River toad *(Bufo alvarius),* the marine toad *(Bufo marinus),* and the poison-dart frogs of central America *(Dendrobates* spp.). These species secrete complex venoms all containing a toxin that mimics the action of cardiac glycosides, which poison the electrolyte pumps of heart muscle. **Batrachotoxin,** the steroidal alkaloid of the poison dart frog, irreversibly blocks sodium channels in neurons and leads to membrane depolarization. The *Bufo* species have parotid glands behind the eyes that secrete **bufotoxin,** a conjugation of bufagin (a digitalis-like toxin) and bufotenine (which produces marked pressor action resembling that of oxytocin). Most poisonings occur in dogs and cats that attack and bite the *Bufo* toads. Young kittens and puppies are especially susceptible and exhibit salivation, cardiac irregularities, ventricular fibrillation, and pulmonary edema.

Tetrodotoxin is concentrated in liver, ovaries, intestine, and skin of many species of puffer fish, which are prized as food in the Orient. Tetrodotoxin binds to sodium channels on nerve axons and suppresses conduction of nerve impulses. Generalized paralysis occurs, followed by convulsions and death. Tetrodotoxin is also produced by the California newt, the Australian blue-ringed octopus, and other amphibians, but poisoning from these species is rare. **Saxitoxin,** a similar toxin, is produced by a genus of plankton, *Gonyaulax* spp., which under favorable conditions multiplies so rapidly that it reaches a density of many millions per liter and creates a "red tide," turning the ocean surface rusty

TABLE 3.6. Toxins in crude snake venom

Venom	Crotalidae (rattlesnake)	Viperidae (gaboon viper)	Elapidae (cobra)	Hydrophidae (sea snake)
Phospholipase A$_2$	+	+	+	+
Phosphodiesterase	+	+	+	+
Hyaluronidase	+	+	+	+
Peptidase	+	+	+	+
Kininogenase	+			
Neurotoxin (presynaptic)				+
Neurotoxin (postsynaptic)			+	
Defibrinating peptides	+[a]			
Antithromboplastin			+[a]	

[a]Some species.

brown by day and luminescent by night. Shellfish that feed in red tide waters concentrate the toxin in their tissues and are poisonous to animals.

Fungal toxins

Fungal toxins (mycotoxins) include a diverse group of fungal peptides. **Aflatoxins**, the best-known mycotoxins, are a group of hepatotoxic metabolites produced by some strains of *Aspergillus flavus*. They are synthesized by fungi growing in feeds, and they poison when these feeds are ingested by the animal. The primary effect of aflatoxin is on the liver, where it causes hepatocyte necrosis, fibrosis, and bile duct proliferation. Hepatocytes around the central vein are most susceptible to the toxin, resulting in **centrolobular necrosis**. Within the hepatocyte, aflatoxin is directly toxic to a DNA-dependent RNA polymerase in the nucleolus, and the end result is a blockade of protein synthesis in the hepatocyte. In **chronic toxicity**, aflatoxin causes liver tumors. The natural occurrence of aflatoxin-induced neoplasia is difficult to prove, but in feeding experiments where aflatoxins are given in small amounts over a long period, hepatomas have been induced in trout and hepatic carcinomas in rats.

Sporidesmin, produced by the fungus *Pithomyces chartarum* (a saprophyte on pasture grass), causes **facial eczema**, a photosensitivity of sheep and cattle. It is a hepatotoxin that causes degeneration of hepatocytes and bile canaliculi, occlusion of bile ductules, periductal edema, and hepatitis. Photosensitivity results from failure of the damaged liver to remove **phylloerythrin** from the blood. Phylloerythrin, a chlorophyll metabolite produced in the rumen, circulates and absorbs energy from the sun as it passes through skin; the release of energy causes necrosis.

Penitrem A, a product of *Penicillium* spp., produces acute neurologic disease: muscle tremor, seizures, ataxia, and death. In dogs fed moldy cheese and in large animals that have eaten moldy roughage, penitrem suppresses **glycine**, the neurotransmitter of some inhibitory neurons. Signs resemble those of **strychnine** toxicity, for strychnine is also a glycine antagonist. Treatment with substances that raise glycine content of the brain (e.g., mephenesin and nalorphine) abolish penitrem-induced tremors.

Ergotism is a classic disease of cattle, horses, and other animals. In medieval Europe, human epidemics of gangrenous necrosis of the limbs resulted from ingestion of ergot-contaminated flour. Ergotism is caused by alkaloids of *Claviceps purpurea,* which turns cereal grains black and misshapen. Toxic compounds of the fungus include **er-**gotamine, a vasoconstrictor, and **ergometrine**, a smooth muscle contractor. Other lysergic acid derivatives are also produced. Gangrene is produced by **chronic vasoconstriction, ischemia**, and **capillary endothelial degeneration** in the extremities. In horses and carnivores, nervous signs and convulsion may be the dominant signs.

A second syndrome of gangrene of the extremities called **fescue foot** occurs in cattle that ingest tall fescue grass *(Festuca arundinacea)* infected by the fungus *Neotyphodium* sp. Infected tall fescue, when eaten in small amounts, also produces a wasting disease in cattle called summer fescue toxicosis.

Fusarium spp. produce two types of toxins that cause disease: estrogenic metabolites and trichothecene toxins. Formed in temperate climates or even in cold weather, they produce a wide variety of clinical syndromes. **Zearalenone**, produced in moldy corn, causes precocious sexual development with vulvar enlargement and mammary development in swine. Affected sows have ovarian abnormalities and proliferation of uterine glands. Offspring are born weak, and there is reduced litter size.

Horses that consume feed containing **fumonesin**, a mycotoxin produced by *Fusarium* spp., develop leukoencephalomalacia. This disease is characterized by areas of liquefactive necrosis of the subcortical white matter of the cerebrum, sometimes with cavitation. Fumonesin consumption by swine is associated with pulmonary edema.

Acute interstitial pneumonitis has been reported in cattle eating sweet potatoes damaged by the mold *Fusarium solani*. The disease can be reproduced with a furan (4-ipomeanol) isolated from the moldy potatoes. Clara cells in the terminal bronchioles contain enzymes that convert this furan to a reactive toxin. Pulmonary endothelium, especially capillaries and small veins, play an important role. Endothelial cells metabolize the exogenous furans to highly reactive metabolites by the cytochrome P-450 mixed-function oxidase system of pneumocytes, leading to lung injury.

Mushroom toxins. Most poisonous mushrooms are not lethal but produce signs soon after ingestion (within 1–2 hours). Some contain **muscarine**, which causes blurred vision, sweating, increased peristalsis, and reduced blood pressure. The liberty cap *(Psilocybe semilanceata)* has been deliberately eaten for its hallucinogenic effects. Indoles of this fungus (e.g., psilocybin and psilocin) alter the concentration of indoles, including serotonin, in the brain and thereby interfere with transmission of stimuli regulating perception.

Mushrooms of the genus *Amanita* are the most deadly. Most human deaths are due to a single species of this genus, *Amanita phalloides*. In contrast to most mushroom poisonings, signs of poisoning from this species do not appear for many hours after ingestion. A full day may pass before abdominal pain, diarrhea, and violent emesis occur. If medically treated, patients recover from the gastroenteritis but succumb later to lethal nephropathy. The two major groups of toxins from *A. phalloides* are the **amanitins** (five amatoxins, all cyclopeptides or ring-shaped amino acids) and the **phalloidins**. In renal tubular epithelium of poisoned animals, the major cellular change begins with disintegration of the nucleolus and nuclei; α-amanitin suppresses protein synthesis by attacking an RNA polymerase that directs synthesis of mRNA.

Plant toxins

Alkaloids

The bitter, soluble, organic, acid-alkaloid salts known as **alkaloids** are common in several plants, and more than 5,000 alkaloids have been partially characterized. Unfortunately, they are often named according to the generic name of the plant from which they were extracted. The alkaloid content varies little with growing season or climate. It is distributed throughout the plant, so that any part may be dangerous to livestock.

Pyrrolizidine alkaloids. Species of *Senecio, Crotalaria,* and *Heliotropium* contain pyrrolizidine alkaloids that are toxic. Toxins are most often associated with chronic liver disease in grazing livestock. Signs of wasting, weakness, and icterus occur up to 2 months after ingestion of plants. Lesions consist of an initial necrosis of hepatocytes, followed by **cytomegaly** of remaining hepatocytes and progressive **cirrhosis**—that is, perisinusoidal fibrosis, proliferation of bile ductules, and regeneration of surviving hepatocytes. These alkaloids act as alkylating agents on DNA, producing cytomegaly by preventing mitosis while permitting cytoplasmic ribosomal synthesis to continue.

Crotalaria metabolites produce endothelial damage in the lung that leads to increased thickening of the media of muscular arteries in the lungs and to pulmonary hypertension. Right ventricular hypertrophy followed by heart failure occurs in some species. Heart lesions include focal cytolysis of myocytes, cell swelling, and fibrosis.

Swainsonine. An indolizidine alkaloid in locoweeds (*Astragalus* and *Oxytropis* spp.) and Darling peas (*Swainsona* spp.) produces an oligosaccharide storage disease caused by its specific inhibition of α-mannosidase in lysosomes. Lysosomes accumulate, making affected cells large, pale, and foamy.

Neurons, myocardium, and renal tubules are most severely affected. Poisoned animals become nervous and may fall backward, walk into objects, or leap over imagined objects. Ingestion is habit forming, and grazing animals seek out the toxic plants. Cattle grazing at high altitudes are likely to die from congestive heart failure, which develops when the effects of high altitude are superimposed on the cardiac lesions.

Poison hemlock *(Conium maculatum)* contains at least five alkaloids and is responsible for the rapidly developing signs of ataxia, reduced cardiac function, dilatation of pupils, and coma in acute toxicity. Gastrointestinal irritation occurs, and vomiting is common. Pigs are most commonly affected and develop ataxia and trembling. Skeletal malformations occur in newborn piglets if sows are poisoned between 43 and 61 days of gestation. Arthrogryposis, lumbar-thoracic scoliosis, and twisted limbs result from the teratogenic alkaloid γ-coniceine.

Glycosides

Cardiac glycosides. The glycosides **digitalis, digitoxin, ouabain,** and **squill** have in common a powerful action on myocardium: they increase the contractility of cardiac muscle (in a dose-dependent manner) by binding to and inhibiting the sodium pump in the membranes of myocytes. These drugs are also potent toxins and lead to severe electrolyte disturbances and injury of the myocardium when given in excessive doses.

Oleander *(Nerium oleander),* a common shrub, contains a highly toxic cardiac glycoside. Dogs and humans have been killed merely by putting a stem of oleander in the mouth. Cardiovascular collapse occurs immediately. Oleander toxins produce myocardial degeneration and other widespread changes in the heart muscle.

Cyanogenic glycosides. Members of the family Rosaceae commonly contain glycosides that yield free cyanide on hydrolysis. The high content of hydrocyanic acid (HCN) in wilted and frozen leaves is due to the hydrolytic effects of plant enzymes activated in the dying leaf. Toxicity of HCN occurs after ingestion and absorption. Once it is in the bloodstream, there is little difference between toxic and lethal levels of cyanide. HCN has a high affinity for iron and reacts with the trivalent iron of mitochondrial cytochrome oxidase, the terminal respiratory catalyst linking oxygen with metabolic respiration. Cell anoxia is immediate. The progression of staggering, prostration, coma, and death may all occur within 15 minutes. Because utilization of oxygen is blocked, venous blood is oxygenated and almost as bright red as arterial blood.

Goitrogenic glycosides. Plant thiocyanates and thiooxazolide mimic the effects of thiouracil and thiourea in preventing the accumulation of inorganic iodide in thyroid follicular epithelium. These glycosides occur in several species of *Brassica*, including cabbage, kale, and rape. Poisoning is associated with signs of hypothyroidism, and affected thyroids are hyperplastic. This toxicity is common in sheep. Pregnant ewes may be asymptomatic, yet their newborn lambs will be unthrifty and have large hyperplastic thyroid glands.

Other glycosides. Hepatotoxicity of swine is associated with ingestion of *cocklebur* sprouts (*Xanthium* spp.). Signs of ataxia, convulsions, and death are due to brain edema and neuronal degeneration. Hepatotoxicity is prominent, and there is centrolobular necrosis, hepatic edema, and serofibrinous ascites. The glycoside carboxyatractyloside uncouples mitochondrial oxidative phosphorylation, producing hepatocyte degeneration and an associated hypoglycemia.

Saponins are large molecules that form colloidal solutions that produce froth when shaken with water. These common plant glycosides are rarely toxins. Most saponin-bearing plants are unpalatable, ingested only when grazing is restricted. They produce gastroenteritis and are absorbed through the injured intestine. A saponin in broomweed (*Gutierrezia microcephala*) is nephrotoxic and hepatotoxic in ruminants in the high plains areas of Texas and is a significant cause of abortion. Anemia and hematuria are often consequences of saponin toxicity.

Several plants produce **calcinogenic vitamin D analogues** that cause hypercalcemia, parathyroid atrophy, hyperostosis, and soft-tissue mineralization. Chronic poisoning leads to progressive debilitation and is peculiar to certain geographic areas (e.g., Manchester wasting disease in Jamaica, enteque seco in South America, and Naalehu disease in Hawaii). In the hyperostosis caused by *Solanum malacoxylon*, toxicity is due to a water-soluble glycoside of 1,25-dihydroxycholecalciferol that stimulates bone formation on trabecular surfaces.

Thiaminases

Bracken fern produces a thiaminase that depletes thiamine reserves in monogastric animals. In grazing horses it causes a neurologic syndrome with encephalomalacia. Thiamine is a component of thiamine pyrophosphate, the prosthetic group of three important enzymes in the nervous system. Cattle, protected from this toxin because of production of large amounts of thiamine in the rumen, succumb to a second toxin in bracken fern that causes bone marrow destruction, thrombocytopenia, and widespread hemorrhages. In ruminants, thiamine-deficiency encephalomalacia occurs in poisoning by the anticoccidiostat drug **amprolium** and, under rare conditions, by overgrowth of thiaminase-producing rumen bacilli. **Sulfates** in large amounts in the diet or in drinking water will inactivate thiamine. Several species of fish contain a thiaminase, and mink and other carnivores that are fed these fish may become deficient in thiamine and develop encephalomalacia.

Fluorescent pigments and photosensitivity disease

Several plants synthesize fluorescent pigments, which are ingested by grazing animals and, when absorbed from the intestine, enter the bloodstream (Table 3.7). Although nontoxic, these pigments localize in skin, where in hairless, nonpigmented areas, they are exposed to sunlight. Action of ultraviolet (UV) light produces fluorescence, the transformation of UV waves to longer wavelength.

TABLE 3.7. Photosensitivity disease types

Exogenous[a]	
Fagopyrism	Pigments from buckwheat, *Fagopyrum esculentum*
Hypericism	Pigments from St.-John's-wort, *Hypericum perforatum*
Phenothiazine	Sulfoxides in tears and aqueous humor (keratitis)
Hepatotoxic[b]	
Plant toxins	Mexican fireweed *(Kochia scoparia)*, lechugilla, ngaio-tree leaves, kleingrass
Mycotoxins	*Pithomyces chartarum* (mycotoxin production)
Congenital[c]	
Congenital erythropoietic porphyria	Uroporphyrinogen cosynthetase defect (cow, cat, pig, squirrel)
Congenital protoporphyria	Ferrochelatase defect (cow)
Syndromes of defective bile excretion	Southdown sheep, Corriedale sheep

[a]Fluorescent pigments ingested, absorbed, enter the bloodstream.
[b]Liver necrosis or bile ductule obstruction that blocks biliary secretion of phylloerythrin, a catabolite of chlorophyll.
[c]A defect in porphyrin metabolism.

Energy released damages capillaries and venules, causing endothelial degeneration, hyperemia, and edema. Ears, nose, and teats are particularly vulnerable and may develop raw ulcers and gangrenous necrosis.

The antinematode drug **phenothiazine** is directly toxic, primarily causing hemolytic anemia with hemoglobinuria and icterus. It also produces photosensitivity keratitis by fluorescence injury. During catabolism in the liver, the intermediate phenothiazine sulfoxide escapes into the circulation to enter the aqueous humor of the eye. It is also excreted in tears and, when exposed to sunlight, fluoresces to cause corneal edema and ulceration.

Primary photosensitization is a cutaneous disorder that results from ingestion of phototoxic substances. Fermentative breakdown of chlorophyll in alfalfa silage can result in production of the phototoxic substance **phylloerythrin**. Hepatic degeneration with secondary photosensitivity has been reported in cattle fed flood-damaged hay that contained phylloerythrin.

Photosensitivity dermatitis is also produced when phylloerythrin accumulates in tissue after liver damage. The sequence of grazing on lush pasture, ingestion of phytotoxins or mycotoxins, and exposure to sunlight is the most common. The liver lesion responsible for biliary stasis and failure to excrete phylloerythrin is usually pericholangitis with fibrosis; in rare instances, photosensitivity dermatitis can result from viral or congenital liver disease.

Drug toxicity

Antibiotics

Antibiotics produce disease in two ways: by direct toxic injury, and by disruption of normal bacterial flora of the gut. Many antibiotics are nephrotoxic, although some produce a wide variety of tissue damage (Table 3.8). Anthracycline antibiotics, used as cancer therapy, intercalate into DNA and kill tumor cells by suppressing transcription of genes and subsequent protein synthesis. **Adriamycin**, the prototype drug, produces lysis of cardiac muscle, and poisoned patients die in heart failure.

Neomycin toxicity is associated with malabsorption diarrhea. In the intestine, fragmentation of microvilli on enterocytes causes malabsorption. **Lincomycin** given orally is toxic to horses, rabbits, and most rodents and causes severe diarrhea, dehydration, and even death. Lesions of hemorrhage and necrosis in the cecum and colon of horses are due to suppression of gram-positive aerobic bacteria and certain gram-negative anaerobes. Subsequent overgrowth of nonsensitive coliform bacteria and clostridia leads to damage of the gut wall.

TABLE 3.8. Drugs that are toxic to animals

Tissue	Toxin	Animals very susceptible
Liver (hepatotoxins)	Acetaminophen	Cat
	Halothane	Pig
	Furazolidone	Turkey
	Reserpine	Horse
Kidney (nephrotoxins)	Oxytetracycline	Ruminant species
	Gentamicin	Birds, horses, dogs
	Sulfonamides	Ruminants
	Aminonucleoside	—
	Anthracycline antibiotics	—
Nervous tissue (neurotoxins)	Phenobarbital	—
	Isoniazid	—
	Succinyl choline	—
	Theobromine (in chocolate)	Dog
Intestine (intestinal toxins)	Phenylbutazone	Horse
	Indomethacin	Dog
	Aspirin	Cat, dog
	Ibuprofen	Dog
	Cyclophosphamide	Small animals
	Lincomycin	
Muscle (myotoxins)	Monensin (heart)	Horse
	Chloroquine	Primates
	Anthracycline antibiotics[a]	—
Blood cells (hematopoietic toxin)	Cyclosporine	—

[a]Adriamycin, daunomycin.

Oxytetracycline toxicity is common in cattle and sheep treated with multiple large doses. Typically, a herd is treated for a respiratory disease first by the owner and then by the veterinarian, who is unaware of the previous treatment. Acute diffuse swelling and tubular necrosis of the kidneys is obvious at necropsy (see Frontispiece, Part 1). The proximal convoluted tubules are most severely affected; the distal convoluted tubules are usually spared.

Sulfonamides

Sulfonamides are used against bacterial infections. At high doses they cause acute nephrotoxicity (sulfonamides also cause a more delayed type of injury by immunologic mechanisms). Acute injury is most common in calves, especially febrile animals that are dehydrated. At necropsy, kidneys are enlarged, congested, and pale; linear deposits of sulfonamide crystals are usually present in the medulla, and crystals may also be in the pelvis and urinary bladder. Histologically, the proximal convoluted tubules undergo acute cell swelling and necrosis. Other parts of the nephron are less affected. A mild but diffuse edema and fibrosis develop in the interstitial areas in the medulla and are most prominent at the corticomedullary junction.

Sulfonamide crystals are apt to be washed away in tissue processing. They must be differentiated from oxalate crystals in ethylene glycol (antifreeze) toxicity and in sheep poisoned by plants that contain oxalate.

Anti-inflammatory drugs

Acetaminophen is a widely used analgesic. Safe at therapeutic levels, it causes fatal hepatic necrosis in large doses, especially in cats. Consistent dose-dependent liver lesions can be reproduced experimentally. Within the hepatocyte, acetaminophen is catabolized to highly reactive intermediates within the smooth endoplasmic reticulum, the organelle of detoxification.

Chronic acetaminophen toxicity and that of phenacetin (which is converted to acetaminophen in the liver) leads to hemolytic anemia, methemoglobinuria, and icterus. In cats, signs also include facial edema and cyanosis. Erythrocyte destruction in chronic toxicity is also related to glutathione depletion, because reduced glutathione maintains hemoglobin cysteine residues in the reduced state and keeps hemoglobin in the ferrous state.

Ionophores

Ionophores are drugs that act as ion channels in cell membranes. They become inserted into the cell surface and carry ions across the plasma membrane. Most of these diverse compounds have a common central ring of liganding oxygen atoms that forms a critical cavity to fit a particular ion.

Monensin is the prototype sodium ionophore. It is used both as a coccidiostat (it inserts into coccidial surface membranes, creating ionic imbalances that cause the coccidia to swell and burst) and an enhancer of rumen production of protein in ruminant food-producing animals. Monensin is particularly toxic for the horse. It causes necrosis of both skeletal and cardiac muscle, and poisoned animals die in acute heart failure.

Environmental pollutants

Metals

Metals interact biologically as soluble salts that dissociate in an aqueous environment to facilitate their transport into tissue. Gastrointestinal absorption is the common route of entry, and absorption is greater when ingestion occurs during fasting. Pulmonary absorption is poor with insoluble compounds because they are cleared rapidly in the upper airways. Metals existing as alkyl compounds in which metallic ions are firmly bonded to carbon pass unaltered across lipid membranes and into the circulation. Thus organometallic compounds such as methyl mercury and tetraethyl lead are highly toxic. The clinically significant lesions of heavy metal toxicity often occur in the brain.

Lead. Lead toxicity occurs after animals ingest flaking lead-based paints or contaminated grasses near lead smelters. Disease produces nervous, hematologic, and gastrointestinal signs. Weakness, periodic convulsions, and anemia appear early and progress to paralysis and death.

In cattle, lead poisoning is an acute disease. Calves are especially affected and progress from muscle tremor, staggering, and falling to convulsions and opisthotonos and may die within 24 hours. Brain swelling contributes to clinical signs but is difficult to define histologically. Absorbed lead is immediately deposited in the liver and kidneys and, in chronic toxicity, in bones. In the kidney and liver, lead-protein complexes form in nuclei of hepatocytes and renal tubular cells.

Lead produces its most marked effects in the **brain**. In the nervous system, lesions are primarily vascular. There is **necrosis of endothelial cells** in capillaries and arterioles, and damaged blood vessels are surrounded by **edema** and **hemorrhage**. The neuropil in affected areas is vacuolated (**status spongiosus**), and there is demyelination and necrosis. Necrotic brain tissue develops in layers, a pattern called **laminar necrosis**. Foci of vacuolation and demyelination are common in the cerebral

FOCUS

Mercury Toxicity

THE DISAPPEARANCE OF SEED-EATING BIRDS and their avian predators was observed by ornithologists in the 1950s. Large amounts of
mercury were discovered in dead and intoxicated birds, and mercurials such as methyl mercury used for commercial seed disinfection
were implicated. Studies of birds from museum collections showed increasing mercury in feathers from about 1890 onward. Methyl mercury is readily absorbed by and stable within the bird. It accumulates in
most organs, with preference for kidney, liver, and oviduct. There is an
intense concentration in egg albumin (females excrete mercury faster
than males). Embryonal development is affected, and there is poor
hatchability of the egg.

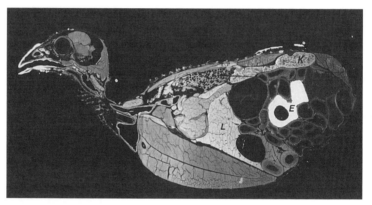

Mercury toxicity: accumulation of radiolabeled mercury *(white areas)* 4 days after
experimental inoculation, whole section of quail. There are heavy concentrations in
beak, egg albumin *(E)*, liver *(L)*, and kidney *(K)*. (Photograph: Jorgen Bäckstrom,
Acta Pharmacol Toxicol 27 [Suppl. 3]:1, 1969, used by permission)

There are three toxic forms of mercury: **elemental mercury** (Hg)
is an inhaled metal distributed to the alveoli and causes chronic toxicity; **inorganic mercury** (Hg^{2+}, as in $HgCl_2$) can be highly soluble and
thus highly toxic when ingested; and **organic mercury** (methyl mercury, ethyl mercury, and the alkyl mercury diuretics) forms salts with
acids and reacts with cell ligands such as sulfhydryl groups to complex
with and pass through membranes. Organic mercury in the environment makes this form the most important animal metallic toxin.

The aquatic environment is contaminated by industrial and agricultural uses of mercurials. Freshwater fish become contaminated
and, if large amounts of mercury are present, will develop gill disease
and die. Rainbow trout exposed to lethal amounts of inorganic mercury develop necrosis of epithelium and fusion of lamellae of affected
gills. Fish gills function not only in respiration but also in osmoregulation, acid-base balance, and excretion of nitrogenous wastes, which
are functions of the kidney in higher animals. Mercury in fish enters
the food chain and is responsible for toxicity in birds and humans. In
Minimata, Japan, a large number of people suffered severe acute neurologic disease from eating fish contaminated with effluents from a
paper mill.

▶

cortex, and in chronic toxicity the cerebral gyri are blunted and atrophic.

Anemia in lead toxicity is due both to suppression of hemoglobin production and to reduction of erythrocyte life span. In stem cells, mitochondria are affected in two ways: defects in uroporphyrinogen synthesis, and suppression of oxidative phosphorylation and citric acid cycles. Other lesions in lead toxicity include hyperplasia of bone marrow, spotty necrosis of skeletal muscle, peripheral neuropathy, and persistence of thick cartilage in trabeculae of the long bones.

Aromatic halogenated hydrocarbons

Hexachlorophene was used as an antibacterial agent in soaps and deodorants in the 1970s and, since it persists in the environment, was detected in surface waters in concentrations as high as 48 ppb. Hexachlorophene concentrates in myelin, and it causes encephalopathy and neuropathy in both humans and animals.

Dioxin. Dioxin refers to the basic structure of a family of chemicals: a pair of oxygen atoms joins two benzene rings, and substitution of chlorine for hydrogen on the rings produces the chlorinated dioxins. For example, 2,3,7,8-tetrachlorodibenzo-*p*-dioxin (TCDD) is a toxic byproduct in the synthesis of the herbicide 2,4,5-T.

An accident in West Virginia in 1949 exposed more than 200 workers to TCDD. Of 122 who developed dermatitis, 121 were followed medically for 30 years. Total deaths in the groups did not differ significantly from the number expected in the population at large, and there were no excess deaths due to cancer. Although some studies have claimed correlations between human abortions and sarcomas and TCDD exposure, most responsible investigations agree that there is no known connection. In

1976 an industrial accident in Italy released a chemical cloud of dioxins and other compounds over a wide area; despite evacuation, there was considerable acute disease in plants, animals, and humans.

Highly toxic to animals, TCDD accumulates in soil from many sources and its long-term effects are not clearly understood. In humans, acute effects include dermatitis, myalgia, and psychiatric disturbances. No case of human death has been associated with TCDD, and there is no unequivocal evidence of chronic sequelae.

Laboratory rodents vary in sensitivity to dioxins. The oral LD_{50} for the guinea pig is 0.6 mg/kg body weight, whereas that for the hamster is 2,000 times greater. At very high doses over long times, dioxins are carcinogenic in rats and mice. However, rats tolerate a daily dose of 1 mg/kg for 2 years without showing toxic effects.

Pentachlorophenol (PCP), a widely used pesticide and defoliant, can be routinely detected in human and animal tissues as a result of contaminated foods. In the 1950s it was associated with the death of millions of chickens in the southeastern United States. Toxicity was traced to components in animal fat used in feed. The fat had been derived from hides preserved with PCP; the toxicity was not due to PCP, however, but to dioxin isomers in the technical grade of PCP used on the hides. Reproduction of dioxin-contaminated PCP disease in cattle induced progressive anemia, thymic atrophy, and villous hyperplasia of urinary bladder epithelium.

Acid water

Depression of pH in lakes causes widespread loss of animal life. Studies in Norway show that even Crustacea are vulnerable to acidification (although *Diptera* are not). Acid precipitation effects have

In large animals, mercury poisoning is associated with ingestion of feeds contaminated with organic mercurial fungicides. In rare cases, inorganic mercurials poison when licked from blister ointments. Acute toxicity is associated with gastroenteritis and ulceration of alimentary mucosa; chronic toxicity is associated with progressive renal disease, colitis, and stomatitis. Horses are more resistant than cattle or sheep and require 8–10 g for clinical signs to appear.

The pathologic lesions in swine chronically poisoned by alkyl mercury develop neuronal necrosis followed by secondary gliosis and capillary endothelial proliferation. Pigs that recover have cerebral atrophy and dilated cerebral ventricles due to loss of brain mass.

been stimulated by addition of sulfuric acid to small lakes in Canada during an 8-year period. The natural balance of animal life was gradually destroyed. The first irreversible disturbances to simple organisms occur before marked changes in pH are apparent; phytoplankton remain relatively constant, but new species appear and numbers of organisms small enough to be eaten by zooplankton decline, adversely affecting zooplankton and their predators. Algae overgrow spawning grounds of lake trout, the normal prey of fish (such as shrimp) die, and trout lose weight and die. Lower vertebrates die from hydrogen ion toxicity and from the secondary effects of parasitism by opportunistic microorganisms.

Inhalation toxicity

Lungs receive constant insults of dust, microorganisms, and toxic gases. The oxygen-exchanging membranes of the alveolar wall are protected from many of these by the mucociliary system of the bronchioles. The ciliated columnar epithelium of the respiratory tract is designed to purify air from the polluted environments for presentation to the respiratory lobule. Warmed and humidified by passage through the upper respiratory tract, the air is cleansed in the bronchioles by the continuous secretion of mucus, which traps and inactivates foreign substances.

Terminal bronchioles are especially equipped to deal with inhaled toxins. Their Clara cells are loaded with enzymes that catabolize inhaled pollutants. These are cytochrome P-450–dependent monooxygenases, bound to smooth endoplasmic reticulum, which catabolize toxic drugs, pesticides, and carcinogens.

Ozone. The current U.S. National Ambient Air Quality Standard for ozone is 0.08 ppm, a level commonly exceeded in metropolitan areas during summer. Alveoli in the proximal acinus are the primary sites of ozone injury.

Sulfur dioxide. Sulfur dioxide (SO_2) is a significant air pollutant in industrial areas that causes loss of cilia on short-term experimental exposure at 100 ppm. Cilia are also susceptible to low levels of ozone and nitrogen dioxide.

Hydrogen sulfide. Hydrogen sulfide (H_2S) gas is produced in large amounts in farm slurries and pit silos. Farm workers in these areas may be unknowingly overcome by heavy concentrations of gas in enclosed spaces. Typically, one worker succumbs, another descends to help and is also affect-

TABLE 3.9. Common agriculture poisons

Group	Compound	Mechanisms of action
Insecticides		
Organophosphates	Parathion, malathion, dichlorvos, diazinon	Inhibition of acetylcholinesterase; signs resemble stimulation of cholinergic nerves
Organochlorines	DDT, methoxychlor, aldrin, dieldrin, chlordane, endrin, heptachlor, toxaphene	Alteration of Na^+ and K^+ transport across plasma membrane of nerve axons (prevents K^+ efflux); signs are tremor, convulsions, and paresthesia; multiple effects on lower vertebrates
	Lindane, mirex, kepone	Blood dyscrasia (chronic) and neural disease (acute)
Botanic insecticides	Pyrethrum, nicotine, rotenone	
Herbicides		
Chlorophenoxy compounds	2,4-D; 2,4,5-T	Myotoxicity
Dinitrophenols	Dinitrophenol, dinitroorthocresol	Suppression of mitochondrial oxidative phosphorylation
Bipyridyl compounds	Paraquat	Lung injury during exhalation (subacute) and myocardiopathy (acute)
Rodenticides		
	Warfarin	Inhibition of coagulation
	Red squill	Cardiotonic glycoside
	Sodium fluoroacetate	Inhibition of citric acid cycle
	ANTU (α-naphthyl thiourea)	Combined with –SH groups, alters carbohydrate metabolism and causes pulmonary edema and hemorrhage
	Strychnine	Lowering of threshold of spinal reflexes by blocking inhibitory pathways; tetanic convulsions
	Reserpine	Depletion of catecholamines

ed, and so on. H_2S, like HCN, inhibits mitochondrial cytochrome oxidase, and death occurs suddenly without overt lesions of disease.

Pesticides and herbicides

Organophosphorus insecticides

TEPP (tetraethyl pyrophosphate), tabun, and sarin were secretly developed in Germany during World War II as possible nerve gas warfare agents. Although useful as insecticides, they were highly toxic to mammals and hydrolyzed in the presence of moisture. Further research led to the synthesis of parathion in 1944. Extensively used in agriculture, parathion has been the pesticide most frequently involved in human fatalities in the past 30 years. It is now being replaced by other, less toxic organophosphorus compounds (Table 3.9).

Parathion is an **acetylcholinesterase inhibitor**. It prevents inactivation of acetylcholine at neural synapses, leading to excessive stimulation of cholinergic nerves. The immediate cause of death from this and other organophosphorus insecticides is asphyxia resulting from respiratory failure. Effects contributing to death arise from three major nerve sites: (1) motor nerves to skeletal muscle (**nicotinic signs** resulting from accumulation of acetylcholine at myoneural junctions are muscle weakness, twitching, and fasciculation); (2) postganglionic parasympathetic nerve fibers (**muscarinic signs**, which occur in cardiac and smooth muscle and exocrine glands, include bronchoconstriction, increased bronchial secretion and salivation, sweating, urination, diarrhea and defecation, and constriction of pupils); and (3) certain central nervous system synapses (accumulation of acetylcholine in brain is associated with restlessness, drowsiness, and other behavioral abnormalities).

In muscle, the cytopathic effects of parathion arise from a combination of presynaptic and postsynaptic events, such as excessive release of acetylcholine, plus repeated binding of unhydrolyzed acetylcholine to receptors, both leading to excessive depolarization of endplate receptors.

Organophosphorus insecticides commonly produce rapid poisoning and in large doses may be fatal. However, they are quickly metabolized and excreted, so that chronic poisoning is not a major problem. Cessation of exposure results in complete recovery.

Organochlorine insecticides

Organochlorine insecticides are neuropoisons that show a wide range of acute toxicities. Unlike the organophosphorus compounds, their mechanisms of action are not clearly defined; they are less acutely toxic and have a greater tendency to chronic toxicity. Organochlorine insecticides are now in disfavor because they persist in the environment and accumulate in animal tissue, especially in fat.

Intense use of **DDT** (dichlorodiphenyltrichloroethane) from the 1940s to 1960s led to chronic exposure of animals and humans, with accumulation of DDT residues in adipose tissue. The significance of these residues is unknown. Despite its widespread use in human antilouse dusting in World War II, there is no record of fatal human toxicity. In contrast, the devastating effects of DDT on wild animals and birds have caused ecologic imbalances and governmental restrictions on DDT use.

In mammals, DDT has primary toxic action on the motor cortex of the brain and on peripheral nerve fibers (both motor and sensory). Manifestations of toxicity (hyperexcitability, tremor, and convulsions) result from prolonged and repetitive action potentials in individual nerves.

Herbicides

Chlorophenoxy compounds. 2,4-D (dichlorophenol) and 2,4,5-T (trichlorophenol), used for control of broadleaf weeds, exert their action by suppressing plant growth hormones. 2,4,5-T is an important herbicide and an ingredient of Agent Orange, used as a military defoliant in the Vietnam war. The action of chlorophenoxy compounds on animals is poorly understood. In large doses they cause cardiac ventricular fibrillation, and in small doses, muscle damage. Lesions at necropsy are those of general toxicity: gastric hyperemia and degenerative changes in hepatocytes and renal tubular epithelium. Chronic exposure in humans has been associated with dermatitis, which probably results from effects of the contaminant dioxin. **Dioxin** is also a major factor in production of the teratogenic effects of these herbicides. In 1970, birth defects in animals were ascribed to 2,4,5-T, but the teratogenic compound was probably a dioxin.

Bipyridal compounds. Paraquat most commonly causes toxicity by accidental ingestion. Acute poisoning in mammals by a single large dose leads to myocardiopathy and transient neurologic signs. Subacute injury is more commonly fatal; the target organ is the lung, regardless of route of entry. Necrosis of pneumocytes and progressive fibrosis of the alveolar septa occur during exhalation of paraquat in the process of elimination of the toxin by the lung.

Carbamate herbicides have low toxicity for animals. Substituted ureas such as diuron and monu-ron are likewise relatively nontoxic. The **triazines** simazine and atrazine, shown experimentally to be slightly toxic for cattle and sheep, will kill in large doses. Amitrol is similar to the triazines but is a potent antithyroid drug; it can produce significant depression of thyroid function and is prohibited for use near animals. Many herbicides that are nontoxic for adult animals can produce subtle teratogenic effects.

Rodenticides

Strychnine. Strychnine is in many rodenticides and in several products for animal and human consumption, including laxatives, sedatives, and tonics. Strychnine excites all of the central nervous system, and its effects clinically resemble tetanus. The important effects result from strychnine's anti-inhibition of spinal cord interneurons. Strychnine competitively antagonizes the inhibitory neurotransmitter **glycine** at the postsynaptic receptor sites of ventral horn motoneurons. Animals that

---

FOCUS

The Hidden Signs of DDT Toxicity

A SWISS RESEARCH CHEMIST, Paul Muller, testing chemicals for insecticidal properties in 1939, discovered the extraordinary effectiveness of dichlorodiphenyltrichloroethane (DDT). It was highly toxic to insects, insoluble in water, and of low toxicity to mammals. By 1941 the Swiss were using the compound successfully to combat the Colorado potato beetle, and it was widely used in World War II to control mosquitoes and body lice. By 1948, when Muller received the Nobel prize for his discovery, DDT was used throughout the world.

Dangers of DDT use had already been recorded in 1945 by biologists of the U.S. Fish and Wildlife Service who warned against using DDT in marshes. By the 1960s, clues began to appear around the world that DDT was accumulating in soils and in tissues of wild animals. Furthermore, the "food chain effect" was proposed: plants accumulate toxins, herbivores get them from plants, carnivores from their food, and finally, humans—if the rate of absorption is higher than the rate of loss. In one well-studied estuarine marsh, accumulation of DDT via the food chain was documented carefully. Marsh water had DDT residues of less than 0.001 ppm; plankton contained residues of 0.01–0.1 ppm; clams, up to 1.0 ppm; fish, a few ppm; and birds, especially carnivorous birds, contained 10–100 ppm. The long struggle to legislate against use of DDT began sometime later, when conspicuous effects were noted; peregrine falcons and osprey began to disappear from their North American ranges along the Atlantic seaboard. DDT caused production of soft-shelled eggs, which were easily broken in the nest. Reproduction failed, and bird populations declined.

Fish are very sensitive to organochlorine pollutants, which inhibit osmoregulation in gill epithelium. Muscle may also be affected by interruption of muscular excitation related to deficient Ca^{2+} uptake by sarcoplasmic reticulum; that is, the insecticide inactivates the Ca^{2+}-dependent pump, causing abnormal Ca^{2+} metabolism in muscle.

Wild marine birds are commonly affected by organochlorine insecticides. Because DDT accumulates in adipose tissues, these carnivorous birds are at the end of the biologic accumulation line. Eggshell thinning results, and increased egg breakage contributes to bird population decline.

survive even for a few hours show profound lactic acidosis, hyperthermia, and rhabdomyolysis.

NUTRITIONAL DISORDERS

When the tissue concentration of a nutrient falls to a critical level, evidence of deranged cellular metabolism occurs, and abnormal metabolites appear in blood, urine, and feces. As the deficiency progresses, microscopic tissue changes develop in rapidly metabolizing tissues such as skeletal muscle, myocardium, and brain. Immature animals are most susceptible to nutritional disease, and the rapidly growing tissues such as bone are also markedly affected. The time required for a nutritional deficiency disease to develop influences the course and character of the tissue changes. Lesions of **acute deficiencies** and **chronic deficiencies** are often different. Swine with acute thiamine deficiency may die suddenly of cardiac failure with few lesions in cardiac muscle, whereas those with chronic deficiency have severe lesions in the heart.

Multiple deficiency is the usual case in animals: that is, a diet of poor quality is apt to be lacking in several important nutrients. When a deficiency of several essential factors occurs, syndromes develop that differ from the combined effects of individual deficiencies.

Nutritional imbalance is more common than a simple deficiency of one particular dietary factor. Some of the delicate interrelationships in nutrition are those of calcium and phosphorus, fat and calcium, and iron and phosphorus. Excess of one dietary component may enhance the deficit of another.

Protein/calorie malnutrition, one of the most common nutritional diseases in animals, is a consequence of a dietary deficiency in total quantity or quality of food. It arises because there is no food available or because animals are unable to feed. Nonnutritional diseases that are prone to be complicated by nutritional deficiency include intestinal malabsorption diseases; increased nutrient loss from diarrhea; increases in demand for nutrients due to excessive heat, cold, or work; and diseases that suppress tissue storage of nutrients (Table 3.10).

Loss of body fat and **muscle wasting** are the dominant signs of calorie deficiency. To determine the nutritional state of sheep, stockmen palpate the longissimus dorsi because the spaces over the back and lateral to the vertebral spines should be filled with this muscle. In progressive atrophy of cachectic sheep, an early change in the longissimus dorsi is loss of type II muscle fibers; the reduced muscle volume results from alternate episodes of atrophy and hypertrophy that cause marked variation in muscle fiber size.

Calorie deficiency: starvation

Food deprivation is characterized by emaciation, loss of musculature, serous atrophy of fat, subcutaneous edema, cardiac muscle degeneration, and atrophy of viscera. The liver and pancreas are markedly reduced in size, and individual hepatocytes are small. After a few days of food deprivation, hepatocyte volume decreases about 50% and the total volume of the energy-producing mitochondria may fall by 50%.

In **starvation**—the long-continued deprivation of food—fatty degeneration of the liver, anemia, and skin lesions develop but often involve mechanisms other than calorie deficiency. Fatty livers are especially common in animals on low-protein diets, in which total calorie intake is near normal but the diet is so deficient in protein that body tissues are broken down and the fats and carbohydrates are transported to the liver to be used to synthesize protein.

There are great age and species differences in death during starvation. Very young and old animals are much less able to withstand food deprivation. Homeothermic animals can withstand starvation for about two weeks (unless hibernating), but poikilotherms can survive several months. Fish, for example, are able to survive long periods of fasting.

TABLE 3.10. Factors that contribute to nutritional deficiency

Mechanism	Examples of disease
Interference with intake	Anorexia
	Gastrointestinal disease
	Food allergy
	Tooth disease
Interference with absorption	Intestinal hypermotility
	Insoluble complexes forming in food (e.g., fat, Ca^{2+})
Interference with storage	Hepatic disease (vitamin A)
	Thyroid disease (iodine deficiency)
Increased excretion	Polyuria
	Sweating
	Endocrine imbalances
	Lactation
Increased requirements	Fever
	Hyperthyroidism
	Pregnancy and lactation
Natural inhibitors	Thiaminases

Intestinal involution occurs early

Fasting has a rapid effect on renewal of epithelial cells of the intestine. Absorptive cells shrink, and their nuclei become pyknotic. Villi become shorter, and the basement membranes underlying the epithelium are markedly thickened. These changes may be due to lack of the hormonal stimulation of gut epithelium that is induced by food. Changes in the intestine closely resemble atrophic changes in other tissues (e.g., the involuting mammary gland at the cessation of lactation).

Atrophy of muscle and fat releases substitutes for food

In early starvation, weight loss is due largely to decreases in muscle mass. Muscle protein breakdown is accompanied by loss of water (associated with loss of Ca^{2+}, K^+, and Mg^{2+}). As starvation progresses, the greater weight losses are accounted for by consumption of body fat, a much richer source of energy than is protein. Cortisol causes adipocytes to increase lipolysis and to liberate fatty acids. Circulating fatty acids are oxidized in the liver to acetoacetic acid and other ketones, and ketosis signals a response to depletion of body glucose. The brain of a starved animal uses ketones as a substitute source of energy.

Gluconeogenesis is an early event in food deprivation

In early fasting, blood glucose drops. **Insulin** levels are low, and **glucagon** levels high (relative to insulin). A consequence of the high glucagon:low insulin ratio is hepatic glycogen depletion. Insulin, a potent inhibitor of adipose tissue lipolysis, is the primary determinant that regulates liver changes in early starvation.

The glucocorticoid **cortisol** helps to maintain blood glucose by stimulating gluconeogenesis, chiefly in the liver. This anabolic effect on liver includes stimulation of enzymes required for gluconeogenesis and for shunting of glucose to glycogen. Cortisol has catabolic effects on skeletal muscle, adipose tissue, lymphoid tissue, and most other tissues.

In muscle, amino acids are produced to provide substrates for the liver. Of the amino acids appearing in plasma, alanine is the principal substrate for hepatic glucose production. Given by injection, alanine can increase synthesis of glucose in the liver. An alanine cycle (the conversion of alanine to glucose and reconversion to alanine) recycles a fixed supply of glucose and is an efficient means of transporting nitrogen to the liver from amino acids liberated by muscle breakdown.

Liver atrophy is followed by marked metabolic alterations

Within 24 hours of food deprivation, glycogen in hepatocytes and glucose in the bloodstream are markedly decreased. Within the liver cells, there are simultaneous increases in glycogen phosphorylase (for glycogen degradation) and decreases of glycogen synthetase (for synthesis). As fasting continues, there are profound changes in other enzyme systems relating to utilization of glucose and fatty acids.

As excessive mobilization of fatty acids from adipose tissue continues in response to the negative energy balance, the liver begins to accumulate fat. Decreased protein synthesis by the atrophic hepatocytes contributes to fat accumulation by reducing the amounts of apoprotein available for secretion of triglycerides into the blood. After entering the hepatocyte, fatty acids are shunted to mitochondria, where they are oxidized to acetyl CoA. Acetyl CoA formed during fatty acid oxidation enters the citric acid cycle, if fat and carbohydrate degradation are balanced. As fat breakdown predominates as the energy source, acetyl CoA accumulates and undergoes a different fate. If carbohydrate is not available, oxaloacetate is reduced and is unavailable for condensation with acetyl CoA. Thus acetyl CoA cannot enter the citric acid cycle and is diverted to acetoacetate and hydroxybutyrate (ketone bodies), which leave the cell and circulate in the bloodstream.

The prime factor leading to **ketosis** in starvation is the **insulinopenia** that develops with fasting. It leads not only to lipolysis but also to changes in hepatic ketogenic enzymes and impairment of mechanisms for peripheral utilization of ketones. All three events act in concert to cause ketones to accumulate in the circulation.

As ketone production rises, ketones are increasingly utilized by the nervous system as alternative fuels to glucose. This permits reductions in gluconeogenesis and sparing of protein and is a crucial adaptive mechanism that prolongs survival in starvation.

Several factors spare energy in starvation

The starving animal attempts to adapt to the low level of caloric intake. Diminished physical activity, loss of metabolically active tissue (with decreased caloric need), and lowering of the basal metabolic rate all play major roles. The metabolic rate is reduced in part by lowering of the serum thyroid hormone T_3 (with concomitant increase in noncalorigenic T_3 metabolites). The decrease in plasma insulin and increase in glucagon also attempt to conserve energy. In prolonged starvation, there is a shift of glucose from liver to kidney cortex; the kidney is able to synthesize glucose from amino acids.

Starvation is accelerated by trauma and infection

Food deprivation that is associated with trauma or severe systemic infection develops more rapidly into a wasting disease. Some of this effect is mediated through the autonomic nervous system. Glucagon secretion is enhanced, insulin secretion is impaired, and the release of epinephrine is increased; free fatty acid release from fat tissue is stimulated, and gluconeogenesis is accelerated. In addition to the marked hyperglycemia, there is an increase in vasopressin and corticosteroid secretion during trauma, which causes decreased water excretion and sodium resorption by the kidneys.

In infections, monocytes release cytokines that selectively enhance muscle breakdown. The protein released from this process is transported to the liver, where it is used both for gluconeogenesis and for synthesis of proteins released as acute phase proteins by the liver.

Brain respiratory centers are depressed in starvation ketosis. Ketones dissociate to yield hydrogen ions, which use bicarbonate and depress plasma pH. At about pH 7.2, the respiratory center in the brain is stimulated. The resulting hyperventilation is an attempt to depress pH (increased loss of carbon dioxide reduces plasma carbonic acid). Further decline of pH is associated with depression of cerebral function, coma, and death.

Vitamin deficiency

There are two groups of vitamins: the fat-soluble ones—A, D, E, and K—and the water-soluble ones, which include the vitamin B complex and vitamin C. The biochemical roles of the water-soluble vitamins are relatively well established, and most of these vitamins are components of coenzymes. For example, vitamin B_{12} (riboflavin) is a precursor of flavin adenine dinucleotide.

Vitamin A

Vitamin A alcohol (retinol) or its precursors, the carotenes, occur in most normal diets. Both are present in plants containing yellow pigments and in animal fats and liver (e.g., cod liver oil). Beta-carotene, the most important, is cleaved in the gut mucosa into two molecules of retinal (vitamin A aldehyde). After absorption, large amounts of retinal are stored in stellate, interstitial cells of the liver (liver disease impairs storage).

Vitamin A exerts a controlling influence on development of epithelial cells. It has a steroidlike effect on nuclear transcription that causes dedifferentiation of cells, followed by redifferentiation along a different pathway.

Vitamin A deficiency. Squamous metaplasia of epithelial surfaces is the dominant lesion in vitamin A deficiency. Throughout the body there are widespread changes of simple types of epithelium to stratified squamous epithelium. This is most easily detected at body orifices but also occurs in viscera such as the pancreas, bladder, and other organs. It is especially important in ductal structures and has been incriminated as a cause of urolithiasis in cats, although this has not been confirmed. In calves, clinically significant changes occur in arachnoid villi of the meninges; outflow of cerebrospinal fluid is inhibited, causing increased intracranial pressure.

In **respiratory epithelium**, goblet cells are eliminated and replaced with keratin-synthesizing squamous cells. Foci of hyperplastic basal cells develop and expand, causing cells to desquamate. As basal cells enlarge, they gradually convert to keratin production.

Teeth are often abnormal in young animals with vitamin A deficiency. Ameloblasts show abnormal differentiation, which in turn adversely affects odontoblast development. Lesions induce hypoplasia of enamel, deficient mineralization of teeth, and retarded eruption.

Vitamin A deficiency in pregnant animals has been associated with stillbirth and abortions, particularly in swine.

Retinol (vitamin A) is the precursor of retinal, the light-absorbing group in visual pigments. Retinol deficiency leads to deterioration of the other segments of rods. Retinal is the prosthetic group of the photosensitive pigment in both rods and cones. The differences between the photosensitive pigments in rods (rhodopsin) and in cones (iodopsin) are in the protein bound to them. Sight involves isomerization in the dark of all-trans retinal to the 11-cis form, which in combination with opsin forms rhodopsin. During light absorption, the 11-cis isomer is converted back to the all-trans form. During this cycle, some retinal is reduced to retinol and lost to the reaction; thus vitamin A must be continually added to this visual reaction. In vitamin A deficiency the retinal used in rod vision is rapidly depleted, and vision in low-intensity light is lost—the explanation for human "night blindness."

Vitamin A toxicosis. Mucous metaplasia occurs in vitamin A excess. Normal squamous epithelium is converted to mucus-producing epithelium. This is brought about not by inducing mitosis but by influencing postmitotic cells to abandon

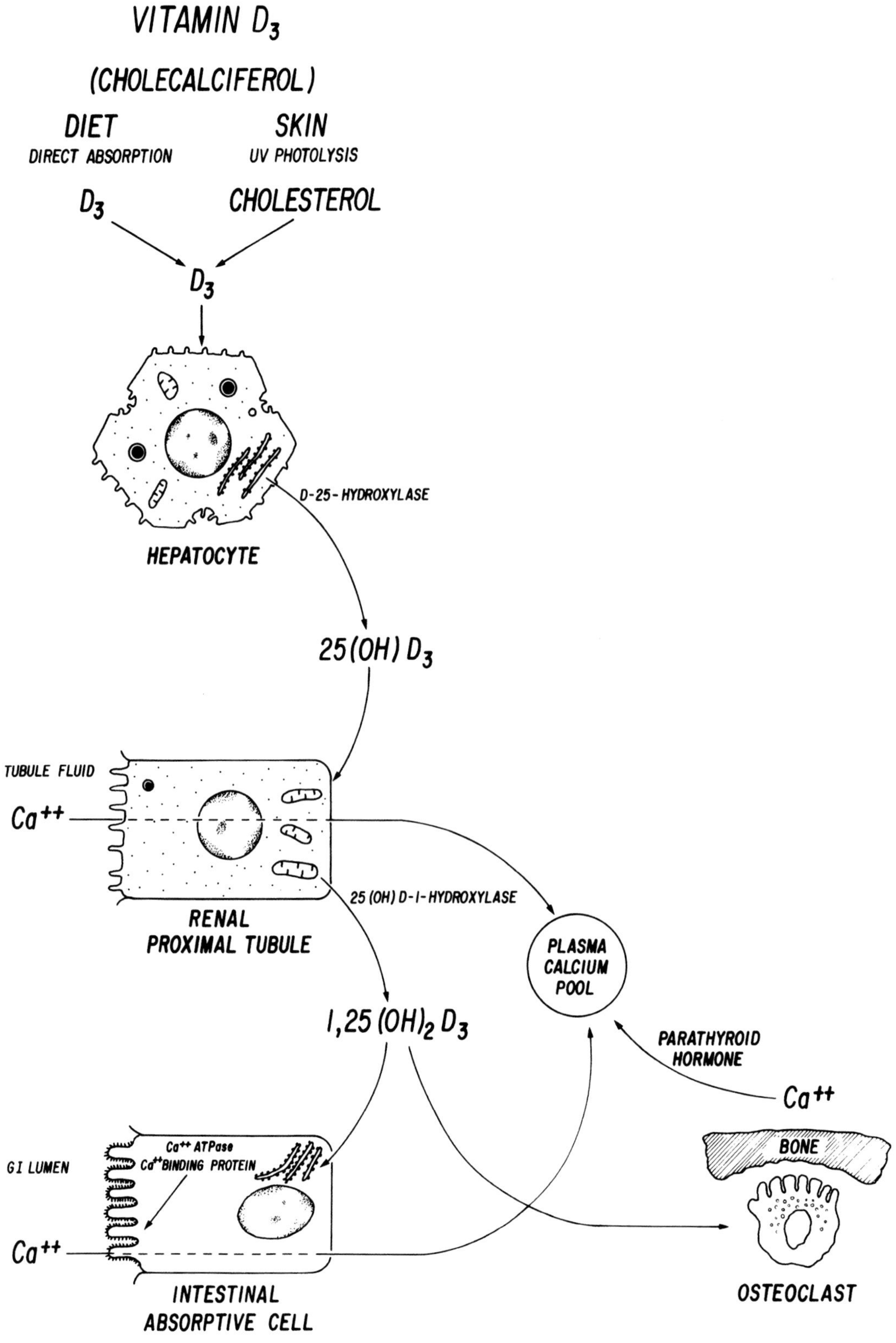

FIGURE 3.13. Vitamin D metabolism: hormonal regulation of Ca^{2+} in extracellular fluids.

keratinization and to differentiate to mucous glandular epithelium.

Vitamin D

Diet is the important source of vitamin D_3 (cholecalciferol) in most mammals and birds, although some is formed in skin by light-induced nonenzymatic photolysis of dehydrocholesterol. In the bloodstream, D_3 is bound to an α_2-globulin and transported to the liver. Vitamin D_3 is hydroxylated to $25(OH)D_3$ in hepatocytes and further hydroxylated to $1,25(OH)_2D_3$ (dihydroxycholecalciferol) in the kidney. Circulating $25(OH)D_3$ serves as a substrate for either 25(OH)-1-hydroxylase or 25(OH)-24-hydroxylase, both of which are in the renal cortex. The steroid hormone and active metabolite $1,25(OH)_2D_3$ is taken up by receptors within cells of target organs (intestine, bone, and kidney). The hormone-receptor complex passes into the nucleus, binds to specific portions of chromatin, and initiates gene expression and protein synthesis. The peptide that results produces the biologic action on calcium.

Vitamin D and its two chief metabolites, $1,25(OH)_2D_3$ and $24,25(OH)_2D_3$, interacting with calcitonin and parathyroid hormone, maintain calcium and phosphorus homeostasis (Fig. 3.13). Both of the biologically active metabolites of vitamin D are produced in the proximal convoluted tubules of the kidney.

The steroid hormone $1,25(OH)_2D_3$ induces Ca^{2+}-binding proteins. In kidney, synthesis of a calcium-binding protein is stimulated in cells of the distal tubule. In small intestine, $1,25(OH)_2D_3$ induces epithelial cells to produce another calcium-binding protein that passes into the microvillous glycocalyx, migrates to the cell surface, and causes Ca^{2+} to pass from lumen into the bloodstream. Vitamin D metabolites produce two effects on **bone**: calcification of osteoid on trabecular surfaces, and osteoclastic resorption for Ca^{2+} mobilization. They also directly interact with **parathyroid** to suppress secretion of parathyroid hormone, which in turn inhibits formation of $1,25(OH)_2D_3$ in the kidney.

The conversion $25(OH)D_3$ —(1-hydroxylase)→ $1,25(OH)_2D_3$ is the rate-limiting step in vitamin D metabolism and explains the delay between injections of vitamin D and a biologic response. Conversion is controlled by secretion of parathyroid hormone and calcium. Parathyroid hormone increases and calcitonin decreases the production of $1,25(OH)_2D_3$. Other steroid hormones, such as estrogens, increase renal hydroxylase action and play roles in special demands for calcium.

Vitamin D deficiency causes rickets in young and osteomalacia in adults. These syndromes are no

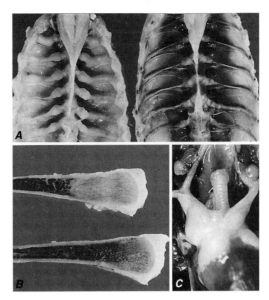

FIGURE 3.14. Vitamin D deficiency, chicken. A. Thorax, distortion of vertebrae and ribs *(left)*; normal thorax *(right)*. B. Tibia, expansion of metaphysis and shortened bone lengths; normal tibia *(bottom)*. C. Parathyroid hyperplasia in response to calcification defect and need to maintain plasma calcium.

longer common but occur when errors are made in dietary formulations or as part of food deprivation during general debilitating disease. Rickets is commonly seen in birds, where it is characterized by retarded growth, hypocalcemia, parathyroid hyperplasia, and fibrous osteodystrophy (Fig. 3.14). There is marked expansion of growth plates, with failure of calcification of cartilage and osteoid. Although osteoclasts are increased, they may be less functional in late disease, a defect probably related to parathyroid exhaustion.

Vitamin E

Vitamin E occurs in eight natural forms—four tocopherols and four tocotrienols. Alpha-tocopherol is the most biologically active and the important metabolite in vitamin E deficiency in animals. Early biochemical studies recognized the antioxidant property of tocopherols; for example, in vitamin E–deficient rodents, body fat was susceptible to oxidation and treatment with E prevented this oxidation.

Major lesions of vitamin E deficiency occur in muscle, brain, and skin. In addition, the reproductive system of some species (especially rodents and swine) requires E for normal function, and reproductive failure has been ascribed to vitamin E defi-

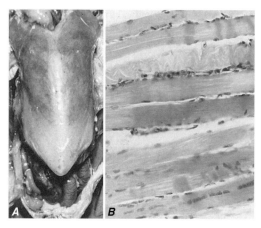

FIGURE 3.15. Vitamin E deficiency, breast muscle, chicken. A. Patchy pallor, or "white muscle disease." B. Myodystrophy, skeletal muscle with disintegration of myofibrils and aggregation of muscle proteins.

ciency in these species. Muscle dystrophy, the best-known disease syndrome associated with vitamin E deficiency, is common in ruminants, swine, and poultry and is rare in carnivores and nonhuman primates.

Myodystrophy. Myodystrophy, or "white muscle disease," was first described as a disease in ruminants. In advanced disease, skeletal muscle becomes irregularly pale with blotches of white among areas of varying pallor. Degeneration of skeletal muscle cells begins in the mitochondria, which in early phases of deficiency enlarge and then, as the myocyte fails, show disintegration. Lesions of necrosis are most prominent in the cerebellum.

In primates, the nervous system is also affected, although clinical signs often arise from lesions outside the brain. Loss of sensory axons in posterior columns, sensory roots, and peripheral nerves leads to a syndrome of **sensory neuropathy**.

Vitamin E deficiency in birds is associated with three clinical syndromes: myopathy, encephalomalacia, and exudative dermatitis (Fig. 3.15). All are variants of the same injury, and all occur to some degree in each case, although the dominance of one usually determines the clinical diagnosis applied. Which form develops is largely controlled by the amount of fats in the diet. Rations high in saturated fats predispose to encephalomalacia because of the increased oxidation stimulated by the fat.

Vitamin K

Vitamin K occurs in three forms: K_1, phylloquinone; K_2, menaquinone; and K_3, menadione. The first two are in green plants and animal tissues and are synthesized by gut microbes. K_3 is a synthetic compound. Since all are fat-soluble, uptake in the intestine requires normal fat absorption, including bile salts and pancreatic enzymes.

Vitamin K deficiency leads to abnormal prothrombin. Vitamin K is required by hepatocytes to synthesize prothrombin (factor II) and also factors VII, IX, and X. Vitamin K deficiency is referred to as hypoprothrombinemia. Abnormal prothrombin is synthesized in the absence of vitamin K. Although its amino acid sequence is normal, the carboxyglutamate amino terminus that binds Ca^{2+} is defective, because the vitamin K is an integral part of the enzymes that carboxylate the glutamate residues.

Vitamin B complex

The B vitamins play roles in energy-releasing mechanisms in mitochondria that provide ATP, especially in cells involved in hematopoiesis. Deficiencies of B vitamins tend to produce changes in tissues with high rates of metabolism.

Thiamine. Thiamine is a component of **thiamine pyrophosphate** (TPP), the prosthetic group of three important enzymes (pyruvate dehydrogenase, α-ketoglutarate dehydrogenase, and transketolase) that transfer activated aldehyde units. Most important, TPP (as a component of the pyruvate dehydrogenase complex) serves as the initial catalytic cofactor in the oxidative decarboxylation of pyruvate: pyruvate + CoA + NAD acetyl CoA + CO_2 + NADH. Blood levels of pyruvate and α-ketoglutarate are abnormally high in thiamine deficiency because of depressed activities of the pyruvate and α-ketoglutarate dehydrogenases. Transketolase activity of erythrocytes is also low; this is the basis for a useful diagnostic test.

Lesions of thiamine deficiency center on early mitochondrial hypertrophy and degeneration. Thiamine deficiency affects metabolically active cells of brain and myocardium, a condition that is reflected in clinical signs of ataxia. Astrocytes and oligodendrogliocytes are the most susceptible; glial swelling is the initial change in experimental disease. Neural lesions, which progress from edema to hyperemia, hemorrhage, and necrosis, are the most prominent in the periventricular gray matter, cerebral cortex, and corpora quadrigemina.

Thiamine deficiency is a disease of ruminants and carnivores, especially foxes, cats, and mink. Deficiencies develop from (1) **dietary deficiencies** (e.g., beriberi of humans, caused by thiamine-deficient diets of polished rice, and Wernicke's encephalopathy accompanying alcoholism); (2) **thiaminases in the diet** (e.g., Chastek paralysis of mink, foxes, and cats, due to the thiaminase in fish muscle; and the central nervous system disease of horses, associated with the thiaminase in bracken fern); and (3) toxicity of **thiamine-splitting drugs**, notably the thiamine analog amprolium, which is used as a coccidiostat and is causally associated with polioencephalomalacia in cattle and sheep.

Riboflavin. Riboflavin (vitamin B_2) is a component of several enzymes, all associated with oxidation-reduction reactions (e.g., cytochrome reductase and xanthene oxidase). Deficiency is associated with malfunction of the nervous system. "Curled-toe paralysis" of chicks is one of the few documented syndromes. Swelling of sciatic and brachial nerves is associated with axonal swelling, Schwann cell proliferation, and demyelination.

Niacin. Niacin (nicotinic acid, nicotinamide) has an essential role in electron transport in the mitochondrion. Deficiency in humans causes **pellagra** (L. *pelle*, skin, plus *agra,* rough) characterized by dermatitis, diarrhea, and dementia. Pigs fed purified diets deficient in niacin lose body weight, become anorexic, and develop diarrhea and anemia. At necropsy the gastrointestinal tract has mucous hyperplasia and in severe cases is congested with tiny hemorrhages.

Pyridoxine. Pyridoxine (vitamin B_6) deficiency has not been established as a clinical disease. Pyridoxine deficit occurs in uremia and is associated with amino acid imbalances in plasma. **Pyridoxine toxicity** is generally considered a laboratory disease. No clinical disease has been reported, but pyridoxine is widely used as a model to study human sensory neuropathies. Recently ataxia and neuropathy have been reported in humans consuming large daily doses of pyridoxine, but the pathologic lesions remain unknown.

Vitamin C

A vitamin C (**ascorbic acid**) deficiency markedly retards fibroplasia, because this vitamin is required as a cofactor for proline hydroxylase. In animals, **scurvy** is seen only in guinea pigs fed on old stale feeds. Affected bones have excessive ground substance and fibroblasts but very few mature collagen fibers. Fibroblasts do not form in parallel arrangement, and the resulting signs of disease are related to delayed wound healing and abnormal bone. In the classic medical literature, human scurvy patients were afflicted with breakdown of very old scars, a fact that emphasizes the active metabolism of collagen that occurs even in dense connective tissue.

ADDITIONAL READING

Physical causes of disease
Bartels KE, Stair EL, Cohen RE. 1991. Corrosion potential of steel bird shot in dogs. *J Am Vet Assoc* 199:856.

Buckley IK. 1960. Tissue injury by high frequency electric current. *Aust J Exp Biol* 38:195.

Finnie JW. 1997. Traumatic head injury in ruminant livestock. *Aust Vet J* 75:204.

Fullington RJ, Otto CM. 1997. Characteristics and management of gunshot wounds in dogs and cats: 84 cases (1986–1995). *J Am Vet Med Assoc* 210:658.

Gleiser CA. 1954. The pathology of total body radiation in dogs which died following exposure to a lethal dose. *Am J Vet Res* 15:329.

Hoopes PJ, et al. 1985. The pathogenesis of radiation nephropathy in the dog. *Radiat Res* 104:406.

Hooser SB, et al. 1989. Atypical contagious ecthyma in a sheep after extensive cutaneous thermal injury. *J Am Vet Med Assoc* 195:1225.

House JK, et al. 1996. Primary photosensitization related to ingestion of alfalfa silage by cattle. *J Am Vet Med Assoc* 209:1604.

Loebl EC, et al. 1973. The mechanisms of erythrocyte destruction in the early post-burn period. *Ann Surg* 178:681.

McChesney SL, et al. 1988. Radiation-induced cardiomyopathy in the dog. *Radiat Res* 113:120.

Powers BE, et al. 1991. Percent tumor necrosis as a predictor of treatment response in canine osteosarcoma. *Cancer* 67:126.

Rodemann HR, Bamberg M. 1995. Cellular basis of radiation induced fibrosis. *Radiother Oncol* 35:83.

Stoner HB, et al. 1985. Trauma and its metabolic problems. *Br Med Bull* 41:201.

Biologic causes of disease
Beverly, SM 1996. Hijacking the cell: parasite in the driver's seat. *Cell* 87:787.

Brownstein DG, Gras L. 1997. Differential pathogenesis of lethal mousepox in congenic DBA/2 mice implicates natural killer cell receptor NKR-P1 in necrotizing hepatitis and the fifth component of complement in recruitment of circulating leukocytes to spleen. *Am J Pathol* 150:1407.

Frost AJ, et al. 1997. The early dynamic response of the calf ileal epithelium to *Salmonella typhimurium*. *Vet Pathol* 34:369.

Hoffmann R. 1974. Tod eines Schäferhundes infolge überfalls durch einen Bienenschwarm. *Berl Münch Tierarztl Wschr* 87:374.

Krakowka S, et al. 1998. Production of gastroesophageal erosions and ulcers (GEU) in gnotobiotic swine monoinfected with fermentative commensal bacteria and fed high-carbohydrate diet. *Vet Pathol* 35:274.

Miller CW, et al. 1996. Streptococcal toxic shock syndrome in dogs. *J Am Vet Med Assoc* 209:1421.

Pérez V, et al. 1998. Mammary and systemic aspergillosis in dairy sheep. *Vet Pathol* 35:235.

Song L, et al. 1996. Structure of staphylococcal

α-haemolysin, a heptameric transmembrane pore. *Science* 274:1859.

Turk J, et al. 1990. Coliform septicemia and pulmonary disease associated with canine parvovirus enteritis: 88 cases (1987–1988). *J Am Vet Med Assoc* 196:771.

Williams KJ, et al. 1998. Cerebrospinal cuterebriasis in cats and its association with feline ischemic encephalopathy. *Vet Pathol* 35:330.

Toxicologic disease

Collins LG, and Tyler DE. 1985. Experimentally induced phenylbutazone toxicosis in ponies. *Am J Vet Res* 46:1605.

Reimschuessel R, et al. 1996. Evaluation of gentamicin-induced nephrotoxicosis in toadfish. *J Am Vet Med Assoc* 209:137.

Spangler WL, et al. 1980. Gentamicin nephrotoxicity in the dog. *Vet Pathol* 17:206.

Stegelmeier BL, et al. 1995. The lesions of locoweed *(Astragalus molissimus)*, swainsonine, and castanospermine in rats. *Vet Pathol* 32:289.

Walton RM, et al. 1997. Mechanisms of echinocytosis induced by *Crotalus atrox* venom. *Vet Pathol* 34:442.

Wilson TM, and Drake TR. 1981. Porcine focal symmetrical poliomyelomalacia. *Can J Comp Med* 46:218.

Nutritional disease

Divers TJ, et al. 1986. Blindness and convulsions associated with vitamin A deficiency in feedlot steers. *J Am Vet Med Assoc* 189:1579.

Floyd EE, and Jetten AM. 1988. Retinoids, growth factors, and the tracheobronchial epithelium. *Lab Invest* 59:1.

Goedegebuure SA, et al. 1986. Morphological findings in young dogs chronically fed a diet containing excess calcium. *Vet Pathol* 23:594.

Kennedy S, et al. 1997. Histopathologic and ultrastructural alterations of white liver disease in sheep experimentally depleted of cobalt. *Vet Pathol* 34:575.

Okada HM, et al. 1987. Thiamine deficiency encephalopathy in foxes and mink. *Vet Pathol* 24:321.

Read DH, and Harrington DD. 1986. Experimentally induced thiamine deficiency in beagle dogs. *Am J Vet Res* 47:2281.

Smith JE, et al. 1984. Serum ferritin and total iron-binding capacity to estimate iron storage in pigs. *Vet Pathol* 21:597.

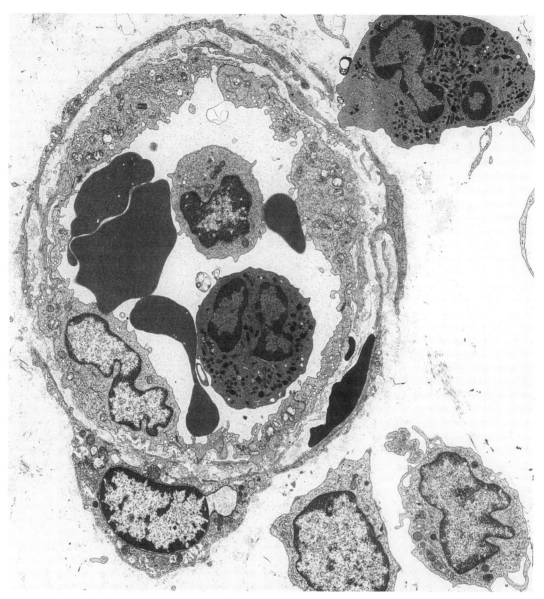

Dilatation and endothelial cell activation in a postcapillary venule, acute inflammation of the skin of a rat. Endothelial cells are vesicular and have irregular surfaces. Erythrocytes are adhered to endothelium, and one *(arrow)* is in the subendothelial tissue. Neutrophil and monocyte are in the lumen. Perivascular spaces are enlarged by edema fluid and contain a neutrophil *(upper right)* and monocytes *(lower right)*.

PART 2

Inflammation and Healing

INFLAMMATION (L. *inflammare*, to set on fire) is a complex progression of vascular and interstitial tissue changes that develops in response to tissue injury. The cardinal signs of inflammation are **redness, heat, pain, swelling, and loss of function**. Vasodilation, which develops promptly when tissue is injured, underlies the cardinal signs. Increased blood flow to the site of injury is responsible for redness and heat, and movement of plasma fluids from the vascular lumen into tissue spaces leads to swelling and stimulation of pain receptors of nerves.

The early phase of acute inflammation is designed to dilute, sequester, and destroy the causal agent of injury and to pave the way for repair in the damaged tissue. Inflammation is a protective process. Because it extends the defense mechanisms existing in circulating blood into the tissues, inflammation enables animals to survive even severe injury. Severe inflammation, however, is also destructive to tissue and, in some exaggerated cases, may be life-threatening.

The first major event in the acute inflammatory response is an **increase in permeability of endothelium of the capillary bed**. This arises from the complex effects of cytokines and other inflammatory mediators, which directly and simultaneously activate both endothelium and leukocytes. Activated endothelium becomes both sticky and then leaky, and this increased vascular permeability leads directly to **leakage of plasma proteins and exudation of leukocytes** from blood vessel lumens into the tissue interstitium. Albumin, fibrinogen, globulin, and other proteins in plasma pour into the tissues.

Neutrophils and monocytes become activated, and by exposing a new spectrum of receptors and adhesion molecules on their surfaces, begin to adhere to the activated endothelial surface. Adherence is transient at first and causes the leukocytes to roll and bounce over the endothelial surface. With increasing expression of adhesion molecule receptors on endothelial surfaces, leukocytes begin to stick firmly to endothelium and then rapidly pass the vascular wall. Here they participate directly in phagocytosis or immobilization of the etiologic agent. As fluid accumulates in tissue spaces, toxins, microbial components, and tissue debris are complexed by specialized proteins, processed by phagocytic cells, and drained away into the lymphatic system.

As the local inflammatory response proceeds, potent cytokines and other humoral factors are released from endothelial cells and circulating neutrophils. As the lesion develops, mast cells, platelets, and macrophages contribute additional cytokines. These soluble signal molecules diffuse through the site of injury promoting the inflammatory response by attracting and activating new leukocytes from the bloodstream. Cytokines also travel systemically in the bloodstream to mobilize body defenses—to activate the mechanisms of inflammation and immunity in order to overcome injury.

Different cytokines act to promote **hematopoiesis** (in bone marrow), **lymphopoiesis** (in lymph nodes), and **synthesis of acute phase proteins** (in the liver). As a result, new leukocytes and acute phase proteins pour into the bloodstream, travel back to the inflammatory site, and enter the tissue to provide appropriate stimulation to enhance the inflammatory process. Some of the acute phase proteins that are released by the liver (fibrinogen, complement, and others) rapidly appear in blood, lymph, and tissue fluids and are strongly **vasoactive**. These peptides mediate inflammation by enhancing the increase in capillary permeability and by specifically directing the migration of circulating leukocytes, a process called **chemotaxis**.

In late stages of acute inflammation, reconstructive processes are initiated that repair tissue damage. **Angiogenesis** (vascular regrowth), **fibrosis** (proliferation of fibroblasts), and **epithelial regeneration** flourish in the protein and growth factor–rich tissue matrix established in early inflammation. Populations of leukocytes, which are often called inflammatory cells, persist to clean up tissue debris and to provide specific mechanisms that remove microorganisms and foreign substances. Newly formed, highly vascularized connective tissue of inflammation is called **granulation tissue**. Excess amounts of granulation tissue are characteristic of skin wounds that fail to heal by primary closure.

Inflammation is closely linked to **hemostasis** (fibrin polymerization and platelet aggregation) and **immunologic reactivity** (antibodies and cell-mediated immune mechanisms), both of which limit the initial spread of tissue injury. Immune reactions are an integral part of inflammation and healing. Attack by specific antibodies and lymphocytes soon dominates the healing phase of acute inflammation.

In the end, inflammation usually brings about recovery. In the higher animals, inflammation is the primary process by which the mechanisms of immunity are implemented. Phylogenetically, the inflammatory process becomes increasingly complex as one progresses from lower forms to the higher vertebrates. It consists largely of nonspecific fluid and cellular mechanisms in lower forms of animal life. Inflammation involves most of the more ancient mechanisms of immunity but also induces specific mechanisms such as production of antibodies and lymphocytes with very selective and precise functions.

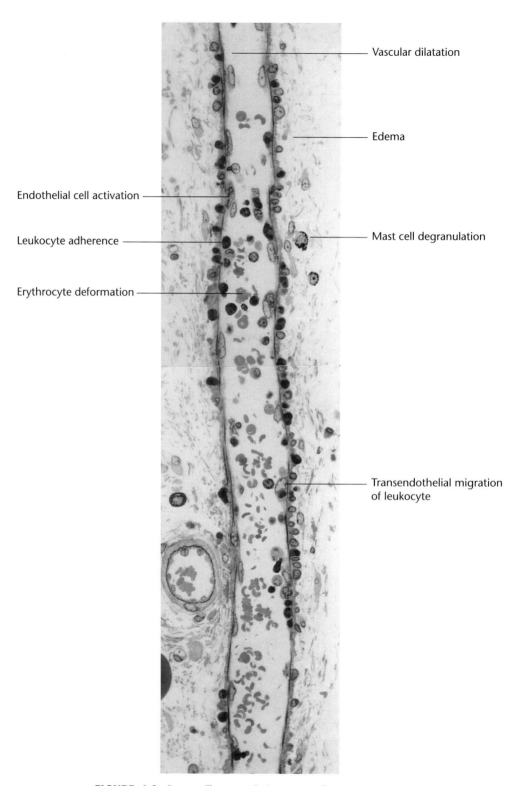

Vascular dilatation

Edema

Endothelial cell activation

Leukocyte adherence

Erythrocyte deformation

Mast cell degranulation

Transendothelial migration of leukocyte

FIGURE 4.1. Postcapillary venule in acute inflammation of skin: vascular dilatation, deformation of erythrocytes, emigration of leukocytes, and edema of perivascular connective tissue.

▦ CHAPTER 4

Acute Inflammation

THE FIRST EVENT: INCREASED VASCULAR PERMEABILITY

The most critical event in the pathogenesis of acute inflammation is increased permeability of capillaries and postcapillary venules. Escape of protein-rich fluids into the interstitium is the hallmark of acute inflammation. Endothelial cell alterations determine the extent of the plasma protein–containing fluid that escapes to the extravascular spaces. Whether capillaries are injured directly by trauma, toxins, or microorganisms, or indirectly by hypoxia, the endothelial cell reacts in much the same way to facilitate the movement of fluids and leukocytes into tissue spaces.

Endothelial cells are activated

Endothelial cell surfaces play an active role in leukocyte migration by secreting proteins that function in adhesion. At the site of injury and in capillaries immediately surrounding the injured tissue, endothelial cells become "activated." Activated endothelial cells enlarge, move frondlike filopodia into the lumen of the capillary, and become sticky to circulating leukocytes. Adhesion molecules, stored in cytoplasmic membranes, are rapidly moved to the surface. Two important adhesion molecules are endothelial-leukocyte adhesion molecule–1 (ELAM-1) and intercellular adhesion molecule–1 (ICAM-1); both act as receptors for ligands on circulating leukocytes and are responsible for binding and moving these cells through the vascular wall.

Autocrine cytokines are also important in injured endothelial cells. For example, endothelium is both a source of and target for **interleukin-1** (IL-1), and the autocrine mechanism of this cytokine is responsible for much of the endothelial stickiness. Endothelial cells also release **nitric oxide**, a potent vasodilator, and **prostaglandins** and **leukotrienes**, which have marked effects on enhancing the inflammatory process.

Capillary lumens dilate

In the early phase of acute inflammation, the dilated blood vessels begin to lose fluid into the surrounding tissue. When early inflammatory lesions are examined by histology, one sees subtle changes in capillary endothelium (Fig. 4.1). Erythrocytes fill the expanding vascular lumen. Leukocytes accumulate in the vascular lumen, and some of these cells can be seen to have emigrated through the vascular wall.

Mast cells release histamine and other pro-inflammatory factors

Mast cells, situated in strategic perivascular locations, act early in inflammation by liberating their granules that contain potent vasoactive factors, such as histamine, serotonin, and leukotrienes, and the anticoagulant heparin. **Histamine** acts directly on endothelium of terminal capillaries and postcapillary venules to cause hyperemia and to increase vascular permeability (Fig. 4.2). It causes gaps between endothelial cells, partly by inducing endothelial cell contraction. **Heparin** is also released by mast cells, and its anticoagulant effect is to prevent the polymerization of fibrinogen into fibrin, thereby sustaining the exudative process.

Arteriolar dilatation increases blood flow

Several factors bring about arteriolar dilatation and affect the inflammatory response by causing vaso-

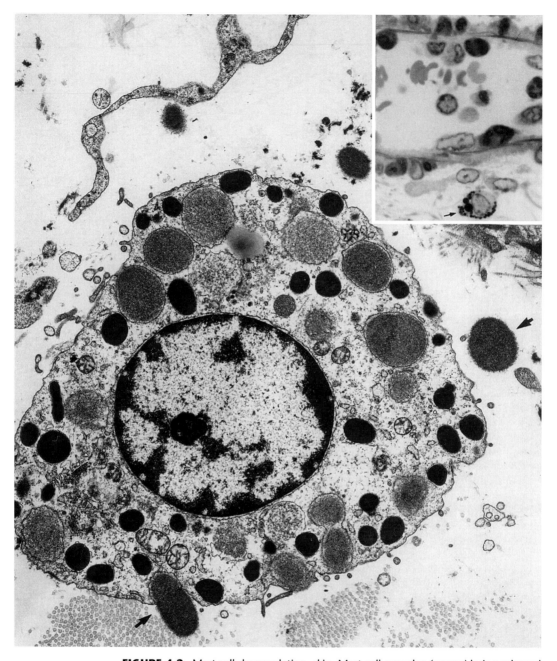

FIGURE 4.2. Mast cell degranulation, skin. Mast cell granules *(arrows)* being released from the cell. Inset: histology of postcapillary venule with transmigrating leukocytes; mast cell *(arrow)*.

dilation upstream from an inflammatory site. The passage of signal molecules between endothelial cells can cause a vasodilatory response that spreads peripherally from the site of injury. Nitric oxide (NO), synthesized and released by endothelial cells, moves peripherally to induce smooth muscle relaxation and vasodilation.

Local tissue injury induces an immediate axon reflex arc (one not traversing the spinal cord of the central nervous system) that is a major cause of arteriolar dilation. After stimulation of sensory nerve endings at the site of injury, a nerve impulse passes centrally along the axon to its division and then peripherally to the arteriole supplying the injured area. Synaptic vesicles within the adrenergic synapse liberate adrenalin, which dilates the peripheral blood vessels. The number and type of receptors on vascular tissues determine how each type of blood vessel responds to adrenalin and other vasoactive agents.

Impulses from the central nervous system can also affect arteriolar blood flow via vasodilator and vasoconstrictor nerves. Experimentally, the sectioning of cutaneous nerves prior to producing skin injury abolished the red flare of the acute response, but not edema at the injury line. Furthermore, the flare was retarded in direct correlation with the presence of wallerian degeneration and death of the nerves sectioned.

Endothelial swelling and hemo-concentration retard blood flow

As plasma leaks from capillaries into perivascular tissue spaces, erythrocytes become increasingly concentrated in blood ("hemoconcentration"). Sluggish movement of this thickened, erythrocyte-rich blood through tissues in an active state of metabolism results in an enhanced depletion of oxygen and glucose. Erythrocytes and leukocytes begin to show altered surface properties, which allow them to interact with endothelial surfaces.

Direct injury to endothelium causes cell swelling, and injured cells protrude into the blood vessel lumen. This retards blood flow in capillaries and may cause stasis. The resulting hypoxia enhances endothelial injury, which affects the cell surface by causing changes in interendothelial cell junctions and in endothelial surface coats that control endothelial-leukocyte interactions. If endothelial injury is severe or if hypoxia is prolonged, erythrocytes may fragment as endothelium disintegrates (Fig. 4.3). When inflammatory lesions are examined by electron microscopy, endothelial cells can be seen to have ruffles and other distortions of both luminal and basal surfaces. Basement membranes are distorted, and there are large numbers of transport vesicles in the cytoplasm. Leukocytes accumulate in vascular lumens and bind to attachment sites on endothelial surfaces (see Frontispiece, Part 2).

Vascular leakage develops by different mechanisms

Vascular leakage begins when endothelial cells are activated or injured. The two major mechanisms, endothelial cell contraction and direct injury, are described below. Minor roles in vascular leakage are also played by two other mechanisms: leukocyte-induced leakage (as neutrophils pass the endothe-

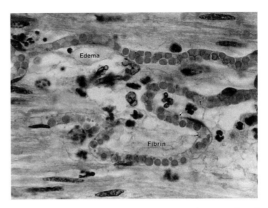

FIGURE 4.3. Degeneration and necrosis of endothelial cells with exudation of fluid (edema), fibrin, and leukocytes into the interstitium. Thrombi are within capillaries *(arrows)*; lamina propria of the intestine, horse, equine viral arteritis.

lial wall, they may induce endothelial damage) and leakage that results from loose, regenerating capillaries in the late stages of inflammation.

Endothelial cell contraction → interendothelial gaps

Leakage via interendothelial gaps created by endothelial cell contraction is the most common form of vascular leakage. It occurs from chemical mediators (histamine, leukotrienes, and bradykinin) acting directly and from cytokines (tumor necrosis factor [TNF], IL-1, and interferon [IFN-γ]) acting via the cytoskeleton. This type of leakage develops rapidly, affects venules of 20–60 μm in diameter, and is associated with increased numbers of receptors on venular endothelium.

Direct injury → endothelial cell death and detachment

The second most common form of leakage is due to endothelial cell death and detachment, resulting from severe direct injury such as burns and trauma. All levels of blood vessels are affected, and this form of leakage is associated with thrombosis.

Leukocytes leave the bloodstream

In normally flowing blood, cells are concentrated in the central zone of the bloodstream. With slowing and stasis, leukocytes **marginate**, attach to the endothelium, and begin to emigrate through the vascular wall. They penetrate endothelial cell junctions and pass through endothelial cell basement membranes into the interstitium. Migration is driven by chemoattractants in inflammatory tissue.

Selectins concentrated in the surface filopodia of neutrophils begin to bind with ligands on the sticky endothelium. Bounding along the endothelial surface, neutrophils begin to be slowed and then finally bind to endothelium firmly and pass the wall:

- Rolling = selectin → selectin receptor
- Binding = integrin → ICAM-1

Neutrophils are recruited to inflammatory sites from the bloodstream by the combined action of many synergistically acting adhesion molecules, cytokines, and chemoattractants. Selectivity in the process comes from the diversity of molecules that mediate each step. Monocytes also penetrate endothelial junctions but are not driven by the strong chemotactic forces that are so effective for neutrophils (Table 4.1).

CLINICAL SIGNS AND LESIONS

The cardinal signs of inflammation tell us about the extent of the inflammatory process in the patient. **Redness** (rubor) is caused by hyperemia that results from vasodilation and increased blood flow to the inflamed area. **Heat** (calor), the increased temperature of inflamed tissue, results from the combined effects of increased blood flow to the inflamed area and the systemic increase in body temperature that is fever. **Swelling** (tumor) is due to accumulation of edema fluid and other exudates as a direct result of increased vascular permeability. **Pain** (dolor) arises from the stimulation of nerve endings by cytokines and other inflammatory mediators of inflammation. **Loss of function** (functio laesa) tells us about

---

TABLE 4.1. Summary of events in acute inflammation (early phase)

1. **Capillaries and postcapillary venules become abnormally permeable:** tissue damage, microbial virulence factors, and other related substances produce a direct effect at the primary site of injury
   a. **Endothelial cells are activated** peripheral to injured site and release . . .
      - Prostaglandins → vasodilation
      - Cytokines (IL-1, TNF, TGF-β) → chemotaxis of leukocytes
      - Procoagulant factors → coagulation
   b. **Mast cells degranulate** and release . . .
      - Histamine → increased postcapillary permeability
      - Heparin → decreased coagulation and stimulation of angiogenesis
      - Serotonin → increased capillary permeability
      - Leukotrienes → pain
   c. **Endothelium becomes leaky** peripheral to the site of injury
2. **Blood flow increases to sites of injury**—after transient vasoconstriction
   - **Arterioles dilate** because of nerve stimuli from axonal reflex arcs
   - **Blood flow stasis** arises from capillary filling and endothelial swelling
   - **Margination of leukocytes** occurs in flowing blood—cells move to periphery
3. **Fluids and cells exude from capillary into perivascular spaces**
   - **Hemoconcentration** as fluid escapes, further slowing blood flow
   - **Plasma proteins exude** into interstitium
   - **Lymph flow is increased** early (it may be suppressed in late stages)
   - **Fibrin polymerizes** from fibrinogen
   - **Leukocytes are activated** and become sticky as surface ligands increase
   - **Neutrophils and monocytes emigrate** and pass vascular walls
4. **Leukocytes degranulate**
   a. **Neutrophils release** . . .
      - Antimicrobial factors (H_2O_2, hydrolytic enzymes, lysozyme)
      - Kinins → vasodilation, vascular permeability, nerve stimulation
      - Proteases → tissue damage
   b. **Platelets aggregate and undergo platelet release reaction**
      - Platelet-activating factor → vascular permeability, platelet aggregation
      - Coagulation factors → blood coagulation
      - Platelet-derived growth factor (PDGF) → angiogenesis
   c. **Monocytes transform into macrophages that synthesize and release** . . .
      - Collagenase, elastase, lysozyme, complement, antimicrobial peptides, and the cytokines IL-1, IFN-γ, TNF-α
      - TNF-α → fever, myalgia, endothelial cell activation
5. **Activation of systemic responses**
   a. Liver releases acute phase proteins (complement, fibrinogen, et al.)
   b. Bone marrow → release of leukocytes and increase of hematopoiesis
   c. Lymph nodes and spleen → lymphopoiesis

Historical Notes on Inflammation

CELSUS, A ROMAN PHILOSOPHER and a contemporary of Christ, enunciated four cardinal signs that are observed grossly in acute inflammation: **redness, swelling, heat,** and **pain** *(rubor, tumor, calor,* and *dolor)*. Rudolf Virchow in 1858 added a fifth: **loss of function.**

With the application of the light microscope to pathology in the middle 1800s, Julius Cohnheim, a German experimental pathologist, revealed the vascular alterations that are the basis of the inflammatory response. By examining mesentery from a loop of intestine pulled through an abdominal incision of a curarized frog, he observed the early changes in blood flow and vascular permeability. Cohnheim recognized that increased capillary permeability was due to direct injury to endothelium and that this explained the initiating reaction in inflammation; that is, hyperemia and the exuding fluid had given rise to redness and swelling.

Cohnheim saw that blood leukocytes migrated through the walls of injured capillaries and small venules to reside in tissue. Like other great pathologists of his day, Cohnheim taught that the observation of these cells filled with bacteria indicated a highly favorable environment for bacterial growth and that leukocytes provided a means of dissemination.

The significance of **intracellular degradation of microbes** was demonstrated by the Russian zoologist Elie Metchnikoff, who investigated the ingestion of particular matter by invertebrate animals. After introducing rose thorns into starfish larvae, he noted that roving cells in the blood localized around the thorns and appeared to ingest and devour them. He termed these cells **phagocytes** (more specifically, **macrophages**) and their process of engulfment **phagocytosis**. His subsequent studies revealed similar activity of "microphages" analogous to the granular leukocytes of vertebrates. These cells have evolved into populations of highly specialized cells (neutrophils, eosinophils, basophils). In the acute phases of inflammation, they migrate through the vascular wall at rates determined by their ameboid potential and their capacity to react to the chemotactic influences that develop in inflammation.

The cardinal signs of inflammation were further explained by Lewis's observations, in 1927, of the **triple response** of skin to a linear stroke produced by a marker. A few seconds after injury, the stroke line was reddened. Slightly later a diffuse pink flare surrounded the red area, and in several minutes a wheal displaced the injury line. Lewis's experiments showed that the initial redness was caused by release of vasoactive mediators such as histamine and leukotrienes that caused capillary dilatation and subsequent endothelial cell disunion. The pink flare surrounding the injury was caused by arteriolar dilation due to an axon reflex arc, and the wheal from exudation of plasma fluids.

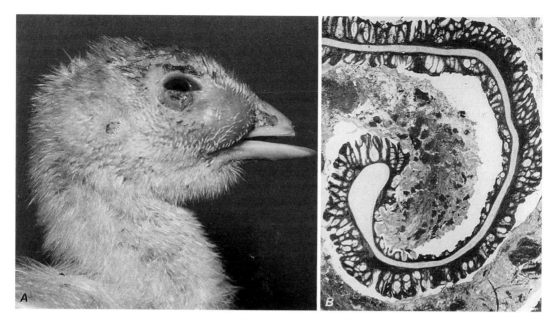

FIGURE 4.4. Severe, diffuse acute serocatarrhal sinusitis, mycoplasmosis. A. Turkey with markedly swollen sinuses. B. Histology of nasal turbinate surrounded by catarrhal exudate.

the extent of injury and leads us to certain types of treatment.

When examining inflammatory lesions, especially of skin, changes should be sought in the lymphatic vessels around the lesion and in the regional lymph nodes. Both provide clues to the seriousness of the inflammatory process. Local infectious processes release microorganisms and inflammatory cells into efferent lymphatic vessels. **Lymphangitis** (inflammation of the lymph vessels) is a serious clinical sign. Efferent lymphatics are red and dilated, and this suggests a more serious inflammatory process that has extended into the regional lymphatic system.

If bacteria escape from an ulcer in the stomach, foci of inflammation may be found in the gastric lymph node. The secondary foci of tissue damage in the lymph node that occur through dissemination of microorganisms are a major connection not to be missed. **Lymphadenitis** (inflammation of the lymph node) is almost always present. Swelling of the lymph node and surrounding tissue may contribute to pain. In severe cases, fibrin polymerizes from fibrinogen within sinusoids of the lymph node and blocks lymphatic drainage.

Serous exudates

The initial exudate in the early phases of most inflammatory lesions is largely serous; that is, leakage has been confined to fluid, albumin, and small amounts of other plasma proteins. The large amount of albumin in the tissue appears histologi-

cally as homogenous eosinophilic granular material. In serous exudates, cells in tissue are spread apart by this albuminous "inflammatory" edema fluid, which serves to dilute the irritant and to ease the migration of inflammatory cells that is soon to follow. Some of the most striking examples of serous inflammation occur in the respiratory tract, such as the severe acute serous rhinitis of upper respiratory viral infections (Fig. 4.4). These lesions rapidly form more complicated exudates, but in early stages the "runny nose" syndrome results from serous exudation.

Blisters begin as serous exudates. Blisters are caused in skin when excessive friction, burns, or chemical toxins damage epithelium and subepithelial capillaries. Epithelium reacts with a general loosening of cell attachments, due to intercellular fluid accumulation. Keratinocytes pull apart, remaining attached only at desmosomes (intercellular bridges). As fluid moves into the epithelium, cell

TABLE 4.2. Differences between transudates and exudates

Characteristic	Transudate	Exudate
Specific gravity	<1.012	>1.020
Protein	Small amount	>4 g/dl
Cells	Few	Many
Capillary defect	Increased capillary pressure or decreased osmotic pressure	Increased permeability

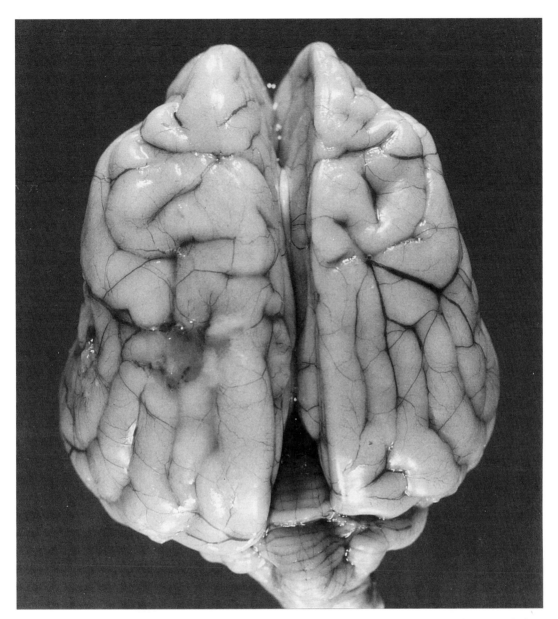

FIGURE 4.5. Inflammation, brain, young dog with severe acute purulent encephalitis. Asymmetry is due to brain swelling; affected left side of brain is swollen (note the rounded gyri) relative to right side. Purulent exudate in the midcortex extends deep into the neuropil. *Escherichia coli* (in large number) and *Corynebacterium* sp. (few) were isolated in cultures of pus from the meninges.

bridges break and serous, intraepidermal microvesicles form. These enlarge and coalesce, forming grossly visible blisters.

In acute inflammation, plasma proteins leak through endothelium at different rates. Differing molecular weights of plasma proteins (albumin 69,000, globulin 150,000, and fibrinogen 340,000) are responsible for the type of exudation and reflect the degree of endothelial injury. The content of plasma proteins in an exudate causes it to differ from the transudates of edema (Table 4.2). Albumin, the smallest and fastest-migrating protein on electrophoresis, is the first plasma protein to leak through the vessel wall. The globulin fractions of serum (α, β, and γ), which also leak early, contain a wide variety of specifically active substances that are highly important in defense, such as **antibodies** (also called **immunoglobulins**).

Progressive tissue swelling leads to pain (Fig. 4.5). When severe injury allows free passage of

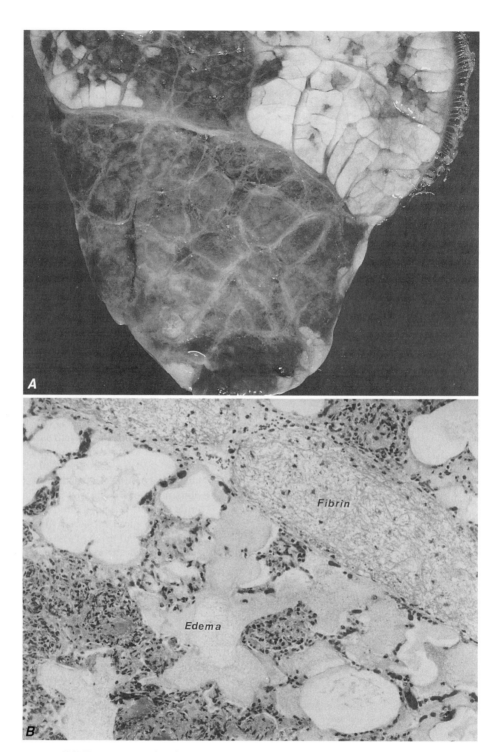

FIGURE 4.6. Focal, subacute, serofibrinous pneumonia, cow with pasteurellosis. A. Septa of the lung contain large amounts of fibrin. Lesions at the periphery are older and are composed of macrophages and fibrous tissue. Lesions deeper in the lobe consist of hyperemia. B. Edema, fibrin, and monocyte infiltrates in alveoli, and large amounts of fibrin strands in interlobular areas. Alveoli are filled with plasma proteins and large numbers of bacteria *(Pasteurella multocida).*

plasma proteins, the equilibrium between hydro-static pressure of the blood and osmotic pressure of the tissue fluid is altered. Extravascular protein abolishes the osmotic suck of the plasma proteins, and more fluid exudes. Increased hydrostatic pressure in dilated arterioles augments fluid loss. The tissue swells, giving rise to pain (two of the five cardinal signs of inflammation). Another pain source is the action of prostaglandin E_2 (PGE_2) and other vasoactive substances on sensitized nerve endings.

Fibrinous exudates

Severe injury to endothelium and basement membranes allows leakage of **fibrinogen**, which polymerizes perivascularly as **fibrin**. Grossly, fibrinous exudates appear as pale tan, stringy, shaggy meshworks on tissue surfaces. In histologic sections, fibrin is bright pink.

Meshes of fibrin around blood vessels impede the escape of plasma proteins. Fibrin also creates a network in tissue spaces that prevents spread of irritants, particularly bacteria (although some bacteria secrete factors that dissolve fibrin). Clotting in lymph vessels suppresses migration of bacteria-laden leukocytes. This effectively slows and often prevents further spread via lymphatics of infectious agents and toxins (Fig. 4.6). Deposition of fibrin also provides the fabric in which the growth of endothelial cells and fibroblasts leads to healing. Fibrinous exudation may be so severe that it is a serious matter for the host.

Mucous (catarrhal) exudates

Liberation of large amounts of glycosaminoglycans and glycoproteins from mucous-secreting cells accompanies inflammation of respiratory and intestinal epithelium. Mucus floods damaged epithelial surfaces. It protects them and provides the tenacious material that, when expectorated, removes much of the debris and irritant. Catarrhal exudates contain not only the mucopolysaccharides of mucus but also many soluble defense factors secreted by leukocytes (antibodies) and epithelial cells (lysozyme).

In the upper respiratory tract, mucus is a stimulus to cilia. Increased ciliary movement propels bacteria, debris, and other materials forward. The irritant effect to sensory nerves induces the cough reflex, which is highly important in diluting and removing irritants and bacteria from the upper airways.

Mucous exudates are antibacterial. Mucus contains many soluble antimicrobial substances. **Lysozyme**, formed by leukocytes and epithelial cells, is secreted onto mucosal surfaces. It occurs in fluids of the respiratory and intestinal tracts and is markedly elevated in inflammation. Lysozyme functions as a mucolytic enzyme (at pH 3–6) on bacterial cell walls and is particularly effective on gram-positive bacteria. Gram-negative bacteria are not lysed, because their cell walls contain lipids as well as mucopeptides.

FOCUS

Traumatic Reticuloperitonitis and Pericarditis

CATTLE, WHICH ARE NOTORIOUSLY unselective in eating habits, are prone to swallow metallic foreign bodies during grazing. Nails, wires, and other sharp objects commonly penetrate the wall of the reticulum and cause traumatic reticuloperitonitis. This event is promoted by contraction of the reticulum and is especially common during the increased abdominal pressure of late pregnancy. Sharp foreign bodies often advance to perforate the diaphragm and pericardium to incite pericarditis.

The pathway of the foreign body through the tissues is accompanied by contamination of ingesta, detritus, and bacteria. Various species of putrefactive bacteria are common in these wounds and stimulate an acute inflammatory response. As the pericardium is penetrated, local fibrinopurulent peritonitis, pleuritis, and pericarditis

▶

Antibodies in mucus inhibit colonization of microorganisms, neutralize toxins, lyse viruses, and generally prevent penetration of antigenic proteins through mucosal surfaces. Secretory antibody (IgA) is the principal mediator of specific immunity.

Purulent exudates

As neutrophils enter an inflammatory site, the transparent serous exudate becomes thick, opaque, and cream-colored. Grossly, these lesions are called **purulent** (or **suppurative**). Microscopically, the exudate can properly be described as **neutrophilic**. In many cases of severe inflammation, exudates are mixed; for example, in the acute, fibrinopurulent meningoencephalitis caused by *Escherichia coli* (Fig. 4.7), fibrin is mixed with the enormous numbers of degranulated neutrophils that accumulate in and distort the ventricles and tissue spaces of the brain.

Bacteria cause most purulent exudates. In infected tissue spaces, bacterial products cause neutrophils to degranulate. Microscopically, neutrophils in pus lack the granules present in normal circulating neutrophils. Most are dead, and many contain bacteria. With time, monocytes migrate into tissue and transform into macrophages as they accumulate in inflammatory foci. Some bacteria survive within the macrophage after being engulfed; for example, bacteria that cause tuberculosis, listeriosis, and brucellosis are known for their capacity to grow within macrophages.

▶

develop. The pericardial space is filled with fibrin, bacteria, and foul-smelling fluid. Adhesions form between the visceral layer of pericardium and the endocardium over the heart surface. If the cow survives, the fibrinous adhesions may resolve somewhat, but it is doubtful that severe cases can return to normal.

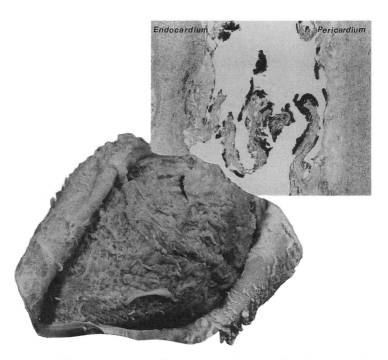

Subacute diffuse fibrinous pericarditis and endocarditis, cow with colibacillary septicemia caused by *Escherichia coli*. Inset: histology; open area is pericardial space between endocardium and pericardium (which are both thickened by inflammatory exudates and fibrosis). The dark material on vegetative growths is fibrin.

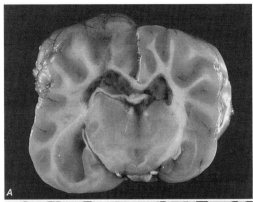

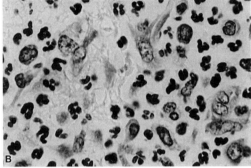

FIGURE 4.7. Acute purulent encephalitis, *E. coli* and *Corynebacterium* sp. isolated from pus in the meninges, young dog. A. Asymmetry of the brain is due to brain swelling. Pus is present on the surface of the brain and extends into the neuropil. Expansion of ventricles and purulent material are seen in the choroid plexus. B. Exudate of neutrophils and macrophages free in the ventricular lumen.

SYSTEMIC SIGNS OF ACUTE INFLAMMATION

Fever

During severe local inflammatory lesions and in generalized infections, neutrophils and other leukocytes release potent cytokines that induce fever by acting on the brain. Fever is a complex systemic response that includes increases in body temperature, respiration, and heart rate. The progression of fever involves pyrogen release by leukocytes, its circulation in plasma and action on the hypothalamus, and suppression of body heat loss by cutaneous vasoconstriction, increased heat production, and shivering.

```
┌─────────────────────────────────────┐
│ Microbes, toxins, antigen-antibody   │
│ complexes, neoplastic cells          │
└─────────────────────────────────────┘
                 ↓
┌─────────────────────────────────────┐
│ cytokines (IL-1, TNF-α) from leukocytes; │
│ hypothalamus stimulation             │
└─────────────────────────────────────┘
                 ↓
      ┌──────────────────────┐
      │ prostaglandin E₂      │
      └──────────────────────┘
                 ↓
      ┌──────────────────────────────┐
      │ vasomotor center of the brain; │
      │ sympathetic nerve stimulation  │
      └──────────────────────────────┘
                 ↓
      ┌──────────────────────────┐
      │ vasoconstriction in skin;  │
      │ heat dissipation           │
      └──────────────────────────┘
```

Normal body temperature is maintained by hypothalamic regulation of the production and dissipation of heat. Stimuli to the hypothalamus originate from superficial thermoreceptors in skin and deep receptors near the hypothalamus that respond to temperature change. During fever, the hypothalamic "thermostat" is elevated by endogenous pyrogens of leukocyte origin. Monocytes and macrophages are also major cells of pyrogen release. The most important pyrogenic cytokines released by leukocytes are the interleukins IL-1β and IL-6, tumor necrosis factor α (TNF-α), and the interferons IFN-β and IFN-γ. In addition, prostaglandin E_2 and other metabolites of arachidonic acids contribute to fever.

Fever is defined as the syndrome of elevated body temperature and associated autonomic and neuroendocrine responses that result from the effect of potent cytokines on the brain (Table 4.3). Fever arises from neurosecretory activity in the hypothalamus and preoptic area of the brain. The most important thermoregulatory mechanism is a

TABLE 4.3. Changes in fever

Metabolic changes
  Acute phase protein secretion
  Skeletal muscle breakdown
  Adipocyte breakdown

Endocrine changes
  ↑ glucocorticoids
  ↑ growth hormone
  ↑ aldosterone
  ↓ vasopressin

Autonomic changes
  ↑ blood pressure
  ↑ pulse rate
  ↓ sweating

↑ = increased, ↓ = decreased

redirection of blood flow from skin to deep capillary beds that is designed to decrease heat loss from the body surface. Characteristic behavior changes in most mammals include anorexia, somnolence, malaise, shivering, and search for warmth (chills).

The effects of pyrogenic cytokines are mediated through the brain's **circumventricular organs**, groups of specialized neurons that encircle the ventricles. These groups of neurons are supplied by capillaries with fenestrated endothelium—endothelial cells lacking the blood-brain barrier that excludes large pyrogenic molecules from other parts of the brain. Neurons in these organs both monitor for and contain substances used as neurotransmitters—for example, angiotensin II in the subfornical organ, cholecystokinin in the area postrema, and cytokines in the organum vasculosum. Neurons in the organum vasculosum and surrounding parts of the brain are activated by cytokines and prostaglandin E$_2$ and send axonal processes into the brain to contact other cell groups to coordinate the febrile response.

Antipyretic drugs can act by (1) interfering with synthesis or release of endogenous pyrogen by leukocytes and other cells, (2) inactivating circulating endogenous pyrogens, (3) interfering with the action of endogenous pyrogen in the brain, or (4) interfering with the effector pathways. Aspirin, the most common antipyretic substance, antagonizes the action of arachidonic pathways in the hypothalamus. Other drugs are known to cause fever (Table 4.4).

Animals become unresponsive to exogenous pyrogen if endogenous pyrogens are depleted. Experimentally, the repeated injections of exogenous pyrogens induce a state of refractoriness termed **tolerance**. The animal no longer responds to further doses of pyrogen by increasing body temperature, because its own endogenous pyrogenic mechanism has become exhausted. Repeated injections of granulocytic pyrogen, however, continue to cause a full response because they act directly on the hypothalamus. Thus animals made tolerant to exogenous substances by exhaustion remain fully responsive to endogenous pyrogen.

TABLE 4.4. Drug-induced fever

Mechanism	Drug
Stimulate heat production	Thyroxin, dinitrophenol
Depress heat dissipation	Epinephrine (vasoconstriction)
Alter thermoregulation	Antihistamines Phenothiazine (inhibits hypothalamus)

Pain

In acute inflammation, pain arises from direct nerve stimulation and from indirect effects of increasing inflammatory exudates on nerves at the site of injury. In early stages, much of this pain is suppressed by endorphins. Inflammatory cells that home to injured tissues release β-endorphin into the developing inflammatory fluids, and this opioid binds to opioid receptors on sensory nerve terminals to inhibit pain and cause analgesia. The central nervous system maintains the pain response after injury; for example, central nociceptive nerve terminals of peptide neurotransmitters such as substance P, combined with release of excitatory amino acid glutamate, play roles in the transmission of pain to the body.

Myalgia (muscle pain) is a common systemic effect of local inflammatory lesions. Cytokines that arise in the early phases of inflammation affect skeletal muscle in several ways. One of the most potent cytokines, tumor necrosis factor α (TNF-α), appears to play the dominant role in myalgia and exerts its effect by inducing breakdown of muscle protein. Other clinical signs that are induced by TNF-α include **sleepiness** and **anorexia** (loss of appetite).

Weight loss

Transient, local inflammatory lesions may be repaired quickly and may not produce noticeable weight loss. However, prolonged inflammation results in decreased body weight. One of the major changes in the systemic **acute phase reaction** is breakdown of fat globules and release of fatty acids by adipocytes, a process mediated by potent cytokines—especially TNF-α. TNF-α, originally called cachectin, was discovered because it caused loss of weight and fat cell breakdown in laboratory animals.

KININS, EICOSANOIDS, AND CYTOKINES IN INFLAMMATORY FLUIDS

Kinins

Kinins are polypeptides in the bloodstream that arise from circulating precursor molecules in plasma. When they are generated at the inflammatory site, kinins sustain and enhance the early transitory capillary alterations begun by histamine and other vasoactive factors.

Bradykinin is the prototype kinin

Bradykinin induces vascular leakage by opening gaps between endothelial cells in postcapillary venules. In sensitive tissues such as skin, it is 10 times more active than histamine. Bradykinin was discovered as an active factor released from an α_2-globulin by incubation with snake venom and was named for the slow, or "brady," contractions it elicited from guinea pig ileum. Although bradykinin can be synthesized in the laboratory, studies on its function are difficult because of the short life span of kinin molecules and the instability of their precursors in the living animal. Kinins are degraded by inhibitors almost immediately as they are generated in serum (usually during passage through the lungs). Inactivation has been attributed to a carboxypeptidase B in serum that removes the D-terminal arginine residue on the peptide molecule. Most kinins are inactivated by enzymes on the surface of the pulmonary capillary endothelial cells and thus do not survive passage through the lung.

Kinins mediate inflammation

Kinins are potent mediators of vasodilation, pain, and increased capillary permeability, the major signs of acute inflammation. Action on arterioles and venules is mediated through contraction of smooth muscle. In the lungs, smooth muscle contraction also causes bronchoconstriction.

Kallikreins activate plasma kininogen

Kinins are released from a circulating α_2-globulin substrate (kininogen) by a plasma enzyme called **kallikrein**. These kinin-generating enzymes are present in neutrophils, which, when lysed, release kallikrein to sustain the inflammatory reaction. "Glandular" kallikreins are common in exocrine glands and their secretions. Renal kallikrein is synthesized by epithelial cells of distal convoluted tubules and collecting ducts and is secreted into urine.

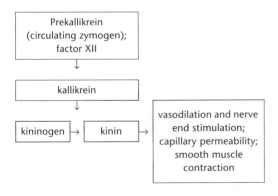

Discovery of plasma kallikrein had origins in the observation that urine, injected intravenously, lowered blood pressure. In the 1930s the hypotensive peptide was characterized and shown to be present in saliva, plasma, and other secretions. Because pancreas was a rich source, it was named kallikrein (Gr. *Kalli*, beautiful, plus pan*kreas*). Later, it was shown that kallikreins act indirectly as enzymes to split a plasma kininogen to form a kinin.

Prekallikrein also regulates coagulation

Prekallikrein influences the rate of activation of factors XI and XII; that is, in the absence of prekallikrein, factor XII is activated more slowly. Kininogen brings prekallikrein and factor XI in proximity to surface-bound factor XII. Reciprocal activation occurs as prekallikrein is converted to kallikrein by factor XII. Factor XII is then cleaved by kallikrein into α and β fractions. The β fraction and kallikrein dissociate from the kininogen on the surface and enter the fluid phase to activate the kinin system.

Prekallikrein deficiency is a rare hereditary defect reported only in the dog. It is usually an incidental finding on hematologic workup. Although dogs have reduced kinin levels, prekallikrein deficiency remains clinically inapparent.

Eicosanoids

Arachidonic acid, produced during degradation of phospholipids in injured cell membranes, is the precursor for prostaglandins and leukotrienes, grouped together as **eicosanoids**. These molecules are important regulators of normal cell activity and participate in inflammation by directly causing smooth muscle contraction, vasodilation, and sensory nerve end stimulation.

Leukotrienes

Leukotrienes (LTs), named because they are produced by leukocytes and have three conjugated double bonds, are progressively altered enzymatically to produce molecules with different activities. The prototype, LTB_4, has potent chemotactic action on leukocytes. LTC_4, after enzymatic removal of one glutamic acid molecule, becomes LTD_4; after removal of glycine, LTD_4 is LTE_4; and so on. LTE_4 increases permeability in postcapillary venules by causing contraction of endothelial cells. Several LTs are active in exudates released into fluids after injury to cause potent smooth muscle contraction.

Prostaglandins

Prostaglandins (PGs) may exert enhancing or depressant effects on tissue, depending on changes in their molecular structure. Much of the effect is caused by enhancement of actions of bradykinin and histamine that pour into inflamed tissue. PGs also stimulate aggregation and degranulation of neutrophils. PGs of the E type are most prominent

TABLE 4.5. Cytokines in inflammation

Tumor necrosis factors	TNF-α (cachectin)
	TNF-β (lymphotoxin)
Interleukins	IL-1
	IL-6
	IL-8
	IL-10
Interferons	IFN-α (leukocyte IFN)
	IFN-β (fibroblast IFN)
	IFN-γ (immune IFN)

in mediating inflammation. Macrophages are important sources of PGE and, when activated, rapidly convert arachidonic acid to PGE. Both the production and effects of PGs depend on the enzyme content of tissue affected. Platelets make primarily thromboxane A_2, whereas endothelial cells form prostacyclin (PGI_2).

Prostaglandins are increased in inflammatory fluids. Efferent lymph-draining inflammatory lesions have increased amounts of prostaglandins within a few hours. PGs also appear in draining lymph nodes. They may facilitate antigen processing, given that their amounts peak when uptake and processing of microbial proteins are maximal.

Aspirin and indomethacin depress inflammation and pain by blocking PG synthesis. Their action is chiefly on cyclooxygenase, the first enzyme to act in the oxygenation sequence of arachidonic acid. Corticosteroids inhibit production of both PGs and

LTs through activation of lipomodulin. Drugs that are now being designed specifically to inhibit LT hold great promise for the future treatment of inflammation.

Cytokines

A family of **cytokines** recruit specific populations of leukocytes to sites of acute injury. The sequential production of these cytokines by macrophages and other cells is essential for inflammation. Acute inflammation is initiated and sustained by the participation of tumor necrosis factor α (TNF-α), interleukin-1 (IL-1), interferon-gamma (IFN-γ), and other pro-inflammatory cytokines (Table 4.5). In contrast, interleukin-10 (IL-10) is a potent anti-inflammatory cytokine, one that is especially important in reducing inflammation in the intestinal mucosa. Cytokines have a marked effect at local sites of secretion. They also enter the bloodstream, where they are complexed with other proteins (α₂-macroglobulin, a plasma proteinase inhibitor, binds several cytokines and thereby inhibits activation). Hepatic Kupffer cells are a major source of cytokines in sepsis and other systemic inflammatory diseases. Other types of cytokines called chemokines (interleukin-8 and others) play important roles in chemoattraction of leukocytes.

Tumor necrosis factor, or TNF, is a potent, broad-acting cytokine produced by activated macrophages and T lymphocytes and released in response to infection. The function of TNF is to stimulate cells

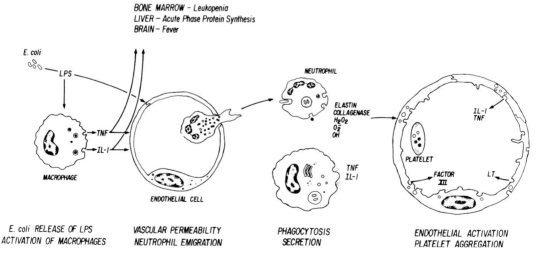

FIGURE 4.8. Release of cytokines from inflammatory cells during the early events in inflammation caused by gram-negative bacteria such as *E. coli*. Release of bacterial lipopolysaccharide (LPS) initiates release of cytokines tumor necrosis factor (TNF), interleukin-1 (IL-1), and leukotriene (LT).

in inflamed tissue to produce pro-inflammatory substances. TNF acts on target cells by activating the transcription factors (such as nuclear factor–κB [NF-κB] and PA-1). This, in turn, leads to induction of pro-inflammation genes and synthesis of pro-inflammatory proteins. In some restricted conditions, TNF can also trigger apoptosis.

TNF-α appears early after tissue is injured. Important systemic effects of TNF-α include induction of fever, increased synthesis of hepatic acute phase proteins, stimulation of endothelial cells to secrete procoagulants, induction of gluconeogenesis, and inhibition of lipoprotein lipase to cause cachexia.

Slightly later, IL-1 is secreted by monocytes and regulates several major events in acute inflammation, such as fever, neutrophilia, and synthesis of acute phase proteins by the liver (Fig. 4.8). If inflammation is severe, IL-1 causes endothelial cells, which normally have anticoagulant surfaces, to secrete procoagulant glycoproteins onto their luminal surfaces, thereby promoting coagulation.

The difference between benefit and injury to the host is blurred for TNF. In severe infectious diseases and toxicities, the release of massive amounts of TNF can cause widespread injury. Shock is a common sequela in animals with gram-negative septicemia.

Platelet-activating factor (PAF), a major mediator of increased vascular permeability, is derived as a breakdown product of membrane phospholipids. PAF is produced largely by activated platelets, neutrophils, and endothelium but can be released by all inflammatory cells. PAF binds to a single G protein–coupled receptor that signals the target cell to become active. PAF is 100–10,000 times more potent than histamine in inducing vascular permeability. The effects of PAF are broad, and at higher concentrations it is also known to stimulate platelets, to enhance leukocyte adhesion to endothelium, and to stimulate smooth muscle contraction, causing vasoconstriction.

ACUTE PHASE PROTEINS

Clinical signs and lesions of early inflammation are associated with the appearance in blood and tissue fluids of certain proteins that sustain the inflammatory process. They are called **acute phase proteins** because they are not normally present in plasma (or are present in very low amounts) and increase markedly immediately after injury. The presence of acute phase proteins in blood is a diagnostic sign of tissue injury and inflammation (Table 4.6).

Most acute phase proteins are synthesized in the liver. Cytokines released by inflammatory leukocytes induce hepatocytes to synthesize and release acute phase proteins. For example, the cytokines interleukin-1 and TNF-α increase hepatic secretion of complement and α$_1$-acid glycoprotein. Interleukin-6 has a wider spectrum of acute phase protein induction, including especially fibrinogen and α$_2$-macroglobulin.

Fibrinogen

Fibrinogen is synthesized in the liver and circulates normally at uniform levels. During the acute phase of inflammation it is released by the hepatocytes and fibrinogen levels in plasma increase markedly. Much of this fibrinogen polymerizes at the site of inflammation to form fibrin. The increase in fibrinogen in plasma also enhances erythrocyte aggregation, which is reflected in an increased **erythrocyte sedimentation rate** in the laboratory.

C-reactive protein

C-reactive protein (CRP) was the first acute phase protein to be described and was used (nonspecifically) in the 1930s to diagnose the presence and extent of inflammatory processes, especially those involving necrosis. CRP is a circulating protein that binds to phosphocholine molecules in surface membranes of macrophages, platelets, and some lymphocytes. Binding causes complement to attach to the cell, which in turn facilitates attachment of bacteria; that is, CRP initiates the complement-dependent opsonization that leads to phagocytosis of microorganisms. CRP reacts with only some types of bacteria. It was discovered because of its strong affinity for the C-polysaccharide fractions of capsules of *Streptococcus pneumoniae*.

CRP-like proteins are found in most mammals, birds, and fish. Composed of five subunits, they have certain specificities and are known to have high affinity for some galactosyl polymers and to

TABLE 4.6. Acute phase proteins

Protein	Function
Fibrinogen	Coagulation—forms fibrin polymers
Complement (C3)	Fulcrum for C cascades—leads to bacterial lysis
C-reactive protein	Initiates C-dependent opsonization
Haptoglobin	Binds hemoglobin, saves iron, has antioxidant effect
α$_1$-Antitrypsin (AAT)	Inhibits serine proteases in serum
Protein SAA	? (forms amyloid fibrils)
LPS binding protein	Binds to monocytes and stimulates TNF-α secretion
Ceruloplasmin	Binds and transports copper

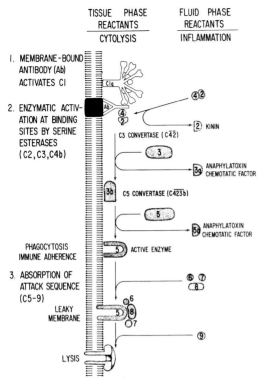

FIGURE 4.9. Complement action on cell surfaces.

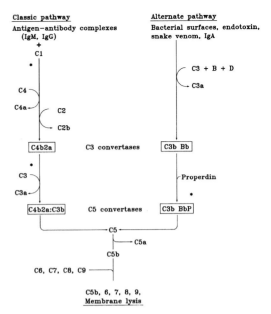

FIGURE 4.10. Classic, alternate, and common pathways of complement (C). Reactions occur as C components in serum attach to molecules on cell surfaces. Pathways are blocked by controlling proteins at certain sites *(asterisks)*.

phosphocholine. Once bound to membranes, CRP then recruits **complement** much like antibody; that is, CRP is a surrogate for antibody in activating the classical pathway. It facilitates the initiation of immune-related activities during the early phases of inflammation, before specific antibody is produced.

During acute inflammation, the amount of CRP can increase 1,000 times within 48 hours. Changes in plasma levels of CRP are nonspecific and occur to the same extent in diverse diseases. Thus CRP measurement provides information similar to an increased erythrocyte sedimentation rate associated with fibrinogen elevations during acute disease. For example, CRP rises markedly within hours of surgery and subsides after a few days (in the absence of infection and severe inflammation or necrosis).

Complement

Complement (C) is a self-assembling, extracellular system of proteins present in inactive form in plasma and body fluids. Most C components are produced in the liver. Smaller amounts are produced in renal tubules, small intestine, brain, thyroid follicular epithelium, and ductal epithelium of the salivary glands. Activation of the C system occurs in a precise sequence (similar to the clotting cascade) on cell or microbial surface membranes (Fig. 4.9). Its consequences are **clumping of bacteria (opsonization)**, enhancement of inflammation through **chemoattraction**, and **cell lysis**.

Lysis (either of cells or of bacteria) occurs when the final products (C5–C9) aggregate to form doughnut-shaped attack sequences that embed in the plasma membranes of the target cell to form pores. Inflammation is promoted by release of vasoactive and chemotactic C fragments cleaved during activation that enter surrounding fluids. Thus, C plays significant roles in inflammation in mediation of the chemotactic attraction of leukocytes, in killing of bacterial cells, and in activation of granule release mechanisms (e.g., histamine from mast cells, procoagulants from platelets). It is essential for antibody-induced lysis of bacteria in which it functions as a nonspecific effector of specific antibody activities.

Complement activation occurs by two pathways. The **alternate pathway** is the more primitive and less specific of the two. The **classic pathway** is specific because of its initiation by antibodies. Both pathways lead to the activation of a critical enzyme, **C convertase**, which activates a final common pathway that generates the **membrane attack sequence** C5–C9 (Fig. 4.10).

Classic pathway

Classic C activation begins when membrane-bound antibody molecules (or antigen-antibody complexes free in plasma) interact with circulating C1. One of the subunits of C1, C1q, recognizes and interacts with the Fc portion of the antibody molecule that is attached to a membrane. The C1's subunit is exposed and mediates cleavage of C4. After attaching to the membrane surface, C4 binds C2 so that it may be cleaved to C2a by C1s. C4 then binds circulating C3 so that it is susceptible to cleavage by C2a. Thus C42 is the **C3 convertase** for the classic pathway. Activation of C1 leads to many C42 complexes capable of cleaving C3 and thus is an amplification step.

Alternate pathway

The alternate pathway includes five plasma proteins that interact to form C3 convertase without participation of circulating components C1, C2, and C4. It is a mechanism to provide protection during early phases of microbial invasion before antibodies are produced. The alternate pathway is initiated when a plasma globulin (factor D, which circulates in active form) binds to particle surfaces, commonly the polysaccharide cell walls of bacteria and fungi. When D cleaves factor B, the molecular rearrangements in B expose an enzyme site that interacts with C3 to form C3bBb, the C3 convertase of the alternate pathway. Properdin, the first complement protein to be identified, stabilizes the C3bBb molecule.

Common pathway

Factors C3–C9 circulate in unassembled but active form. C3 convertases (C42 or C3bBb) attract and cleave circulating C3 into C3a and C3b. C3a is released into fluids to act as an **anaphylatoxin**, a substance that induces mast cell degranulation with release of histamine (thereby increasing vascular permeability). C3b, depending on the type of cell or particle involved, may continue the C cascade or act as an **opsonin**, a substance that renders bacteria susceptible to phagocytosis. To continue C activation, C3b binds C5 and cleaves it into an active enzyme on the membrane (C5b) and a fragment (C5a) that is both an anaphylatoxin and a potent chemotactic factor for neutrophils. C5a aggregates the terminal components of C into an attack complex, which burrows into the membrane to form a transmembrane channel, allowing electrolytes and water to enter the cell. Bacteria affected by this process then swell, and the plasma membrane may rupture.

Neutrophils have specific C3b receptors

Membrane-bound C3b is also the major opsonic protein (it can be assisted by C5b). It is a signal for adherence of neutrophils and monocytes to C-coated surfaces. The attachment of bacteria coated by C3b with specific C3b receptors embedded in the neutrophil surface causes adherence and promotes subsequent phagocytosis. C3b receptor molecules are proteins embedded into the plasma membranes of neutrophils (C3b receptors also occur on monocytes and B lymphocytes).

C3a and C5a play significant roles in inflammation

The C3a and C5a fragments cause (1) histamine release from mast cells, (2) chemotaxis and degranulation of neutrophils, and (3) smooth muscle contraction. The net effect is that neutrophils and other leukocytes are induced to migrate through highly permeable capillaries into a progressively expanding inflammatory focus. The complement system interacts with the kinin and fibrinolytic systems (Fig. 4.11).

C3a and C5a are rapidly inactivated soon after they are formed. Plasma carboxypeptidases rapidly inactivate anaphylatoxins. These "anaphylatoxin inhibitors" act like pancreatic carboxypeptidase B, cleaving carboxy termini of basic amino acids. Activities of kinins and fibrinolytic peptides are also inactivated by these enzymes.

Hypocomplementemia may suppress inflammatory responses

Excessive consumption of complement during some severe infections may result in hypocomplementemia. This occurs when large numbers of antigen-antibody complexes are formed (the complexes bind avidly to complement). C3 is particularly important in opsonizing bacteria. The serum of patients with hereditary C3 deficiency cannot sustain bacterial opsonization, and these patients are susceptible to repeated bacterial infection despite normal amounts of immunoglobulins.

Suppression of complement inhibits tissue injury

Complement can also contribute to undesirable tissue damage. Although effective and necessary in infectious processes, the action of complement in severe burns, ischemia, and autoimmune diseases does more harm than good to the host. In these diseases, aberrant C activation in tissue or bloodstream causes tissue injury and inflammation. C fragments and complexes induce release of inflam-

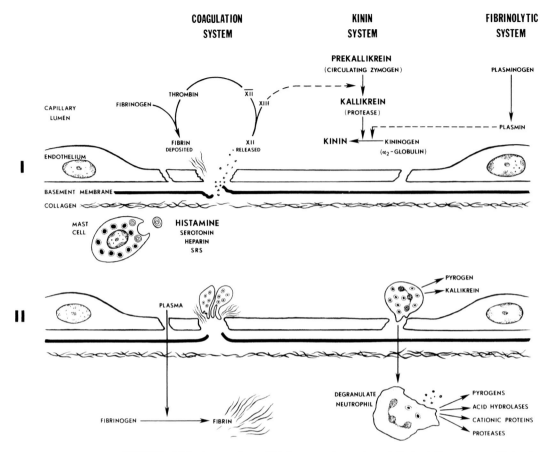

FIGURE 4.11. Interaction of kinin, complement, and fibrinolytic systems. Kinins increase capillary permeability and cause vasodilation.

matory mediators from leukocytes. Inflammation can be suppressed in these diseases by inhibitors of the complement system, especially by using regulatory proteins that block enzymes that activate C3 and C5. For example, experimental animals treated with cobra venom to deplete C3 and C5 are protected from severe tissue injury. The severity of experimental ischemia has been reduced by injection of soluble C receptors (also known as CD35) into rats with experimental myocardial infarcts.

Lysozyme

Lysozyme (muramidase) is a small ubiquitous cationic enzyme that catalyzes the hydrolysis of peptidoglycans in the cell walls of bacteria. It digests cell wall debris of bacteria killed by other mechanisms. Lysozyme is present in large amounts in body fluids, notably milk, tears, saliva, and genital secretions. Lysozyme is found in granulocytes, monocytes, and macrophages, and serum lysozyme levels reflect its liberation from these cells. Lysozyme also

is produced by epithelial cells of mucosae and glands of respiratory and intestinal tracts. It occurs in granular pneumocytes of the lung, in thymic corpuscles, and in intestinal Paneth's cells. In the reproductive tract, the concentration of lysozyme in mucus cells varies in response to hormones. In vaginal mucus, the concentration of lysozyme is lowest at midgestation and highest in the early follicular and late luteal phases.

Interferon

Interferons are soluble proteins induced and released by host cells on stimulation by microbes and other foreign substances. Interferon is one of the first host defense mechanisms to appear in viral infection. It diffuses to surrounding cells and enters those cells that have receptors for interferon on their surfaces. Once inside the cell, interferon suppresses viral replication. The spreading virus thus meets an intracellular barrier to continued replication. Interferon does not inactivate viruses but blocks intracellular viral replication by inducing antiviral proteins in the cell that inhibit production of proteins in the ribosomes.

Considerable amounts of interferon appear in the bloodstream after an appropriate stimulus. Interferonemia rapidly disappears because of loss via the renal glomerulus (Fig. 4.12). Interferonuria develops rapidly, and levels of interferon are often higher in urine than in blood. Salivary secretion also occurs and may be significant in oral infections.

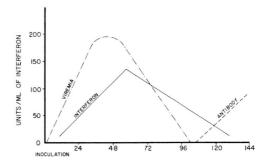

FIGURE 4.12. Rise and fall of interferon in circulating blood relative to viremia and antibodies in an acute infection with an interferon-inducing virus.

Fibronectin

Fibronectin is a glycoprotein associated with fibroblast surfaces and basement membranes. Present in serum as a dimer, it is deposited in tissue as a multimer. Plasma fibronectin (an α_2-glycoprotein) is an opsonin; that is, it enhances bacterial aggregation and promotes phagocytosis. Fibronectin plays a very important role in stimulating Kupffer cells of the liver to remove circulating bacteria. Fibronectin occurs in normal canine plasma at about 240–340 μg/ml; it decreases in plasma during the first phases of acute inflammation because it enters injured tissue sites and because it is used to coat bacterial surfaces. It disappears especially rapidly during bacteremia.

Fibronectin accumulates in inflammatory lesions and plays a role in adhesion of cells during healing. Normally absent in dense connective tissue, it appears coincident with invading fibroblasts and disappears as collagen matures. Fibronectin functions as a matrix for organization of new collagen and promotes cell migration and adhesion.

Ceruloplasmin

The copper-containing α_2-glycoprotein **ceruloplasmin** increases in acute inflammation. It has antioxidant activities and suppresses the damaging effects of oxygen radicals on cells, probably by its ferroxidase activity. Fe^{2+} can promote lipid peroxidation through reaction with oxygen radicals, and ceruloplasmin converts reduced iron (Fe^{2+}) to oxidized iron (Fe^{3+}). **Transferrin**, the normal iron-binding protein of serum, may act similarly, although it is reported that **lactoferrin**, which also binds iron, can potentiate tissue damage during neutrophil granule release by releasing its iron.

Haptoglobin

Haptoglobin is a glycoprotein in normal plasma. It is produced in the liver (the major inducer of haptoglobin synthesis is interleukin-6). In blood and tissue, haptoglobin binds free hemoglobin with high avidity. In so doing, it stimulates hepatocytes to take up the haptoglobin-hemoglobin complex by endocytosis, a process that uses specific receptors on hepatocytes. Clearance of hemoglobin prevents tissue damage by hemoglobin-driven lipid peroxidation.

α_1-Antitrypsin

α_1-Antitrypsin is synthesized in and released from hepatocytes in response to inflammatory stimuli, and serum levels of this enzyme are elevated in acute inflammation. α_1-Antitrypsin inhibits proteases and neutralizes elastases and collagenases released by neutrophils—enzymes that otherwise might have a persistent tissue-damaging effect. Deficiencies of α_1-antitrypsin attributed to a single amino acid substitution of α_1-antitrypsin are associated with chronic liver disease in dogs and with emphysema in humans.

α_1-Acid glycoprotein

Abundant in normal plasma, α_1-acid glycoprotein is an acute phase protein that rises abruptly in acute inflammation because of release by the liver. It closely resembles cell membrane sialoglycoprotein (it is 24% sialic acid) and may function as a nonspecific competitor for cell surfaces. In malaria it blocks the binding of *Plasmodium falciparum* to surfaces of erythrocytes.

Iron-binding proteins in inflammation

Iron in the animal body is both intracellular (as ferritin, hemosiderin, or heme) and extracellular (bound to high-affinity, iron-binding glycoproteins). **Transferrin** is the normal iron-binding protein of plasma and lymph. In birds, the protein ovotransferrin is deposited in the egg and functions to bind iron in a fashion similar to that of transferrin in plasma.

Hyposideremia of inflammation

The plasma concentration of ionic iron and iron-transferrin complexes declines in severe inflammation. The immediate cause of inflammatory **hyposideremia** is the release of lactoferrin from degranulating neutrophils. **Lactoferrin** is an iron-binding glycoprotein that removes iron from iron-transferrin complexes in inflammatory exudates. The acidic environment of the exudate causes transferrin to release iron and lactoferrin to accept it. The neutrophil is stimulated to degranulate and release lactoferrin by the cytokines IL-2 and TNF, which originate from macrophages that have been stimulated by bacteria. Macrophages play another role in hyposideremia by taking up iron-lactoferrin complexes and shunting iron into synthesis of ferritin. Ferritin synthesis diverts labile iron into ferritin stores, reducing its availability for release from tissue into plasma. Macrophages have receptors for lactoferrin on their surfaces, enabling these cells to clear complexes efficiently from the circulation. Reduced serum iron and transferrin saturation are sustained in chronic inflammation by this mechanism.

Hyposideremia withholds iron from bacteria

Hyposideremia is a biologic mechanism of the host to withhold the essential nutrient iron from pathogenic bacteria. Iron concentration in plasma and tissue is less than that required for growth of some bacteria. Thus animals with low plasma iron may be less susceptible to some bacterial infections. Conversely, animals with increased plasma labile iron may have increased susceptibility to these same bacteria.

To circumvent the antibacterial effect of low plasma iron, enteric bacteria such as *Escherichia coli* produce iron chelators called **siderophores**, which remove iron from iron-binding proteins. Called enterochelin (or enterobactin), they are synthesized only during iron-restricted growth and efficiently transport iron into the bacterial cell. Other organisms, such as *Neisseria gonorrhoeae,* remove iron from iron-binding proteins directly via a mechanism by which surface receptors on the bacteria combine with the iron-binding protein.

THE NEUTROPHIL

Neutrophils are mobile, aggressively phagocytic cells. They are the first line of defense against invading microorganisms and in the initial removal of dead cells, fibrin fragments, and necrotic debris that occur in burns, trauma, and other physical injuries. Distinctions of these cells are (1) rapid ameboid movement, particularly in response to chemoattractants; (2) intense phagocytic activity; and (3) elaboration of granules bearing potent enzymes capable of extensive intracellular digestion. Neutrophils have the ability to degranulate and spew enzyme-laden granules into tissue at local sites of inflammation. Although highly mobile, they lack stability and cannot withstand the low pH and high temperature of severe inflammatory lesions.

Neutrophils have two major types of granules: azurophil (primary) granules and specific (secondary) granules. **Azurophil granules** are small, primary lysosomes. In most mammals they contain lysosomal digestive hydrolases, mucosubstances, and peroxidase, most of which function at pH optima in the acid range. Azurophil granules have nearly all of the myeloperoxidase, one-third of the lysozyme, and some lactoferrin. The larger and more numerous **specific granules** contain alkaline phosphatase, cationic proteins, lactoferrin, and most of the leukocyte's lysozyme. Specific granules also contain proteolytic enzymes that act on collagen and elastin, and some lipases, which are lacking in most macrophages (Fig. 4.13). The membranes of secondary granules also contain integrins and other adhesion molecules that move to the cell surface during activation.

Neutrophil chemotaxis

Chemotaxis is the directed movement of leukocytes in response to chemoattractants, the diffusible chemical mediators of inflammation. Neutrophils are highly responsive to chemoattractants; macrophages and eosinophils, moderately so; and lymphocytes, only slightly. Neutrophils respond to many chemoattractants (Table 4.7).

The capacity to react to chemical attractants is an essential character of the neutrophil. Cinematographic studies of leukocytes in vitro reveal rapid movement of neutrophils toward microbes. Under the influence of bacterial chemoattractants in early inflammatory exudates, circulating neutrophils move to the periphery of the capillary and stick to the endothelium.

Most chemoattractants are derivatives of normal plasma peptides. Substances that are cleaved from normal proteins in foci of injury and are (directly) strong chemoattractants for neutrophils include **complement fragments, fibrinopeptides, collagenolytic products,** and **soluble cytokines** released by antigen-stimulated lymphocytes. **Platelet-activating factor**, a potent heparin-binding protein released from α-granules when platelets adhere at sites of vascular injury, is also a strong neutrophil chemoattractant.

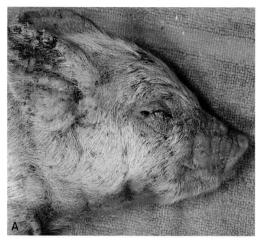

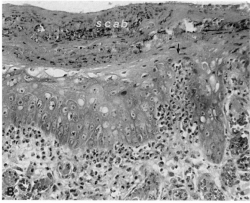

FIGURE 4.13. A. Severe multifocal subacute purulent dermatitis caused by *Streptococcus epidermidis,* pig. B. Neutrophilic leukocytes have extended through the epidermis *(arrow)* into the surface of the scab. Note the vacuolation of keratinocytes.

Chemotaxis is mediated by different classes of receptor molecules on the neutrophil surface. To start the signaling cascade that triggers locomotion, chemoattractant receptors on the neutrophil bind molecules such as C5a. Binding is coupled to phosphoinositide hydrolysis, which leads to an increase of free Ca^{2+} in the cell and then to activation of protein kinase C, which stimulates the cytoskeleton to begin cellular movements.

Pathogenic bacteria are chemotactic for neutrophils

Most pathogenic bacteria will slowly attract neutrophils directly by releasing soluble products in infected tissue. Among the most potent of bacterial **chemotactic factors** are certain hydrophobic peptides released by bacteria. The peculiar feature that imparts chemotactic characteristics resides in the N-terminal amino groups of these peptides. Ex-

perimentally, the tetrapeptide N-formyl-methionyl-leucyl-phenylalanine (called **F-Met-Leu-Phe,** or FMLP) is synthesized and used to induce chemotaxis in vitro.

Complement fragments are strongly chemotactic

Reactions that initiate the C cascade with the attendant liberation of **complement chemotactic fragments** C3 and C5 will attract neutrophils. Enzymes that act in this way (via complement fragments) include bacterial proteases, plasmin, trypsin, thrombin, and other tissue proteases. The complement system is especially potent in dealing with microbes. During infections, chemotaxis is markedly accelerated when complement adsorbs to microbial surfaces, a reaction most efficiently activated via the classic pathway by antibody. The complement system is so effective because it liberates chemotactic fragments directly into tissue fluids and because the mature neutrophil has specific surface receptors for the C4b-C3b complex (immune adherence receptors) that cause the migrating neutrophil to attach to the complement-coated microbe.

Opsonins: substances that adsorb to bacterial surfaces

In infection the processes of opsonization, release of complement chemotactic fragments, and phagocytosis are interrelated. When a bacterium is deposited in tissue, it becomes coated with various proteins that circulate and percolate through tissue. **Immunoglobulins** (antibodies) and **complement fragments** are the most potent **opsonins.** They bind to specific receptors on neutrophil surfaces to initiate movement in the subsurface cytoskeleton of the cell and thus cause phagocytosis and degranulation.

Neutrophil transendothelial migration

Transendothelial migration is the process whereby neutrophils emigrate though vascular walls. The process begins as inflammatory stimuli activate both endothelial cells and leukocytes to express new surface adhesion molecules. Adhesion mole-

TABLE 4.7. Chemoattractants for neutrophils

Complement fragments—C5a and C567
Fibrinopeptides—fibrin split products
Collagenolytic products
Cytokines—IL-1, IL-8, platelet-activating factor (PAF)
Kallikrein
Bacterial components—endotoxin, N-formyl-methionyl
    peptides
Leukotrienes

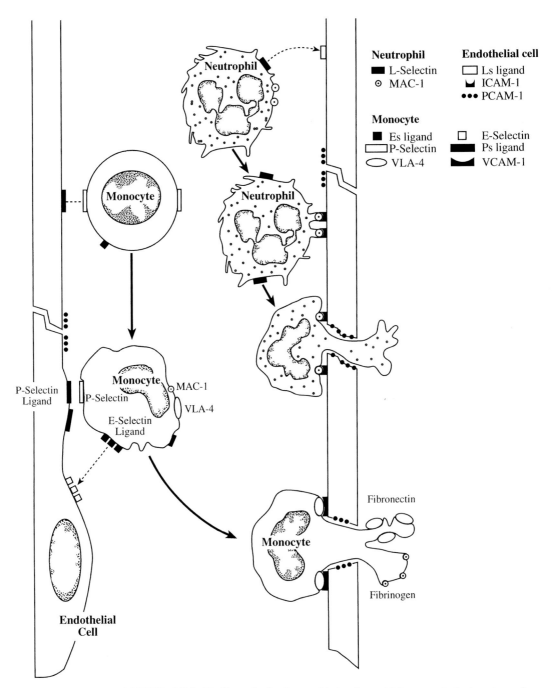

Neutrophil
■ L-Selectin
⊙ MAC-1

Monocyte
■ Es ligand
☐ P-Selectin
◯ VLA-4

Endothelial cell
☐ Ls ligand
⌣ ICAM-1
••• PCAM-1

☐ E-Selectin
■ Ps ligand
⌣ VCAM-1

Neutrophil

Neutrophil

Monocyte

Monocyte

MAC-1

VLA-4

P-Selectin
Ligand

P-Selectin

E-Selectin
Ligand

Fibronectin

Monocyte

Fibrinogen

Endothelial
Cell

FIGURE 4.14. Binding of selectins and integrins, which promote leukocyte emigration through capillary walls. Inflammatory stimuli to neutrophils initiate expression of selectins, which bind to selectin ligands on endothelial surfaces. Transient selectin binding of circulating neutrophils causes them to bounce and roll along endothelial surfaces. Subsequent binding of integrins (neutrophil MAC-1 to endothelial cell ICAM-1) causes adherence sufficient for transmigration. As the neutrophil moves through the vascular wall, MAC-1 and other extracellular matrix ligands bind to connective tissue fibronectin, pulling the neutrophil into the interstitial space. Monocytes follow a similar pattern of transient selectin and firm integrin binding to endothelium.

cules act in sequence to allow leukocytes to contact endothelium and to leave the circulation.

Selectins, which increase on surfaces of activated endothelial cells as a result of inflammatory stimuli, mediate early adhesion without neutrophil activation (Fig. 4.14). Chemoattractants then direct neutrophils to a particular extravasation site of inflammation and stimulate cells to activate their integrins. Once outside the vascular wall, leukocytes interact with extracellular matrix components through **integrins** which mediate strong adhesion and promote diapedesis. These receptors interact with the cytoskeleton, "integrating" the extracellular environment with the interior of the neutrophil.

Selectins are a unique family of cell adhesion molecules

Selectins control many aspects of inflammatory cell movement by interactions involving carbohydrate recognition. **L-selectin** is concentrated in filopodia of activated neutrophils and presents its oligosaccharides to the inducible ligands on endothelium. When endothelial cells are activated, **P-selectin** (stored in secretory granules) is moved to the cell surface and released. **E-selectin** is produced more slowly, requiring 4–6 hours to be expressed on cell surfaces.

Rapid neutrophil binding to activated endothelium is mediated by P-selectin, an interaction that promotes the rolling of neutrophils along the endothelial surface. Rapid mobilization of P-selectin to endothelial surfaces allows it to recognize its carbohydrate ligand on the leukocyte surface. Adhesion of the rolling neutrophil is slowed by the increasingly strong adhesiveness brought about by activation of the β_2-integrins LFA-1 and MAC-1. β_2-mediated adhesion results from increased integrin avidity during neutrophil activation, a change that is due to conformation change in the integrin molecule as it is activated.

Binding affinity of the selectin is relatively low, but sufficient to serve as a brake, making the leukocytes decelerate by rolling along the activated endothelial surface. While rolling, leukocytes become activated by chemoattractants, and this greatly increases the affinity of their β_2-integrin adhesion with ligands on the newly activated endothelial surface.

As neutrophils migrate across endothelium, they enhance capillary permeability and hyperemia begun by direct injury and histamine release, probably by releasing prostaglandins and leukotrienes. There is direct movement through intact endothelium without its disruption, chiefly by way of intercellular junctions.

Some enzymes in tissue (including elastase, collagenase, and cathepsin G) can actually retard neutrophil chemotaxis by splitting the chemotactic fragments C3 and C5 to render them inactive. These enzymes thus contribute to lowered opsonic activity and to prolonged inflammation. Streptococci and some other bacteria contain proteins on their surfaces that bind fibrinogen, and the protein-fibrinogen complex impedes access of complement components to the bacterium and thus suppresses chemotaxis and neutrophil attachment.

Neutrophil phagocytosis

As a prelude to phagocytosis, striking surface projections develop on the surface of the neutrophil and rapidly surround the target particle. Long tentacles form at a polar position and invaginate at the tips to form large phagocytic cups. As the phagocytic **vacuole** (also called an **endosome**) forms, oxidases are internalized as the surface membrane folds in on itself. The enzymes immediately begin to catalyze the formation of acid, and eventually superoxide anions and hydrogen peroxide, which are important in intracellular killing. Degradation of bacterial and cellular debris begins as lysosomes rapidly begin to fuse with the phagosome to form **phagolysosomes**, large dense structures in which bacteria are degraded by potent hydrolytic enzymes.

Intracellular killing and digestion

Defensins

Defensins, "antibiotic" cationic peptides present in neutrophil granules, are discharged into phagolysosomes when neutrophils phagocytize bacteria. They have a potent antimicrobial effect. Defensins are also released into circulating blood as neutrophil granules are discharged. Deposition of defensins in blood vessels is thought to increase clotting and thrombosis during acute inflammation.

The respiratory burst

Contact of neutrophils with stimuli that initiate phagocytosis results in activation of an oxygen-consuming metabolic pathway that is dormant in unstimulated cells. Characteristics of the pathway are increased oxygen consumption, increased glucose utilization, and production of oxygen-related toxic agents: superoxide anion, hydroxyl radical, and singlet oxygen. These events grouped together are referred to as the **respiratory burst**, and they are a consequence of the early activation of the particulate enzyme NADPH oxidase. Activation of the

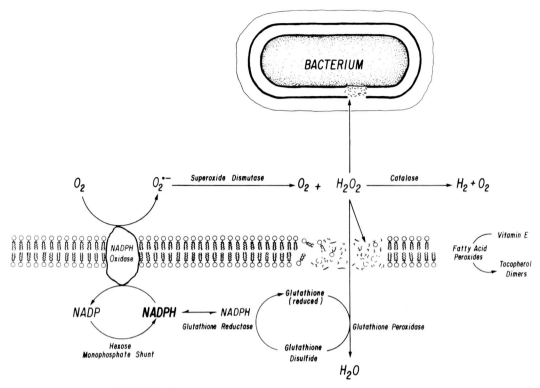

FIGURE 4.15. Production of toxic oxygen radicals and their metabolism.

enzyme NADPH oxidase catalyzes the reduction of oxygen to superoxide anion:

$$2O_2 + NADPH \rightarrow 2O_2^{\bullet-} + NADPH^+ + H^+$$

NADPH oxidase is located within the lipid bilayers of membranes and is partly exposed to the cytoplasm, which utilizes NADPH (produced by the hexose-monophosphate shunt) as a substrate. Hydrogen peroxide released during the burst originates from the dismutation of the superoxide produced by the enzyme superoxide dismutase (SOD). Subsequent reaction between $O_2^{\bullet-}$ and H_2O_2 produces the bactericidal hydroxyl radical.

$$2O_2^{\bullet-} + 2H^+ \xrightarrow{SOD} 2O_2 + H_2O_2$$

$$O_2^- + H_2O_2 \rightarrow OH^{\bullet} + OH^- + O_2$$

Increase in the hexose-monophosphate shunt activity reflects an increase in NADPH turnover due to the nucleotide requirement for the O_2-forming reaction and, in part, due to the activity of the glutathione peroxidase–glutathione reductase cycle, a metabolic pathway that detoxifies H_2O_2 diffusing back into the cytoplasm (Fig. 4.15).

The respiratory burst is a self-limiting phenome-

non. It declines within 1 hour because of loss of activity of the O_2-forming enzymes. This limitation does not adversely affect bactericidal activity, because bacterial killing requires only agents produced during the burst. Furthermore, damage inflicted by these toxic agents on tissues would be limited by termination of the burst after a short period.

Neutrophils kill phagocytized microorganisms through one or a combination of toxic systems, both oxygen-dependent and oxygen-independent. Among the former, myeloperoxidase-H_2O_2 is the most potent; but hydrogen peroxidase (by itself), superoxide, hydroxyl radicals, and singlet oxygen are also antibacterial. The oxygen-independent agents include lysozyme, lactoferrin, phospholipases, and the granule-associated cationic proteins. Chymotrypsin-like cationic proteins of the primary granules are most effective on gram-positive bacteria.

Superoxide dismutase degrades superoxide anion

Superoxide anion ($O_2^{\bullet-}$), a free radical form of oxygen, is generated in phagosomes during early autooxidative processes of the respiratory burst. The enzyme superoxide dismutase protects the cells from

$O_2^{\bullet-}$ toxicity but may also inhibit bactericidal activity. Superoxide anion and H_2O_2 accumulate in the phagosome, where they interact with bacteria and also generate $OH^{\bullet}$ and other oxidants. Superoxide dismutase and catalase do not interfere with them within the vacuole, yet these enzymes protect the remainder of the cell from destruction.

Hydrogen peroxide is microbicidal

Within the newly forming phagosome, superoxide and hydrogen peroxide are generated around the ingested bacterium at very high rates. Hydrogen peroxide kills most organisms in the absence of a catalyst but only in high concentrations. It is most effective in association with neutrophil peroxidase. Hydrogen peroxide may contribute significantly to antimicrobial activity. For example, streptococci produce H_2O_2 (they lack catalase). Conversely, microbial **catalase** inhibits H_2O_2 function and may protect some bacteria. Catalase-rich strains of staphylococci are more virulent than are low-catalase strains.

Myeloperoxidase enhances hydrogen peroxide killing

Myeloperoxidase (MPO), the peroxidase of neutrophils, is critical for oxidative killing. It is in azurophil granules (it is responsible for the green color of pus). Like other peroxidases, MPO catalyzes the oxidation of substances by H_2O_2. MPO, H_2O_2, and an oxidizable halide cofactor such as chlorine combine to form a highly potent antimicrobial system. This MPO-mediated mechanism is effective against microbes at pH 4.5–5.0 and is inhibited by catalase.

MPO reacts with H_2O_2 to form an enzyme-substrate complex with strong oxidative capacity. The cofactor is converted from a weak to a strong antimicrobial agent. When iodide is the cofactor, iodination of bacteria occurs by direct halogenation of bacterial proteins and other groups in or on the bacterium. Hypochlorous acid (HOCl) appears to be the primary lethal agent produced by myeloperoxidase, which oxidizes chloride ions to the strong nonradical oxidant HOCl—the most bactericidal oxidant produced by the neutrophil.

$$MPO + H_2O_2 \rightarrow HOCl \rightarrow OH^{\bullet} + R\text{-}NH_2 + {}^1O_2$$

Nitric oxide (NO)

The cytokines TNF-α and IFN-γ cause leukocytes, endothelial cells, and epithelial cells to produce an enzyme, nitric oxide synthase. NO synthase leads to production of NO, which has antimicrobial properties. The effect in the animal of NO is not entirely clear, but in cells infected with bacteria in rodents, NO has been shown to diminish the severity of infection.

Degranulation of neutrophils

Neutrophils regurgitate lysosomal enzymes into the microenvironment as they become activated (massive amounts of these hydrolases are released when the neutrophil dies). Release of granules is particularly important when the neutrophil is in contact with very large particles, especially when these particles are coated with antibody. Neutrophil surface receptors specific for the Fc part of the immunoglobulin molecule can act as effector cells in killing antibody-coated microorganisms. In addition to killing bacteria by this mechanism, they also rapidly kill virus-infected cells that have become coated with antiviral antibodies; antibody-dependent cytotoxicity tests in cell cultures are indicators of neutrophil function.

Microorganisms and injured cells that become coated with antibodies and then activate the complement system are rapidly attacked by neutrophils. C5a is the major chemotactic component. C3b, the major opsonic component, combines with specific receptors embedded in the neutrophil surface to initiate movement required for both phagocytosis and granule release. When complement activation is limited and the target is very large, lysosomal enzymes and azurophilic granules are released without altering neutrophil viability.

Azurophil and specific granules of the neutrophil are released at differing times during the degranulation process. Specific granules are immediately reactive after stimulus, whereas the lysosomal azurophil granules discharge more slowly. The rapid drop in pH that occurs in bacteria-containing phagosomes is responsible for the sequential discharge of granules. The initial alkaline environment favors specific granule activity, and the later acid pH allows lysosomal enzymes to be more effective (Fig. 4.16).

Tissue injury

Unfortunately, the microbe-killing activities of neutrophils are also directed against normal cells in inflammatory foci. Oxygen radicals cause direct injury by forming hydrogen peroxide (H_2O_2) and other oxygen metabolites such as $OH^{\bullet}$. For example, H_2O_2 and $OH^{\bullet}$ are responsible for much of the neutrophil-induced endothelial injury in lungs during acute pneumonia.

Oxygen radicals can also induce tissue injury by generating additional chemotactic factors, by depolymerizing glycosaminoglycans in interstitium (especially hyaluronate), and by inactivating leukocyte protease inhibitors. Serum enzymes such as

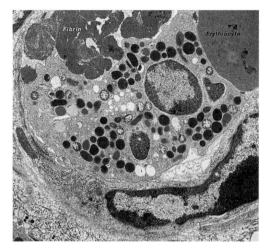

FIGURE 4.16. Electron micrograph of a neutrophil exhibiting degranulation and phagocytosis of virions and fibrin, infectious bovine rhinotracheitis, cow. Vacuoles and lipid are seen in the neutrophil.

α_1-antiprotease normally suppress damage by neutrophil granule elastase and are inhibited by oxidation reactions of inflammation.

Massive conversion of circulating fatty acids to toxic molecules can occur in activated neutrophils and can lead to toxicity. A **leukotoxin** from linoleic acid oxide formed by cytochrome P-450 monooxygenase in leukocytes (linoleic acid is an abundant fatty acid in the diet) is important in severe and extensive injuries such as burns, in which leukocytes are recruited to burned skin of victims and produce leukotoxin. Acting as a protoxin, leukotoxin is converted by epoxide hydrolases to highly toxic diols.

Enzymes from **neutrophil lysosomes** also damage normal tissue. In tissue undergoing acute inflammation, neutrophils generate kinins, cleave complement, initiate clot formation, and synthesize and release peptides that cause fever. They activate mast cells and platelets to liberate histamine and directly attack endothelial cells and basement membranes to sustain increased capillary permeability. Destruction of tissue is also caused by neutrophil lysosomal **proteolytic enzymes** that degrade collagen, basement membranes, and elastin and by **basic proteins** that increase capillary permeability.

In chronic inflammation, the long-term effect of release of neutrophil enzymes may be irreversible tissue destruction. Prolonged elastase release from degenerating neutrophils will gradually destroy elastic fibers in the alveolar wall in chronic lung inflammation, a mechanism that underlies emphysema. The circulating enzyme α_1-antitrypsin suppresses the effects of neutrophil elastase; humans deficient in this enzyme are especially prone to emphysema.

Corticosteroids suppress tissue injury

Therapy is occasionally needed to control the deleterious effects of inflammation. Corticosteroid hormones, when injected into an animal, reduce inflammation by various mechanisms. These include delaying extravasation of inflammatory cells, stabilization of lysosomal membranes in leukocytes, and inhibition of neutrophil granule movement and intracellular digestion. Corticosteroids also inhibit chemotaxis.

Corticosteroids cause leukocytosis by suppressing production of adhesion molecules on endothelial cells and leukocytes and of glycocalyx material for the cell surfaces. By reducing the stickiness of the neutrophil, they prevent its ability to adhere to endothelium and to migrate into tissue.

Toxic neutrophils

In severe bacterial infection, neutrophilic leukocytosis is the usual hematologic finding. The increase in leukocytes is due both to **premature expulsion of neutrophils** from sites of formation and to **enhanced leukopoiesis**. Because demand often exceeds supply, these new cells are usually immature. The appearance of increasing numbers of immature neutrophils in the circulation is called a "shift to the left" (based on the Schilling index of neutrophil maturity) and indicates a relatively severe disease process.

Toxic neutrophils appear in circulating blood during severe infection. These cells have cytoplasmic vacuoles and "toxic granules" (dense azurophil granules). The chemotactic activity of toxic neutrophils is markedly reduced, and their bactericidal effect is less than that of normal neutrophils. Severely burned animals have toxic neutrophils with markedly diminished chemotactic responsiveness a few days after injury, and this promotes septicemia, a common consequence of severe burns. **Döhle bodies**, which are light blue amorphous regions in the cytoplasm, may also be present in toxic neutrophils.

OTHER INFLAMMATORY CELLS IN THE EARLY PHASE

Monocytes

Monocytes enter inflammatory lesions with neutrophils

Substances chemotactic for neutrophils have no specific effect on monocytes, so that these cells do not appear in large numbers in early stages of acute inflammation. Furthermore, monocytes are not as aggressively ameboid as neutrophils; their numbers in circulating blood are much lower, and their reproduction and release are stimulated at a much slower rate. Once in tissue, monocytes avidly attach to microorganisms and either phagocytize them or, in the case of larger fungi, release soluble substances that are lethal for the microorganism.

Bone marrow is the source of promonocytes, and the sequence of promonocyte, monocyte, and macrophage occurs as these cells move from bone marrow to bloodstream and then into tissue. Monocytes are circulating, immature phagocytes. When activated, they emigrate through the capillary wall into inflammatory lesions (Fig. 4.17) and promptly transform into macrophages. Early evidence of synthesis of new degradative enzymes can be detected in monocytes as they adhere to endothelium.

Monocytosis

Monocytosis is elevation of monocytes in circulating blood beyond the range considered normal. It is seen in recovery phases of bacterial infections and is characteristic of acute stages of certain diseases. Only under severe conditions do monocytes phagocytize while in the bloodstream to become circulating macrophages.

In some forms of severe intravascular hemolysis, monocytes become phagocytic, absorb erythrocytes, and degrade hemoglobin. Their role in erythrophagocytosis is related to the capacity of their plasma membrane to attach to immunoglobulins and complement on erythrocyte surfaces.

Monocytes release cytokines that mediate inflammation

Release of **interleukin-1** (IL-1), a polypeptide that induces many features of the acute phase response of inflammation, occurs as monocytes are activated. IL-1 acts as a hormone and circulates to affect distant organs. Its functions include (1) stimulating neutrophils to circulate and release granules by a direct effect both on the bone marrow and on circulating neutrophils, (2) activating T and B lymphocytes, (3) stimulating fever and prostaglandin E_2 synthesis in the **hypothalamus**, (4) increasing synthesis of acute phase proteins in liver, and (5) increasing catabolism of skeletal muscle to provide amino acids for use by the liver.

In the late stages of inflammation, IL-1 acts as a growth factor for fibroblasts and other cells involved in repair. For example, in brain it is a potent mitogen for astroglia (it has no effect on oligodendroglia), and the brain content of IL-1 rises after injury.

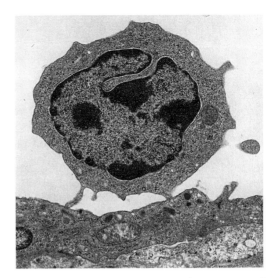

FIGURE 4.17. Monocyte. Ultrastructure of circulating monocyte in process of emigration through capillary wall during inflammation. Note the long processes on cell surface and their attachment to the endothelial cell.

Eosinophils

Eosinophils are large, ameboid, sluggishly phagocytic cells. Their unique granules hold the key to the specialized functions. Like neutrophil lysosomes, they function in phagocytosis to degrade substances. **Eosinophil basic protein** is especially toxic to parasite larvae (it can also cause host tissue damage). When released from eosinophils migrating into epithelium of the respiratory tract, eosinophil basic protein causes ciliastasis and degeneration of bronchial epithelium and may play a role in allergic respiratory disease.

Eosinophils respond to chemotactic factors

Eosinophils respond to antigen-antibody complexes in much the same way as neutrophils. They are less responsive to most other chemotactic factors, however, including complement components. Interleukin-5 (IL-5) is an important cytokine in the induction of eosinophilia. Eosinophil chemotaxis occurs in various inflammatory lesions but is especially noted in parasitic infections of the skin and intestine and in the nasopharynx during some allergic diseases.

The role of immune complexes in eosinophil chemotaxis is critical. These complexes of antigen and antibody activate the complement system to produce factors that attract eosinophils. Chemotactic factors specific for eosinophils include histamine (mast cells are often associated with eosinophil exudates). Mast cell tumors usually have many eosinophils.

Blood eosinophilia

Elevation of eosinophils in circulating blood is common in parasitic infections. Eosinophilia has not been correlated with specific parasite components or with antibody levels. It has, however, been proposed as an immune phenomenon; that is, the ability of animals to respond to parasite infection with eosinophilia was associated with interaction of parasite and lymphocytes. Soluble factors that stimulate eosinophilopoiesis arise from the lymphocyte secretions.

Eosinophils kill parasites by several mechanisms

Most metazoan parasites produce marked tissue eosinophilia, especially in invasive and migratory phases of infection. Eosinophilic activity is generated both by release of chemoattractants by the parasite and by chemotactic activity of the host's inflammatory response.

Eosinophils kill by degranulating onto surfaces of parasites. This is done by depositing **eosinophilic basic protein** (contained in eosinophil granules) onto the parasite cuticle. Eosinophilic basic protein has a direct killing effect in the parasite.

Other mechanisms are superimposed on the activity of eosinophilic basic protein. Parasites coated with antibody and complement attract eosinophils. In schistosomiasis, larvae that enter immune animals are damaged as they penetrate the skin because aggregates of eosinophils firmly adhere to the antibody-coated parasite. Eosinophils contain specific receptors for complement and immunoglobulins on their surfaces. After they attach to the antibody-complement complexes on the parasite surface, they secrete **peroxidases**. Focal lesions are produced in the parasitic tegument, causing it to separate from the body of the parasite.

Damage also results from activation of the alternate complement pathway (eosinophils adhere to complement-coated parasites through their C3 receptors), but this is not an important mechanism for killing parasites. Recently, soluble factors (called **eosinophil cytotoxicity enhancing factors**) released by monocytes and lymphocytes have been found to aid in some unknown way in killing parasites.

When large numbers of parasites are killed by chemotherapy, enormous amounts of eosinophilic basic protein that coats the dying parasites are released into the tissue lymph and bloodstream and may result in clinical disease. Syndromes of erythema, edema, and urticaria have been reported in animals treated with parasiticides (e.g., diethylcarbamazine). Called the Mazzotti reaction, it occurs strikingly in some species.

Lymphocytes

In most mammals, lymphocytes make up 20–40% of the leukocytes in blood and more than 90% of the cells in thoracic duct lymph. Lymphocytes are tiny round cells with a narrow rim of cytoplasm. Dense azurophil granules (5–15 per cell) and clear vacuoles are often present in the cytoplasm. Nuclear chromatin is densely packed, particularly at the periphery of the nucleus. The smallest lymphocytes are resting cells, and the reactions of ameboid movement, phagocytosis, and chemotactic responses are weak or absent. Larger lymphocytes found in smears of normal blood usually represent transformed cells. They are blast cells with intensely basophilic cytoplasm. Increased numbers of these cells are found in recovery stages of pyogenic infections and some viral diseases and are, in fact, immature plasmacytes.

Lymphocytosis, the increase in numbers of lymphocytes in circulating blood, is seen in transient responses to severe muscular exercise, fever, and other stress. Lymphocytosis of long duration is less common.

Lymphopenia, a decrease in numbers of lymphocytes, occurs in viral diseases in which the virus attacks the lymphoid system (e.g., canine distemper, hog cholera, and bovine viral diarrhea) and during therapy with such lympholytic agents as cortisone, radiation, and immunosuppressive drugs.

Basophilic leukocytes

Basophils are present in blood in such small numbers that increases, when noticed, are seldom meaningful. Under specific chemotactic influences, basophils migrate into tissue spaces. They localize in perivascular sites where their degranulation has a maximal effect on vascular permeability. Although tissue **mast cells** play a greater role in acute inflammation, basophils migrating into tissue are more important in chronic inflammation.

Basophils are often a component of chronic lesions arising from immune reactions. They are attracted by lymphocyte cytokines. Basophils have surface receptors for complement fragment C3, which enhances phagocytosis and the ability of basophils (and mast cells) to adhere to parasites that have become coated with complement.

ADDITIONAL READING

Endothelium

Doré M, Sirois J. 1996. Regulation of P-selectin expression by inflammatory mediators in canine jugular endothelial cells. *Vet Pathol* 33:662.

Frenette PS, Wagner DD. 1996. Adhesion molecules—part II: blood vessels and blood cells. *New Engl J Med* 335:43.

Walker DH, et al. 1997. Cytokine-induced, nitric acid–dependent intracellular antirickettsial activity of mouse endothelial cells. *Lab Invest* 76:129.

Clinical signs

Berg DJ, et al. 1998. Rapid development of severe hyperplastic gastritis with gastric epithelial dedifferentiation in *Helicobacter felis*–infected IL-10$^{-/-}$ mice. *Am J Pathol* 152:1377.

Flier JS, Underhill LH. 1994. The neurologic basis of fever. *New Engl J Med* 330:1880.

Machelska H, et al. 1998. Pain control in inflammation governed by selectins. *Nat Med* 4:1425.

Kinins, eicosanoids, and cytokines

Bazzoni F, Beutler B. 1996. The tumor necrosis factor ligand and receptor families. *New Engl J Med* 334:1717.

Caspi D, et al. 1987. C-reactive protein in dogs. *Am J Vet Res* 48:919.

Premarck BA, Schall TJ. 1996. Chemokine receptors: gateways to infection and inflammation. *Nat Med* 2:1174.

Acute phase proteins

Asghar SS, Pasch MC. 1998. Complement as a promiscuous signal transduction device. *Lab Invest* 78:1203.

Neutrophils

Ackermann MR, et al. 1996. Passage of CD18$^-$ and CD18$^+$ bovine neutrophils into pulmonary alveoli during acute *Pasteurella haemolytica* pneumonia. *Vet Pathol* 33:639.

Baracos V, et al. 1983. Stimulation of muscle protein degradation and prostaglandin E_2 release by leukocytic pyrogen (interleukin-1). *New Engl J Med* 308:553.

Barnathan ES, et al. 1997. Immunohistochemical localization of defensin in human coronary vessels. *Am J Pathol* 150:1009.

Bertram TA. 1985. Neutrophilic leukocyte structure and function in domestic animals. *Adv Vet Sci* 30:91.

Brogden KA, et al. 1996. Isolation of an ovine pulmonary surfactant-associated anionic peptide (SAAP) bactericidal for *Pasteurella haemolytica*. *Proc Natl Acad Sci* 93:412.

Caswell JL, et al. 1998. Expression of the neutrophil chemoattractant interleukin-8 in the lesions of bovine pneumonic pasteurellosis. *Vet Pathol* 35:124.

Eaton KA, Radin MJ, Krakowka S. 1995. An animal model of gastric ulcer due to bacterial gastritis in mice. *Vet Pathol* 32:489.

Hampton MB, et al. 1998. Inside the neutrophil phagosome: oxidants, myeloperoxidase, and bacterial killing. *Blood* 92:3007.

Perlmutter DH. 1991. The cellular basis of liver injury in α_1-antitrypsin deficiency. *Hepatology* 13:172.

Stolzenberg ED, et al. 1997. Epithelial antibiotic induced in states of disease. *Proc Natl Acad Sci* 94:8686.

Wilhelmsen CL, Pitt MLM. 1996. Lesions of acute inhaled lethal ricin intoxication in rhesus monkeys. *Vet Pathol* 33:29.

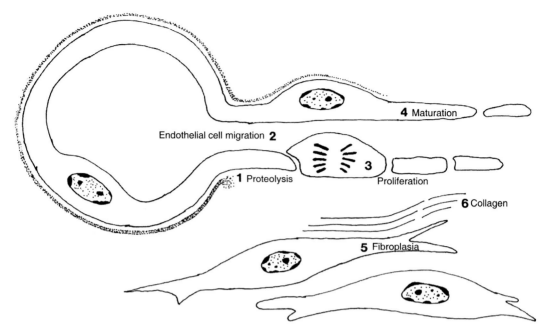

FIGURE 5.1. Angiogenesis and fibroplasia in formation of granulation tissue. 1. Proteolytic degradation of basement membrane of the parent vessel. 2. Migration of endothelial cells toward angiogenic stimuli (fibroblast growth factor, vascular endothelial growth factor). 3. Endothelial cell mitosis with proliferation behind the leading front of migrating cells. 4. Endothelial cell maturation and remodeling into tubes and mature blood vessels. 5. Fibroblast migration and replication, triggered by growth factors (controlled by transforming growth factor from platelets and macrophages). 6. Collagen production by fibroblasts.

::: CHAPTER 5

Healing and Chronic Inflammation

THE HEALING PHASE OF ACUTE INFLAMMATION

Repair begins rapidly after injury. As acute inflammation subsides in damaged tissue, processes associated with repair begin to dominate the wound. This involves alterations in the extracellular matrix, phagocytosis of necrotic cells and debris by macrophages, and formation of granulation tissue. **Granulation tissue** is the clinical hallmark of healing. The term is derived from the soft, pink, granular appearance of wound surfaces. Histologically, granulation tissue is characterized by new blood vessels and fibroblasts. New blood vessels are leaky, and the escape of fluid makes granulation tissue soft and spongy. **Angiogenesis** (invasion by new capillaries) and **fibrosis** (fibroblast replication with deposition of collagen) provide a scaffold for future reorganization and regeneration of the injured tissue.

Wound fluids are mixtures of plasma proteins and ground substance. They provide the milieu in which tissue reconstruction takes place. Ground substance, the amorphous, gel-like material separating cells and fibers, is composed of glycosaminoglycans bound to protein. In inflammation, the long-chain polymers that impart the gel consistency to ground substance are broken by depolymerization, and the gel becomes fluid. Bacterial enzymes, such as clostridial hyaluronidase, hasten this process. As acute inflammation progresses, there is rapid formation of hyaluronic acid in the ground substance of connective tissue. Ground substance becomes rich in glycosaminoglycans, and regeneration of connective tissue is initiated. Fibroblasts are the source of glycosaminoglycans, and mast cells contribute. Hyaluronic acids and hexosamine disappear as fibroblasts secrete collagen.

All damaged cells at the site of injury secrete cytokines that stimulate and sustain the healing process. Some of the important cytokines are **fibroblast growth factor, platelet-derived growth factor, angiogenic growth factor, epidermal growth factor**, and **transforming growth factors** α and β. This battery of growth factors acts in paracrine and even autocrine pathways to stimulate cells that will repair tissue. Some of the major effects of cytokines are to initiate **angiogenesis**, and some are potently chemotactic and mitogenic for endothelial cells. Other cytokines stimulate fibroblasts to produce collagen, and still others act on epithelial cells to regrow over damaged epithelial surfaces.

Angiogenesis

At the surviving borders of injured tissue, vascular endothelial sprouts appear from surviving capillaries. As the capillary sprout first develops, endothelial cell secretions digest the surrounding basement membrane and the extracellular matrix to facilitate invasion and migration into the site of injury. The advancing endothelial cell sprout must invade and migrate through the clot matrix of the wound. The new vascular sprouts and syncytia fuse and canalize and gradually establish a network of patent capillaries.

Migration of endothelial sprouts is guided by the chemotactic influence of potent cytokines released from platelets and leukocytes (Fig. 5.1). Cytokines such as **fibroblast growth factor** (FGF) activate endothelial cells, causing them to express increasing numbers of integrins on their surfaces. In wound healing, the initial angiogenic stimulus is supplied by FGF and is followed by a subsequent and more prolonged angiogenic stimulus provided by vascular endothelial growth factor (VEGF). Activated endothelial cells produce new adhesion molecules. The αvβ3 integrin is heavily expressed on activated endothelial cell surfaces, has a broad range, and can attach to receptor sites on fibronectin, vitronectin, and other components of the clot matrix.

In addition to cytokines, other physiologic stimulants to vascular growth include hypoxia, products from injured tissue, blood pressure differentials, and changes in the connective tissue stroma. The combination of these stimuli causes vascular syncytia (cords of cells) to form and to differentiate rapidly to create channels for blood flow.

Endothelial cell mitosis and proliferation are most intense in areas lacking epithelium. When wounds become covered with epithelial surfaces, endothelial mitotic activity decreases. **Heparin** released from mast cells has a significant secondary role in the stimulation of capillary endothelial proliferation.

Fibrin provides a scaffold for vascularization

In the healing wound, new endothelial buds move into the wounded tissue along strands of **fibrin**. Fibrin is absorbed during vascular ingrowth. It persists beyond the disappearance of neutrophils and is not entirely removed until vascular invasion is accomplished. The newly formed endothelial cells are fibrinolytic. Unlike fibroblasts, they contain an activator of plasminogen. Removal of fibrin polymers is necessary as capillary buds migrate into the wound. In this phase of healing, both fibroplasia and vascularization are retarded in conditions of nutritional deficiency or other severe systemic disease. In vitamin C deficiency, for example, endothelial cells are abnormal and do not enter wounds at rates comparable to those for wounds of normal animals.

Platelets and coagulation factors contribute to healing

Platelet-derived growth factor is a mitogenic peptide secreted by platelets trapped at sites of inflammation. It stimulates both angiogenesis and proliferation of fibroblasts and smooth muscle cells. **Factor XIII**, one of the terminal products of the clotting cascade, not only catalyzes cross-linking of fibrin molecules but also promotes cross-linking of fibrin to the connective tissue matrix and to fibronectin on the surfaces of mesenchymal cells in the healing wound.

Newly formed blood vessels and fibroblasts form granulation tissue

Early in the repair process, proliferating fibroblasts align perpendicular to invading capillary buds and begin to secrete collagen. **Transforming growth factor** β, a family of closely related peptides released by inflammatory cells, exerts a differential effect on fibroblasts, endothelium, and epidermis to bring about healing. All TGF-βs act by binding to receptor complexes on target cells. In granulation tissue of healing skin wounds, these receptors increase markedly on fibroblasts and endothelial cells and decrease as granulation tissue is remodeled.

Fibrosis

Fibrosis, the formation of fibrous tissue (syn: fibroplasia), begins early after injury. The critical events in fibrosis are activation of fibroblasts and production of collagen. As collagen is released from the cell, it assembles into collagen fibrils, which cross-link to form collagen fibers. As healing is completed, modified fibroblasts contract to form the scar. In the early healing wound, fibrocytes are the source of new fibroblasts, although the pluripotentiality of vascular endothelial cells and pericytes indicates that these cells may also provide collagen. Fibroblasts consist of subsets of cells much like lymphocytes; different subsets display differing phenotypes and secrete differing cytokines. Stem cells circulating in the bloodstream are a source of both fibroblasts and endothelial cells in the healing wound.

In uninfected, uncomplicated skin wounds, fibroblasts multiply and new cells migrate into the wound along strands of polymerized fibrin. Collagen is synthesized, and collagen fibers aligned until the wound is completely bridged. In small linear wounds, this process occurs in 5–7 days. In the subsequent 2–3 weeks, the wound is repaired. Fibrosis increases as scar tissue is organized. By 4 weeks, when collagenization and fibrosis are largely completed, elastic fibers begin to appear in the wound (Fig. 5.2). Elastic fibers consist of globules of elastin complexed with a hydrated glycosaminoglycan. The elastic fibers weave among the collagen fibers, giving the newly formed connective tissue stretchability and elasticity. Large amounts of basement membrane material and reticulin are deposited in wounds and can be demonstrated by special stains.

Collagen directs capillary growth

Collagen does not lie as an inert bridging material but is constantly re-formed to strengthen a wound. It plays an inductive role in new capillary formation, and when collagen synthesis in a wound is inhibited, capillary ingrowth is markedly delayed. Experimentally, when collagen is added to endothelial cells growing on the surface of a gel, cells reorganize into a network of branching and anastomosing capillary tubules.

Fibrous connective tissues of wounds are constantly being remodeled as healing occurs.

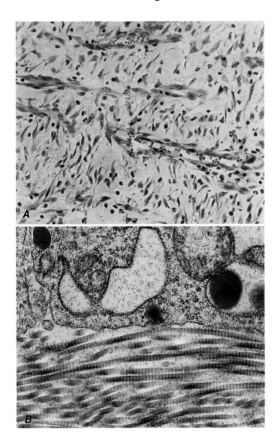

FIGURE 5.2. Fibroplasia in healing wound, surgical incision in a cat. A. Endothelial cell invasion with extension of fibroblasts parallel to endothelial cell buds (1 week after incision). There are collagen deposits with few neutrophils. B. Electron micrograph of collagen fibrils adjacent to a collagen-producing fibroblast. Large groups of collagen fibrils *(bottom)* make up collagen fiber. The fibroblast cytoplasm *(top)* contains ribosomes and endoplasmic reticulum that synthesize collagen.

Macrophages secrete collagenase, elastase, and plasminogen activators that mediate hydrolysis of connective tissue proteins extracellularly. Local conversion of plasminogen to plasmin allows elastase easier access to its substrate, elastin. After the initial hydrolysis, macrophages endocytose protein matrix fragments that are completely degraded within lysosomes.

Remodeling of the wound is regulated by the differential expression of growth factors. In the massive granulation tissue of deep wounds and burn scars, the number of TGF-β receptors remains very high. Excessive scarring is associated with a failure to eliminate TGF-β receptors, overproducing fibroblasts in the wound.

As the scar is formed, the process of wound contraction depends on specialized fibroblasts. After about 1 week of wound growth, peculiar modifications of fibroblasts develop. These new cells, called **myofibroblasts**, have increased cytoplasmic contractile microfilaments and surface attachment sites that facilitate the role of these cells in wound contraction.

Fibrogenesis

Increased formation of collagen fibrils in connective tissue occurs in such diverse conditions as inflammation, healing, atrophy, and degeneration. Chronic progressive fibrosis may develop if collagenases and elastases are missing or abnormal. Fibrosis of the lungs, myocardium, and liver may in fact contribute significantly to disease and death. The point of irreversibility in **cirrhosis** of the liver has been correlated with disappearance of liver collagenase.

Collagen forms the building blocks for connective tissue fibers and nonfibrous structures such as cartilage and basement membranes. Mammalian tissues produce more than 20 collagen types, each designed for different construction work outside the cell. There are, however, 2 major collagens that form most of the extracellular collagen: **collagen I**, which polymerizes into fibrils that aggregate to form collagen fibers of connective tissues, and **collagen IV**, which forms granular aggregates that in turn form basement membranes.

The common property of all collagens is the triple helix, a unique coil of three polypeptide chains wound together in a helix to form a rodlike molecule. Within each type of collagen, heterogeneity occurs, because variations in hydroxylation, glycosylation, and cross-linking of the molecule are dependent on tissue type, age, and hormonal status. For example, collagen type I in the Achilles tendon is highly cross-linked, whereas that of the tail tendons is much less so.

Hepatic fibrosis

Fibrosis in the liver occurs secondary to severe liver injury. Collagen is laid down in the Disse's spaces. Although interstitial fibroblasts are credited with releasing much of the collagen, it is clear that hepatocytes can synthesize and release collagen. Type IV collagen (for basement membranes) is synthesized early, whereas types I and III are produced later in hepatic injury. Fibroplasia in chronic liver injury is an important component of cirrhosis.

Cirrhosis is characterized by **diffuse fibrosis** and parenchymal **nodular regeneration** (hepatocellular necrosis, an antecedent to cirrhosis, is sometimes listed as a third component). Cirrhosis is the

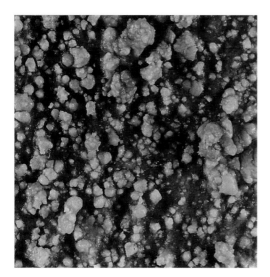

FIGURE 5.3. Multifocal, granulomatous peritonitis, cow with tuberculosis.

result of abnormal reconstruction of liver architecture and is usually a scarred, end stage of chronic inflammation of the liver with an attempt to regenerate without a tissue framework for repair. Collagen fibers are deposited around the vascular sinusoids in connective tissue septa that link the portal and central zones. Thus fibroplasia is both a result of and a contributor to vascular obstruction. Because of postsinusoidal portal hypertension, there is increased hepatic lymph flow, and portal lymphatics are dilated.

Pulmonary fibrosis

Pulmonary fibrosis is a sequel to severe, acute injury to the lungs and is a significant cause of morbidity and mortality in animals. In pulmonary fibrosis that accompanies cardiac failure in the dog, ischemia, parenchymal cell degeneration, and hormonal factors combine to sustain progressive collagen deposition. Excess collagen fibrils and their associated connective tissue microfibrils and thickened basement membranes are characteristic. Basement membranes become attached to underlying collagen by specialized anchoring fibrils and to the plasma membranes of overlying pulmonary epithelium by hemidesmosomes. The final lesion is thus due to a complex interaction with collagen and glycoproteins of the interstitial ground substance.

Diffuse pulmonary fibrosis may result from inhalation or expiration of toxins. Prolonged low levels of noxious chemicals in inspired air produce slow progressive degenerative changes accompanied by extensive diffuse fibroplasia of the alveolar wall interstitium. Aerogenic toxicity involves vacuolation in pneumocytes and endothelium. Hyperplasia of

granular pneumocytes occurs as a reparative process. If toxicity continues, there is progressive deposition of glycosaminoglycans, basement membranes, and collagen.

Collagen is produced by interstitial fibroblasts and deposited in the proteoglycan-rich matrix of the alveolar septae. Macrophages are prominent in fibrotic alveolar walls, probably to degrade and recycle collagen and, in chronic microbial infections, to process antigens.

Granulomatous inflammation

Granulomatous inflammation is a chronic inflammatory process that involves macrophages and newly formed blood vessels. Granulomatous lesions lack the cardinal signs of acute inflammation. On gross examination, granulomatous tissue may be focal or a continuous layer of granular, vegetative growths that cover serosal surfaces of body cavities. Granulomatous inflammation does resemble neoplastic processes, and the clinical differentiation from neoplasms is often a problem that must be resolved by biopsy and microscopic examination.

Granulomatous inflammation is dominated by activated monocytes and macrophages. These cells compose the lesion and continue to infiltrate granulomatous inflammatory sites in immense numbers. Bacteria, fungi, aberrant parasites, and inert particles such as silica and asbestos are notorious initiators of granulomatous lesions. All contain components that macrophage lysosomes cannot degrade. Macrophages become large and foamy because they accumulate both the causal agents and the debris from injured tissue. These foamy macrophages, called **epithelioid cells**, are the hallmark of granulomatous inflammation (Fig. 5.3).

Macrophages

Macrophages are large, pale cells designed for phagocytosis and intracellular digestion. They constitute a second line of defense. They are not rapidly attracted by chemotactic substances that attract neutrophils and are less discriminating in the material they phagocytize. Whereas neutrophils degranulate and spew proteases and oxygen radicals into inflamed tissue, macrophages function more slowly to engulf particulate material. Uptake is slower, and degradation is less complete. Digested debris accumulates in large membrane-bounded lysosomes called **residual bodies**, which may, by exocytosis, be shunted outside the cell.

In normal tissue, macrophages are continually involved in degradation of aged erythrocytes, cholesterol, fibrin polymers, pulmonary alveolar secretion, and other proteins. They clear and process dead cells and debris. In the atrophy of the involuting uterus following pregnancy, macrophages take up massive amounts of collagen, which is removed for the return of the uterus to normal size.

The unequaled ability of macrophages to process foreign proteins in a slow, limited manner (without enzymatically destroying protein) allows them to fulfill a vital role in processing and retaining antigens for specific lymphoid immune reactions.

Macrophages are activated by particulate material. Activated (stimulated) macrophages are distinguished from inactive forms by increased numbers of lysosomes, phagosomes, and mitochondria. Activated forms have increased amounts of hydrolases in their lysosomes, hypermobility of cell membranes, and markedly increased synthesis of lysozyme and cytokines, and they secrete complement, interferon, plasminogen activators, and, probably most important, the multifunctional cytokine interleukin-1 (Table 5.1).

The functional capacity of the **monocyte-macrophage system** can be calculated from the clearance of carbon particles injected intravenously. The **phagocyte index** (PI) can be formulated where C_0 and C_t are the concentration of carbon in the blood at 0 time and at time t.

$$PI = \frac{\log C_0 - C_t}{t}$$

Blockade of the monocyte-macrophage system can be transiently induced by overloading its macrophages with substances such as carbon. Macrophages are temporarily unable to phagocytize additional particulate material. Paralysis of macrophages accompanies some severe infectious dis-

TABLE 5.1. Products secreted by macrophages

Antimicrobial	Lysozyme
	Complement components
	Interferon
	Microbicidal peptides
	Defensins
Cytokines	Interleukin-1
	Tumor necrosis factor α
Enzymes	Lysosomal hydrolases
	Collagenase
	Elastase
	Plasminogen activators

eases. Substances such as the capsular material of anthrax bacilli inhibit cell membranes of macrophages, thus rendering them incapable of phagocytosis. Surfaces of fungi such as *Cryptococcus neoformans* also produce this direct inhibitory effect on macrophages.

Viral infections of the monocyte-macrophage system also predispose the animal to bacterial infection. Any blockade of this system increases an animal's susceptibility to infection, shock, and intravascular coagulation. Blockade is traditionally viewed as physical saturation of macrophages with particulate material. It also involves depletion of fibronectin and serum proteins (opsonins) that interact with particles to promote phagocytosis.

Granulomas

Granulomatous lesions develop more slowly than do purulent lesions. The lesions of tuberculosis or histoplasmosis take weeks or months to cause dis-

FOCUS

Granulomas in Tuberculosis

PRIOR TO THE DEVELOPMENT of systems of public health laws and of sanitary engineering in the early 1900s, tuberculosis was one of the dominant plagues of animals and humans. The early milestones in medicine and veterinary medicine alike were often milestones in tuberculosis research.

Tubercle bacilli (*Mycobacterium* spp.) produce characteristic lesions no matter where they localize in tissue. The **tubercle**, or mature lesion, is a nodule of caseous necrotic tissue surrounded by macrophages and walled off by chronic granulation tissue that contains plasmacytes, lymphocytes, and fibroblasts. Bacilli are taken up by macrophages where they survive to stimulate the granulomatous reaction. Trapped within phagolysosomes inside the macrophage, most

▶

ease, whereas pyogenic streptococci can cause acute purulent reactions in 24 hours. Most microbes that cause granulomatous inflammation are not strongly chemoattractive to neutrophils. Monocytes are attracted to sites of infection and ingest but do not kill or degrade all of the invading microorganisms. Additional blood monocytes migrate to the lesions, transform to macrophages, and rephagocytize the agents and its associated cell debris. New macrophages collect in progressively expanding foci

▶

bacilli are killed. A few survive, however, and are able to propagate within the lysosome despite the potent hydrolases that kill most other bacteria.

When tubercle bacilli first enter the respiratory or intestinal tract to initiate primary infection, they may be confined within small foci of infection and ultimately destroyed. If host macrophages cannot handle the initial infection, however, dissemination of mycobacteria occurs. Secondary foci of infection develop by extension or, upon erosion of lymph or blood vessels, by lymphogenous or hematogenous distribution.

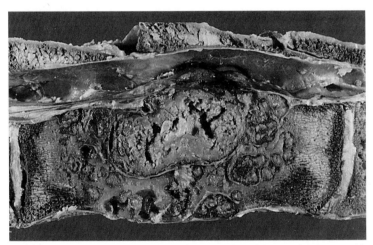

Chronic focal granulomatous spondylitis (inflammation of the vertebrae), cow with tuberculosis caused by *Mycobacterium bovis*. Many small granulomas surround a large granuloma with a necrotic center, which protrudes into the spinal canal, compressing the spinal cord (missing).

Tubercles begin as small aggregates of neutrophils and macrophages that sequester and ingest bacilli. If macrophages take in bacteria but do not kill them, they themselves are killed. Foci of necrotic cells become surrounded by a mantle of new macrophages. The lesion progressively expands because of the continuous entry of "immune" monocytes. These cells phagocytize dead macrophages and their viable bacteria and are, in turn, destroyed. At the periphery of the lesion, monocyte activity is most intense, and large, plump macrophages known as **epithelioid cells** are prominent. These cells contain markedly undulant and interwoven cell surfaces, and fusion of their plasma membranes leads to formation of the giant cells that characterize tuberculosis. The massive necrosis and cavitation in pulmonary tuberculosis in some mammals are due less to the virulence of bacterium than to the hypersensitivity of macrophages in that particular host.

called **granulomas**. Although the bacterium or fungus may not be destroyed, the granuloma provides an effective means of localizing the agents and allowing other inflammatory and immunologic mechanisms to act for longer periods of time. When fully developed, the granuloma may contain a necrotic center, a peripheral zone of macrophages and other cells, and an outer rim of fibrotic tissue.

Immune reactions contribute to granulomas

The induction phase of infectious granulomas is a macrophage response to persistent insoluble material; neither antibody nor cell-mediated immunity plays a role in evolution or resolution of the early lesion. As the granuloma expands, however, it becomes increasingly complex. Although the dominant cell type remains, the macrophage, lymphocytes, plasmablasts, and other cell types invade, and the granuloma becomes altered by the interaction of these cells. **Lymphocytes** release cytokines and other mediators, which attract and activate new monocytes and macrophages. In some lesions, **plasmacytes** are common, indicating a role, even though ineffective, of these antibody-containing

cells in attempting to overcome the organism involved.

Giant cells are common in granulomas

Fusion of monocytes and macrophages gives rise to huge, multinucleate cells called **giant cells**. Fusion occurs in regions of extensive macrophage surface interdigitation and results in cells with multiple nuclei. Nuclei may be clustered in the center of the cell or arranged in rings around the periphery. The finding of giant cells in lesions suggests the possibility of disease involving fungi, mycobacteria, or foreign bodies and is a valuable aid in diagnosis (Fig. 5.4).

In most infectious diseases, giant cell formation occurs by **fusion of monocytes and macrophages**. The stimulus for fusion is the cytokines released from lymphocytes that migrate into the granuloma. That is, when stimulated by specific antigens, T lymphocytes produce a soluble protein that causes circulating monocytes to fuse and form giant cells.

Giant cells also form by **division of nuclei without cytoplasmic division**. This mechanism occurs rarely in granulomatous inflammation. However,

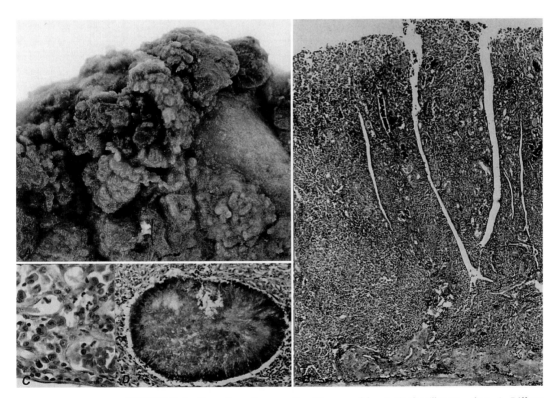

FIGURE 5.4. Granulomatous peritonitis caused by *Actinobacillus* sp., dog. A. Diffuse granulomatous growth on surface of diaphragm. B. Fronds of granulation tissue project from muscle of diaphragm *(bottom).* C. Large macrophages in spaces between blood vessels. D. "Sulfur granule," a large mass of bacteria and bacterial secretions among granulomatous tissue.

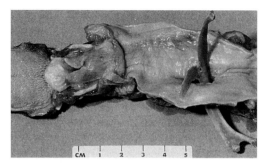

FIGURE 5.5. Perforating esophageal ulcer, aged dog. Rib bone (avian) has penetrated the esophageal surface.

the fungal metabolite **cytochalasin** produced by some aspergilli affects cell division by altering microtubules of macrophages. It inhibits cytokinesis (cytoplasmic division) without affecting karyokinesis (nuclear division), and the giant cells found in granulomas of the lungs in aspergillosis may arise from this mechanism.

Inflammatory cells in late inflammation

Lymphocytes

Lymphocytes are found in tissues undergoing recovery from acute inflammation and repair. Small lymphocytes are resting cells that carry immunologic memory—their role in immunity is a sign that an immune response is occurring in tissue. **Lymphopenia**, a decrease in numbers of lymphocytes in blood, occurs in viral diseases in which the virus attacks the lymphoid system (e.g., canine distemper, bovine viral diarrhea) and during therapy with lympholytic agents such as corticosteroids, radiation, and immunosuppressants.

REPAIR

Repair is a fundamental process of all living things. It begins soon after injury and utilizes both the fluids and cells that have exuded into the tissue during the acute phase of inflammation. Repair involves fibrous reconstruction, ingrowth of new blood vessels (angiogenesis), and hyperplastic regeneration of epithelium. The large differences in repair processes among different animals result from the regenerative capacity of the species involved, cleanliness or contamination of the site of injury, and the tissue in which repair is occurring.

Epithelialization

In epidermis, basal cells of the surviving epithelium at the periphery of the wound begin to slide across the bare, fibrin-covered wound surface soon after injury. Migrant epithelial cells have blunt pseudo-

pods that project, by ameboid movement, into fibrin strands. As epithelial cells cover the wound, they form intercellular bridges and secrete collagen IV and glycosaminoglycans that form a new basement membrane. Epithelial cells also cover gaps in epidermis by growing up from skin appendages such as hair follicles, providing these structures remain intact after injury.

Acute tissue injury causes circulating platelets and leukocytes to produce autocrine and paracrine factors that promote reepithelialization and healing in the wounded tissue. **Epidermal growth factor** (EGF), **transforming growth factor** (TGF), and other platelet-produced growth factors have a powerful influence on migrating epithelial cells. As healing begins, cells in connective tissue adjacent to the wound, largely endothelial cells and fibroblasts, take over this function and become the major, sustained source of growth factors.

Small wounds may be covered in 12 hours. Mitosis begins in migrant epithelial cells, and new cells rapidly fill in the gaps in the new surface. New keratinocytes develop intercellular junctions that bind with other epithelial cells and with the basement membrane to complete the repair process. To increase attachments, neighboring epithelial cells form adhesion plaques that bind firmly to E-cadherins, catenins, and other molecules.

Epithelial cell proliferation ceases when cells contact one another. **Contact inhibition** is the poorly understood phenomenon involving cell recognition and establishment of normal intercellular communication. Information causing epithelization to cease is somehow transferred from cell to cell (probably through specialized gap junctions); cell proliferation does not cease if mechanical barriers are placed in the path of advancing cells.

New epithelial surfaces lack appendages, such as hair follicles and glands, and are usually poorly pigmented. Mammalian skin heals in a well-defined sequence, but there are marked species differences in wound healing among lower vertebrates. Fish skin contains large numbers of extraordinarily large "alarm cells" interspersed among keratinocytes and containing an aqueous substance that causes other fish to move away; alarm cells are not present in new epithelium over wounds.

Mucosal surfaces regenerate rapidly

Mucosal epithelial surfaces regenerate more quickly than does epidermis. In small experimental wounds of the rat trachea, injured mucosa is covered by new epithelium in 48 hours; cilia and goblet cells appear in 14 days. Similar experimental wounding of the cat duodenum has shown equally rapid growth. Simple epithelium covers the clot-filled defect in a few days and subsequently remodels to form new villi and glands.

Granulation tissue is required for epithelization

Massive wounds will heal progressively, provided that a proper base of granulation tissue is present. In some patients, surgical incisions are deliberately left unsutured to promote drainage and to avoid pockets of infection below the suture line. If infection is controlled, these wounds heal efficiently. When an **ulcer** erodes through the wall of an organ so that a base of granulation tissue cannot form, the epithelial margins of the wound do not grow together (Fig. 5.5). The stimulus provided by collagen is missing, and the wound edges will not coalesce.

CONTAMINATION OF WOUNDS

Healing of a clean, incised wound: first intention

Surgical incisions are generally sharp and free from large numbers of bacteria and tissue debris. Because blood vessels have been ligated and wound edges approximated, they contain little free blood. Repair is rapid (Fig. 5.6). Fibroblasts generally bridge the area in 12 hours. Capillary buds invade, allowing a framework of blood vessels to form and assisting fibroplasia and collagen deposition that impart tensile strength to the wound. Within 4–5 days, epi-

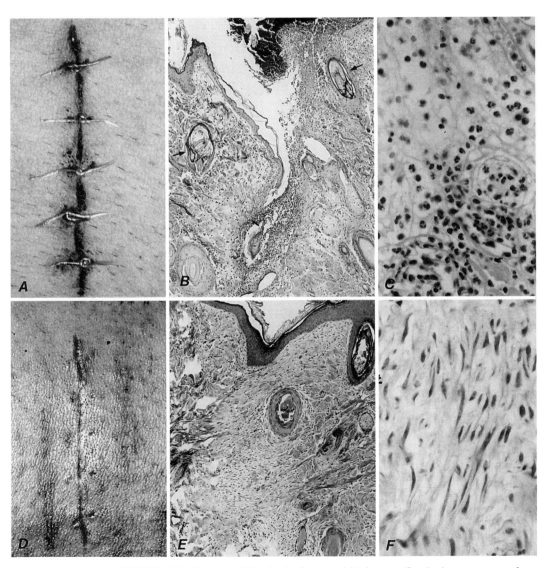

FIGURE 5.6. Gross and histologic (low- and high-magnification) appearance of sutured skin incisions in abdominal skin, dog. A–C. Biopsy at 2 days after a surgical incision. D–F. Biopsy at 14 days. Compare neutrophils in C with fibroblasts in F.

thelium has grown over the wound, acute inflammation has ceased, and repair is sufficient to allow movement of the injured area. General expectations for healing of a surgical incision in the skin by first intention are as follows:

- 24 hours—Clot is formed in spaces of incision; neutrophils appear at margins of incised tissue; mitotic activity occurs in basal cells of epithelium remaining at wound margin.
- 3 days—Macrophages are prominent in the wound; granulation tissue formation with collagen deposition has begun; epithelial cells have migrated over the wound surface.
- 5 days—Blood vessels and fibroblasts fill the incision site; angiogenesis is at its peak; epithelial layer covers the wound surface, and keratinization has begun.

At the end of the first week, all components of healing are in place, but wound strength is about 10% of normal, unwounded skin. By the end of the second week, fibroplasia is maximal. Formation of myofibroblasts and their subsequent contracture give the wound a blanched, or white, appearance.

Healing of an open wound: second intention

Lacerations of tissue that are not sutured must heal by new tissue formation at the base of the wound. They are usually filled with tissue debris, free erythrocytes, and dead bacteria. Although bacteria usually do not persist, continual recontamination has the same effect, prolonging the phase of chronicity. The regularly spaced invasions of capillary buds into this tissue give it, when freed of exudate, a granular appearance—hence the term **granulation tissue**. Microscopically, new granulation is composed of invading endothelial cells and capillary buds from which, in parallel arrangements, fibroblasts and collagen fibers are formed.

Organization: uniform bridging by connective tissue

As resolution of the wound occurs and resorption of exudates takes place, angiogenesis and fibroplasia dominate. Organization begins to form a scar, or **cicatrix**. As collagen production increases, the fibroblasts become less active. The scar appears white and glistening because of the dominance of collagen.

Collagen is constantly remodeled

Collagen does not lie as an inert bridging material but exists in a dynamic state in which synthesis and removal is slowly occurring. With time, collagen fibers become progressively stronger by increased bonding among the fibrils. Collagenases, the enzymes that degrade collagen, occur in

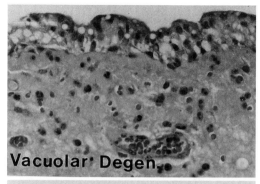

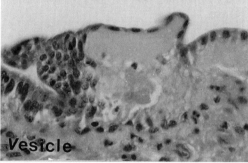

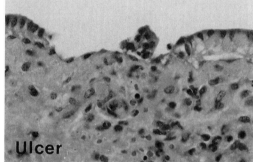

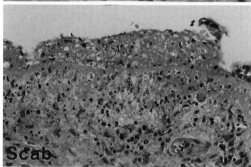

FIGURE 5.7. Sequence of changes in epithelium of the bovine teat cistern during staphylococcal mastitis: vacuolar degeneration in epithelium; microvesicle formation by exuding plasma; ulcer; and scab.

wounds several years old. Even though wounds may be completely healed, they may break down if the animal experiences a severe systemic disease that represses collagen synthesis for long periods.

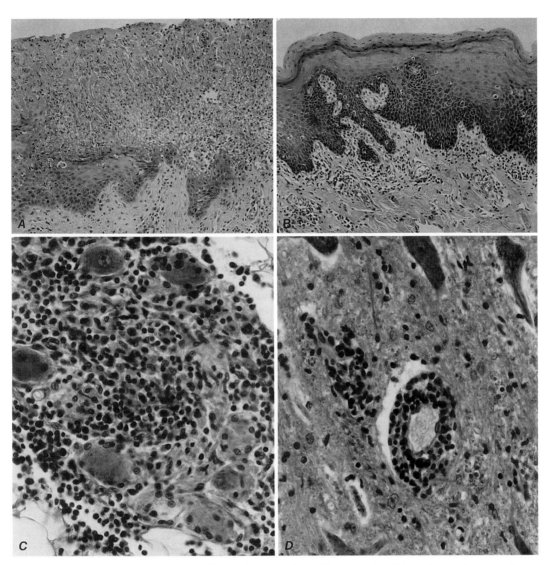

FIGURE 5.8. Healing lesions, monkey with herpesvirus B infection. A. Scab over lip ulcer, 7 days after appearance of first lip lesion. B. Healed epithelium with subepithelial lymphocytes, 12 days. C. Lymphocytic ganglionitis, trigeminal ganglion, 21 days. D. Lymphocytic perivasculitis, trigeminal ganglion, brain.

Scabs retard epithelization

Scabs form in wounds exposed to the air (Figs. 5.7 and 5.8). Although the dry exudate is a protective cover against pathogenic bacteria on the skin, it may also inhibit wound healing. The advancing epithelial cells do not attach to the scab and must grow beneath or circumvent the necrotic material. This is accomplished more quickly if the wound is kept moist and free of bacteria.

Systemic disease and local factors inhibit healing

Aging, protein deficiency, vitamin C deficiency, and endocrine deficiencies (especially in diabetes

mellitus) can seriously inhibit wound healing (Table 5.2). Fibroplasia, extremely active in neonates, is delayed in aged animals. In aged animals, elastic fiber degeneration (senile elastosis) can be seen histologically as splitting and granulation of collagen fibers. Deposition of collagen and matrix material is restricted in cartilage and bone, which seriously affects wound healing in these tissues in aged animals. Fibroplasia in wounds is also inhibited by tissue debris and bacteria. Less important factors are decreased temperature, irradiation, and foreign bodies such as talcum powder granules. Clinically, fibroplasia is enhanced by elevated body temperature and by debridement, the surgical removal of necrotic tissue.

TABLE 5.2. Factors that retard wound repair

1. Contamination
   - Pathogenic bacteria or fungi
   - Foreign body debris
2. Inadequate blood supply
3. Systemic hormonal disorders
   - Diabetes mellitus
   - Hyperadrenocorticalism
4. Inadequate nutrition
   - Vitamin C
   - Protein
5. Movement or failure of restraint
6. Old age
7. Chemotherapeutic drugs and radiation
8. Immunodeficiency diseases

Wounds of starved animals heal slowly

In starvation and protein depletion there is an impairment of collagen synthesis and granulation tissue formation. This seems to be most critical with regard to proteins containing methionine and cystine. These sulfur-containing amino acids are important in the intermediate forms of collagen.

Cold inhibits wound healing

Generally, wounds heal more slowly in cold weather, and experiments on poikilotherms have shown that the rate of wound healing is proportional to the temperature of the environment at which they are kept. A rise of 10°C results in a 2-fold increase in the speed of wound healing. In hibernating squirrels at 5°C, epithelization of granulation tissue is totally inhibited.

Wound dehiscence

Dehiscence (the bursting open of a wound) is especially important in surgical incisions of the abdomen. Weakening of the sutured wound results from severe inflammation. Edema puts marked tension on sutures, which, if not properly placed, will fail to hold fascial planes and peritoneum. **Movement** delays healing by persistent trauma; it also appears that exercise can delay healing through an effect on adrenal corticosteroid secretion. Vomiting, coughing, and any straining movement that puts pressure on the wound may precipitate dehiscence. In most animal species, biting and chewing of sutured wounds also leads to wound dehiscence.

Mortality is high after wound dehiscence, largely because of bacterial infection, aided by contamination of the wound by soil and organic matter. **Peritonitis** (inflammation of the peritoneum) is often fatal and makes further attempts at wound suturing more difficult.

CHRONIC INFLAMMATION AND ABNORMAL HEALING

Hyperplasia

Stimulation of tissue growth that accompanies acute and chronic inflammation is stopped as tissue returns to normal. In some instances the irritant persists, causing tissue overgrowth that requires clinical attention.

Occasionally, in some species such as the horse, granulation tissue has a tendency to become excessive and may restrict function. This **keloid**, or "proud flesh," proliferates massively, often resembling tumor formation.

Epidermal hyperplasia is protective

Hyperplasia of epithelium is a response to chronic irritation. In skin, this response is common in parasite infestations. Grossly, the skin becomes thickened, hairs disappear, and the expanded stratum corneum causes the epidermis to scale (Fig. 5.9). This barrier prevents a parasite and its toxins from interacting with subcutaneous tissue.

In viscera, hyperplasia of epithelium may lead to proliferative lesions that reduce normal function. Hyperplasia of the epithelium of the terminal bronchioles in pneumonia can produce lesions that inhibit normal lung function. Several diseases of the intestine involve excessive proliferation of mucosal epithelium. Proliferative enteritis of pigs and hamsters is associated with thickened intestinal walls made largely of reduplicated mucosal epithelium (Fig. 5.10).

Atrophy

Destruction of tissue or suppression of epithelial regeneration during acute inflammation may lead to atrophy. A common response to enteric infection is atrophy of intestinal villi. Villi shrink from the normal, slender, elongate forms to short, stubby protuberances. The marked reduction of mucosal absorptive surface area results in malabsorption. **Villous atrophy** is due both to destruction of epithelium and to contraction of smooth muscle in the lamina propria of the villus, which pulls the villus toward the base of the gut wall. In transmissible gastroenteritis of piglets, the infecting virus has a tropism for epithelium of the upper villus; destruction causes the core of the villus to retract, resulting in shortened villi. In contrast, panleukopenia virus of cats, which replicates in crypt epithelium (killing off the progenitor cells that are destined to populate villous surfaces), also causes severe villous atrophy.

FOCUS

Parasites in Gastric Ulcers

TO PREVENT SPREAD OF PROCESSES such as necrosis, inflammation, and neoplasia, biological mechanisms have evolved to sequester causal agents in foci of initial contact. For example, as some parasites attach to gastrointestinal mucosa, they produce small foci of necrosis and ulceration. These foci become underlined first by acute and then by chronic inflammatory tissue. Chitinous oral hooks of parasites produce erosions and ulcers surrounded by hyperplastic squamous epithelium and chronic focal fibrosing gastritis with many plasma cells. The surface of the pit contains many aerobic and anaerobic bacteria. Opportunistic bacteria attach to the site of epithelial damage, but this threat is largely neutralized by invasion of the tissue by plasmacytes that produce and release antibodies that initiate the process of bacterial uptake and killing.

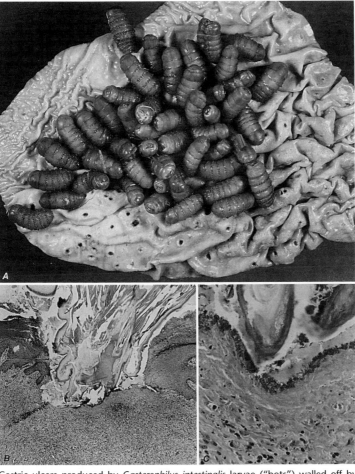

Gastric ulcers produced by *Gasterophilus intestinalis* larvae ("bots") walled off by chronic inflammation. A. Detachment of larvae leaves ulcers on the gastric surface. B. Histology of attached parasite. C. Layer of bacteria between parasite hooks and inflammatory disease.

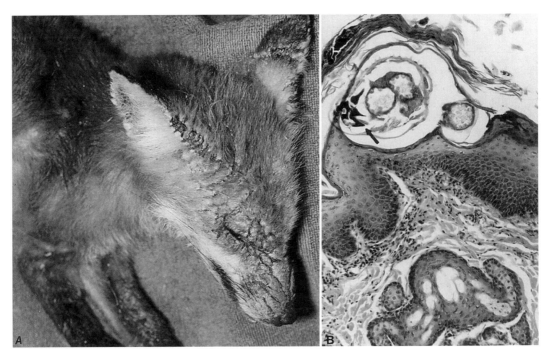

FIGURE 5.9. Severe diffuse chronic dermatitis, fox with sarcoptic mange caused by *Sarcoptes scabiei*. A. Extensive epidermal hyperplasia is responsible for thickening of skin. B. Parasite is present in cornified layers (note hooks, *arrow*).

Turbinate atrophy

Atrophy of the bony and connective tissue components of the nasal turbinates is a consequence of chronic rhinitis. For example, gray collies with cyclic hematopoiesis suffer recurring episodes of chronic mucopurulent rhinitis. After a few episodes, the nasal turbinates have become smaller than those of normal dogs. **Atrophic rhinitis** is a major disease of swine (Fig. 5.11); tissue destruction is due to soluble toxins secreted by bacteria that colonize the turbinate surfaces (*Pasteurella multocida* and *Bordetella bronchiseptica* are the most often implicated).

REPAIR IN SPECIAL TISSUES

Bone

In the simple traumatic fracture of a long bone, the broken ends of the bone are misaligned, and adjacent soft tissues are torn. Blood vessels are ruptured. **Hemorrhage** occurs throughout the fracture zone, and if blood seeps past the torn periosteum, it occurs in muscle. **Coagulation** of blood soon forms a clot that fills the spaces of the fracture. **Necrosis** occurs because of vascular damage; this develops in bone because the osteocyte, which depends on nutrients from canaliculi of the haversian system, is deprived of its precarious source of nutrition. Peri-

osteum and marrow are better vascularized normally, so that necrosis is much less evident in those tissues. As trauma-induced **inflammation** develops, monocytes pass into the fracture area and transform into macrophages that play a major role in bone repair (Table 5.3).

Fracture is repaired by callus formation

Within 48 hours after fracture, the blood clot is invaded by osteogenic cells of the deep layer of the

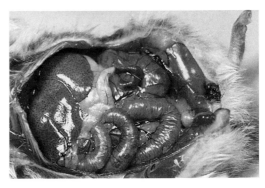

FIGURE 5.10. Chronic diffuse enteritis with dilatation of the intestinal lumen and thickening of the gut wall, hamster with proliferative ileitis.

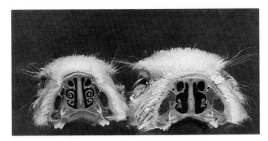

FIGURE 5.11. Tissue destruction and atrophy, pig with atrophic rhinitis (normal nose, *left*). Purified toxin given intranasally produced rapid atrophy of nasal turbinates. (Photograph: Mark Dominick, *Am J Vet Res* 47:1532, 1986)

periosteum, the endosteum, and the marrow. These cells proliferate at the margins of the fracture and quickly invade the clot and adjacent necrotic areas.

The **callus** is the tissue mass that connects fractured bone ends. Early, when the mass is granulation tissue, it is a "soft callus"; later, when formed of cartilage and bone, it is a "hard callus." If bone ends are inadequately immobilized, as is common in animals, the granulation tissue phase is prolonged and formation of hyaline cartilage is favored over bone formation in the callus (Fig. 5.12).

Cartilage is formed early

By 1 week, proliferating cells have begun to differentiate into chondroblasts, and cartilage is laid down. Matrix material released from the surface of chondroblasts is deposited in a halo surrounding the cell. In calcifying cartilage, tiny matrix vesicles are released that possess enzymes (alkaline phosphatase and enzymes for ATP-dependent calcium transport) that increase the local concentration of orthophosphate and lead to hydroxyapatite formation. At 7–10 days, the pH in the callus increases, and this "alkaline tide" favors deposition of calcium salts.

The cartilage that forms has only a temporary existence and is eventually replaced by woven bone, which is remodeled, in time, to lamellar bone. The intercellular matrix calcifies, which causes the chondrocytes to die.

New bone is formed as cartilage disintegrates

New trabeculae of bone are firmly cemented to old bone, even though the old bone ends may be dead. Osteocytes develop from pluripotential mesenchymal cells and fibroblasts and deposit **osteoid**. As dead calcified cartilage disintegrates, it is removed, and osteoblasts lay down osteoid that calcifies to form bone.

As the provisional bony callus is removed, osteoblasts lay down osteoid in a more orderly arrangement. The collagen molecules orient around blood vessels to form haversian systems.

Phagocytic cells are important in removal and rearrangement of the new bone. Osteoclasts, phagocytic cells derived from monocytes, adhere to surfaces of bone trabeculae to resorb bone. The cancellous bone that is first laid down is gradually altered to form compact bone, and the callus continues to remodel itself. Eventually, with good apposition and minimal callus response, the original alignment of the bone is restored, and the thickened callus cannot be detected by palpation.

Osteomyelitis

Bacterial infection of the bone marrow arises from severe local trauma or from septicemia with localization of bacteria in the bone marrow. It commonly leads to progressive debilitating inflammatory disease and lameness. **Osteomyelitis** is often resistant to antibiotic therapy and persists until dead and infected bone chips are removed. Bacterial infection of bone can become sequestered by fibrosis and new bone, which make the delivery of antibiotics difficult. These lesions often require surgical intervention to complete healing and recovery.

Traumatized and dead pieces of bone are especially likely to become colonized with bacteria (and so do orthopedic prostheses). "Polymicrobial" infections are common and usually involve symbiosis of aerobic and anaerobic bacteria, all held together in a matrix of bacterial polysaccharides. Adherence

TABLE 5.3. Wound healing in an uncomplicated fracture

Immediate	Hemorrhage and hematoma formation
	Clotting at fracture line
	Invasion of macrophages, which begin to remove debris, RBCs, fibrin
	Necrosis of osteocytes at fracture lines (hypoxia)
Days 1–5	Edema and fibrin deposition in soft tissues around fracture
	Granulation tissue invasion of the clot
	Chondroblast and osteoblast proliferation from periosteal and endosteal margins
Days 3–7	Provisional callus formation as bone is bridged by granulation tissue and islands of cartilage
Weeks 1–4	Bridging of provisional callus by network of osteoid trabeculae produced by osteoblasts; formation of bony callus by calcification
Weeks 4+	Remodeling of bone: continued osteoclast removal and osteoblast formation; removal of external callus; hollowing of internal callus to form bone marrow

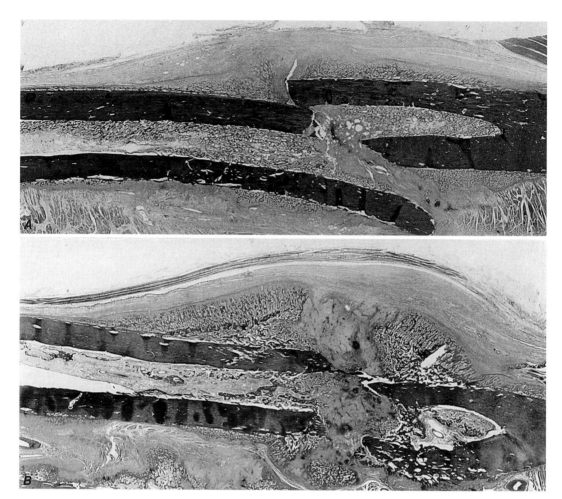

FIGURE 5.12. Prolonged healing of bone due to improper alignment, bone fracture, dog. A. Ten days after fracture: swelling, increased vascularity, and residual hemorrhage. The bone is not properly aligned. Resorption of old bone is limited. Trauma line contains a zone of debris (crushed tissue, extravasated blood, fibrin, bone fragments, and residual marrow). Callus (proliferating tissue) is formed by two sources: activated periosteum and activated endosteum. B. Large callus, 28 days after fracture. Callus is calcified, and there is layering of periosteal cells. Excess new bone formation. (Sections: American College of Veterinary Pathologists, Scientific Seminar, 1958)

of most bacteria in microcolonies in tissues is through highly hydrated anionic exopolysaccharide polymers that bind to teichoic acid polymers (of gram-positive bacteria) or to lipopolysaccharides (of gram-negative bacteria).

Joint capsule

The **joint capsule** of synovial joints consists of an outer fibrous layer, continuous with the periosteum of the bone, and the synovial membrane or inner-layer synovial membranes line the joint everywhere except over articular cartilage. Disease of the synovial joints is a cause of lameness and disability. **Arthritis**, inflammation of the joint, cripples in both acute and chronic phases. Acute fibrinous arthritis

is particularly important in swine, in which mycoplasmas, streptococci, and *Erysipelothrix* bacilli are common causes of acute arthritis when they localize in the synovial membrane and joint cavity.

The extensive exudation in most acute forms of arthritis distorts and effaces the architecture of the synovial membrane. When bacteria gain entrance to the joint cavity, they are phagocytized by synovial lining cells. Pyogenic arthritis is initiated by development of hyperemia and fluid exudation. Long filopodia develop on synovial cells, and they avidly take up bacteria. This is followed by rapid and intense neutrophil exudation.

Chronic arthritis involves fibrosis and synovial cell hyperplasia of the synovial membrane. These lesions tend to be irreversible and self-sustaining; proliferative lesions into the synovial cavity provoke not only pain but also a superimposed subtle inflammatory response.

Brain

Inflammation of the brain, meninges, and spinal cord is called **encephalitis, meningitis, and myelitis**, respectively. The earliest events of inflammation (those that are involved in fluid accumulation) are critical in the brain because this organ cannot expand beyond the limits of the cranium. Even minimal swelling in the brain may cause neurologic signs. If swelling occurs in highly sensitive areas in the brain stem, death may occur.

Acute inflammation (encephalitis)

Fluid accumulation within the brain substance, or neuropil, is separated classically into **brain swelling** (intracellular accumulation of fluid, within glial cells) and **brain edema** (accumulation of fluid in the extracellular spaces). In most cases, fluid is present at both sites. Astrocytes are most severely involved, and marked swelling of the cell and its processes leads to secondary changes in adjacent myelin sheaths.

Purulent encephalitis is commonly caused by bacteria

Exudation of inflammatory cells leads to serious consequences in the brain. **Purulent encephalitis** is nearly always due to bacterial infection. Neutrophils actively pass out of the capillary wall and accumulate in the neuropil. Bacteria most often arrive by way of the bloodstream, commonly during pyemia as metastatic emboli.

Purulent exudate in the neuropil tends to accumulate in microabscesses. If the animal survives, these abscesses become walled off by a capsule of connective tissue and lymphoid cells. Caseous necrotic material remains in the center of the abscess.

Lymphocytic encephalitis is characteristic of viral infection

Acute lymphoplasmacytic encephalitis (also called nonsuppurative or aseptic encephalitis) is usually of viral origin. Most neurotropic viruses replicate in vascular structures prior to spreading to glia and neurons, but others arrive hematogenously or via nerve sheaths and affect neurons directly. The lymphoid response leads to accumulation of lymphocytes and often monocytes in perivascular spaces. Called **perivascular cuffing**, these inflammatory cell populations are often mixed; as disease progresses, plasmacytes appear. Plasmacytes can and do enter infected neurons, although this process does not play a major role in recovery.

Repair

Repair in the brain occurs by proliferation of fibroblasts and glial cells along vascular networks. When the neuropil is punctured by a sterile instrument, the lesion heals by **astrocytic gliosis** and **fibrosis**. The lesion becomes filled with a fibrous core derived from the meninges and perivascular adventitia.

Astrocytes respond to injury

The glial reaction to brain injury is rapid. Astrocytes are less vulnerable than are nerve cells and, if they are not destroyed during injury, react progressively to form a dendritic network around the wounded neuropil. Necrotic brain tissue initiates reactive astrocytosis. The **reactive astrocytes** (also called fat astrocytes or gemistocytic astrocytes) are very large cells with homogeneous, acidophilic cytoplasm. They are stimulated by edema and ischemia and are most common in slowly progressing and diffusely sclerotic lesions. They develop at the margins of a lesion, and their cell processes extend into the affected area. Reactive astrocytes are phagocytic and play a dominant role in the repair of brain tissue, especially in large defects.

Microglia are phagocytic

Microglia are migratory, actively phagocytic cells of the neuropil. They engulf lipids and remnants of necrotic dendrites and neurons. In the process, they accumulate large amounts of lipids and are referred to as **foam cells** (also gitter cells, or lipid phagocytes). **Neuronophagia**, the phagocytosis of nerve cells by microglia, should be distinguished from **satellitosis**, which is the residence of oligodendrogliocytes around neurons. In the process of reacting to injury in the brain, microglia undergo enlargement, hyperplasia, and autophagy. Nodules of hyperplastic microglia, called **glial nodules**, are characteristic of some rickettsial and viral encephalitides. **Monocytes** also enter the neuropil. Most of the macrophages found in inflammatory lesions in the brain in late stages of encephalitis originate from circulating monocytes.

Oligodendrogliocytes are involved in demyelination

Oligodendrogliocytes undergo acute swelling in injured areas. Their nuclei become pyknotic, and the cytoplasm is vacuolated. These cells bear the same relation to myelin as do the Schwann cells to peripheral nerves, and they are most reactive in lesions characterized by extensive demyelination. The presence of several oligodendrogliocytes around a nerve cell body is referred to as **satellitosis**.

ADDITIONAL READING

Antoniades HN, et al. 1993. Expression of growth factor and receptor mRNAs in skin epithelial cells following acute cutaneous injury. *Am J Pathol* 142:1099.

Clark RAF, et al. 1996. Transient functional expression of αvβ3 on vascular cells during wound repair. *Am J Pathol* 148:1407.

Kipar A, et al. 1998. Immunohistochemical characterization of inflammatory cells in brains of dogs with granulomatous meningoencephalitis. *Vet Pathol* 35:43.

Majno G. 1998. Chronic inflammation: links with angiogenesis and wound healing. *Am J Pathol* 153:1035.

Rhyan JC, Saari DA. 1995. A comparative study of the histopathologic features of tuberculosis in cattle, fallow deer (*Dama dama*), sika deer (*Cervus nippon*), and red deer and elk (*Cervus elaphus*). *Vet Pathol* 32:215.

Rothschild KJ, et al. 1983. Polypeptide transforming growth factors isolated from bovine sources and used for wound healing in vivo. *Science* 219:1329.

Sacco RE, et al. 1996. Cytokine secretion and adhesion molecule expression by granuloma T lymphocytes in *Mycobacterium avium* infection. *Am J Pathol* 148:1935.

Schmid P, et al. 1998. Enhanced expression of transforming growth factor-β type I and type II receptors in wound granulation tissue and hypertrophic scar. *Am J Pathol* 152:485.

Smith RS, et al. 1997. Fibroblasts as sentinel cells. *Am J Pathol* 151:317.

Squier CA, Kremak DR. 1980. Myofibroblasts in healing palatal wounds of the beagle dog. *J Anat* 130:585.

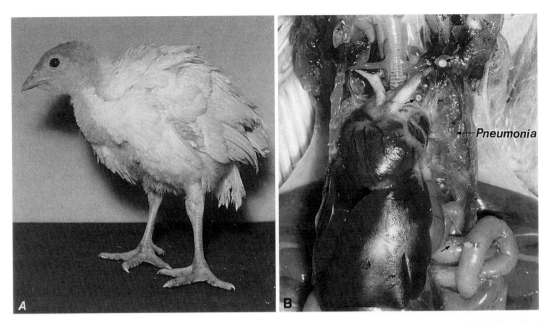

FIGURE 6.1. Aspergillosis, turkey. A. Emaciation, lethargy, and anorexia. B. Purulent airsacculitis and colonies of fungi *(arrows)* in the air sacs.

CHAPTER 6

Immunopathology

In the broadest sense, **immunity** is resistance to disease. An animal is considered immune when it is resistant to a disease process. The word originated to describe immunity to some of the great animal and human plagues, many of which are still serious causes of death, especially in young animals. Although common usage of the term *immunity* often implies resistance to **infectious disease**, the mechanisms that make an animal immune play critical roles in the control of abnormal growth, in neoplasia, and in other pathologic processes.

All living animals must recognize and eliminate foreign material to survive in a hostile environment. Lower animals depend heavily on nonspecific mechanisms such as encystment, phagocytosis, and intercellular digestion. Mammals possess the most complex immunologic apparatus and, in general, have three major ways to resist pathogenic microorganisms: barriers in skin and mucous membranes, cellular and humoral factors that affect immunity by nonspecific mechanisms, and systems of lymphocytes and plasma cells that have both specificity and memory.

When born into an environment of reasonable temperature, given adequate food and water, and not exposed to predators, young animals are at greatest risk from infectious diseases. Biologic mechanisms for resistance have evolved to deal with pathogenic microbes. These same mechanisms also operate against toxins, tissue grafts, and neoplasms.

DISORDERS ASSOCIATED WITH REDUCED IMMUNITY

The consequences of reduced immunity are infectious diseases that are rarely, if ever, seen in animals with normal immune functions. For example, horses with hereditary combined immunodeficiency of-ten suffer acute respiratory disease due to an equine adenovirus or to the protozoan *Pneumocystis carinii,* two agents not known to affect foals that receive proper colostral antibodies and have intact lymphoid systems. Fungi are notorious for causing disease in immunosuppressed animals, particularly those with cold stress and heat stress (Fig. 6.1). Birds are particularly susceptible, and the fungal disease aspergillosis is common in newly hatched cold-stressed chicks and in penguins housed in warm environments.

Chemical and physical barriers of body surfaces

Epithelial barriers of the skin, gut, and respiratory tract are bridged continuously with opportunistic bacteria that the host eliminates with remarkable efficiency. Normal animals breathe in dust bearing large numbers of fungal spores without ever suffering disease. These situations change markedly when the immune system is crippled. No longer eliminated, these microorganisms of low virulence play an important role in causing disease. Chemical barriers on epithelial surfaces include antimicrobial proteins in mucus, lipids in cornified layers of skin, and hydrochloric acid in the gastric lumen. Movement of surface hairs and of respiratory cilia prevent stable contact of microbes with tissue surfaces.

Defects in normal bacterial flora

All body surfaces and orifices have characteristic normal resident microflora, the secretions of which prevent overgrowth of pathogenic bacteria. For example, nonpathogenic bacteria colonize skin, teeth, urogenital tract, and intestine. These normal microbial populations reduce the growth rates of some pathogenic bacteria through competition for nutrients and adhesion sites.

Defects in ciliary movement

Suppression of ciliary movement in cold environments or through inhalation toxicity can lead to depressed ciliary function and infection of the respiratory tract. This is especially important in birds, which shift from poikilothermy (cold-blooded) at hatching to homeothermy (warm-blooded) soon after hatching.

Congenital defects in the structure of cilia, called the **immotile cilia syndrome**, result in prolonged retention (delayed clearance) of inhaled particulate material in the lungs. Canine patients with this syndrome have widespread evidence of abnormal cilia in the nasal cavity, ependyma, and spermatozoa. Disease is manifest as chronic sinusitis, bronchiectasis, and (in males) infertility. The basic defect is absence or abnormality of the dynein arms in ciliary axonemes. Movement of cilia is slowed and random rather than rapid and directed as in normal cilia.

Defects in secretions

All body secretions contain antimicrobial substances. Saliva, urine, tears, milk, and the secretions of respiratory, intestinal, and urinary tracts all contain potent substances for controlling microorganisms. Antibodies play a major role in defense in these secretions. Hereditary **lysozyme deficiency** occurs in dogs, rodents, and humans. Most instances of lysozyme deficiency are not associated with clinical disease. Some strains of rabbit have leukocytes that are deficient in this antimicrobial protein, yet the rabbits show no marked susceptibility to bacterial infection.

Defects in neutrophils

Phagocytosis and killing by neutrophils and other granulocytic leukocytes, by monocytes and macrophages, and by at least one subpopulation of small lymphocytes are potent nonspecific systemic defense mechanisms. In addition, nonspecific protection is achieved by the actions of lysozyme, lactoferrin, and many other antimicrobial substances in serum and body fluids.

Acquired neutrophil defects

Any depression of neutrophil function leads to an increased susceptibility to disease. Transient effects are common but are of such short duration that no significant clinical disease results. In other cases, an effect on neutrophils is produced, but the suppressive effects on specific lymphoid-induced immunity are even greater, and this system dominates the clinical picture.

Toxic chemicals and radiation induce suppression of **granulocytopoiesis** and predispose animals

to infections. **Corticosteroids** used therapeutically have a suppressant effect. Although most markedly affecting lymphocytes, corticosteroids also inhibit neutrophil expression of integrins and other receptors that promote passage of neutrophils across the vascular wall during inflammation. Studies of bovine neutrophils suggest that corticosteroids reduce neutrophil surface stickiness and attachment of neutrophils to endothelium, thus suppressing their margination and diapedesis, even though bacterial killing may remain unaffected.

Neutrophil dysfunction and metabolic change. In dogs with diabetes mellitus, high blood glucose has a suppressive effect on neutrophil function, and this makes diabetic patients susceptible to some infection by bacteria, particularly staphylococci. Hormones that appear during estrus may have an inhibitory effect on neutrophils, which is sometimes translated into bacterial infections of the female reproductive tract.

Bacteria suppress neutrophils and macrophages. Components of pathogenic bacteria that cause disease can also actively suppress neutrophils and macrophages. Polysaccharides of bacterial **capsules** and **cell walls** markedly inhibit phagocytosis of neutrophils. Some bacteria secrete **exotoxins** that are directly antiphagocytic—for example, the streptolysins of streptococci. Polysaccharides produced by *Cryptococcus* sp. and other fungi inhibit both neutrophils and macrophages, and lesions caused by these fungi are notorious for their lack of cellular exudation.

Viruses suppress neutrophils. Systemic viral infections such as canine distemper and bovine viral diarrhea have suppressive effects on neutrophil function. Although these effects promote secondary bacterial infections, the viruses have a more profound effect on specific lymphoid immune mechanisms.

Congenital abnormalities of neutrophils

Some rare but intriguing genetic abnormalities in neutrophils illustrate the essential role of leukocytes in perpetually monitoring the blood for microbes. **Cyclic hematopoiesis** (cyclic neutropenia) is an inherited disease in collie pups that have a coat color mutation (the gray collie). The bone marrow defect involves cyclic depression of neutrophil maturation, with consequential disappearance of mature neutrophils from the bloodstream every 11 days. Affected dogs develop periodic bacterial infections that coincide with phases of neutropenia. The defect involves insufficient stem cell production and can be corrected by bone marrow transplantation.

Chédiak-Higashi syndrome. The disorder known as Chédiak-Higashi syndrome is characterized by the presence of anomalous giant granules in neutrophils (and in all granule-containing cells), defective pigmentation, and increased susceptibility to infections. Chédiak-Higashi syndrome occurs in partially albino Hereford cattle, killer whales, inbred (beige strain) mice, white mutant tigers, and Persian cats. The primary granules of neutrophils are defective, and although phagocytosis occurs normally, bactericidal activity is diminished. The defect in cattle involves abnormal bactericidal ac-

tivity associated with the hexose-monophosphate shunt and delayed degranulation. Recurrent infections lead to early death. The Chédiak-Higashi defect in the Aleutian mutant strain of mink is the basis for the remarkable susceptibility of these animals to the virus-induced plasmacytosis known as Aleutian disease.

Leukocyte adhesion deficiency. The leukocyte adhesion deficiencies are rare, autosomal recessive disorders caused by a lack of leukocyte integrins. Leukocyte (β_2) integrins are glycoproteins that are essential for normal leukocyte-endothelial

---

FOCUS

Cyclic Hematopoiesis

THE GRAY COLLIE SYNDROME is a lethal hereditary disease associated with abnormal hair pigmentation, cyclic depression of circulating neutrophils, and bilateral ocular scleral ectasia. Neutrophils disappear from the peripheral blood at intervals of 10.5–11.5 days, although intervals between neutropenic phases vary with the severity of disease. Episodes of fever, diarrhea, gingivitis, respiratory infection, lymphadenitis, and lameness (bone necrosis) follow neutropenic phases. Most untreated affected dogs die within a few days of birth, yet some survive only to succumb in early adulthood. The life span of those surviving puppyhood is markedly lengthened if they receive supportive clinical treatment; even so, they eventually develop lymphoid exhaustion, reticuloendothelial hyperplasia with monocytosis, anemia, and amyloidosis.

The wide spectrum of clinical signs and lesions in canine cyclic hematopoiesis is due largely to one basic defect: **cyclic neutropenia**. The basis for periodic cycling of blood cells is unknown, although in normal animals these changes occur in a very subtle manner.

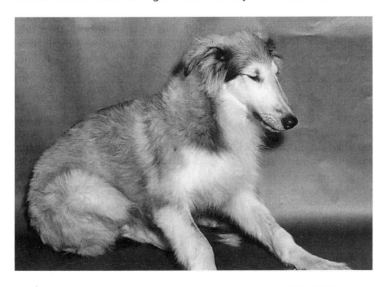

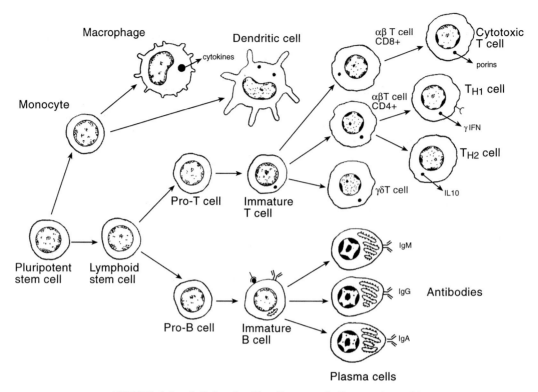

FIGURE 6.2. Cells involved in efferent and afferent wings of immune responses.

cell adherence and emigration. In bovine leukocyte adhesion deficiency (BLAD), affected calves develop recurrent bacterial infections, persistent leukocytosis, and severe lymphoid hypoplasia. Calves have recurrent pneumonia, ulcerative and granulomatous stomatitis, enteritis, periodontitis, and delayed wound healing. Leukocytes from affected animals lack the α subunit (CD11b) of MAC-1, the integrin component that mediates the tight adherence of leukocytes to activated endothelium.

Deficiency of complement

Hypocomplementemia that occurs in inflammation most often results from a consumption of complement during systemic microbial infection. Antigen-antibody reactions use complement to kill bacteria, and the component C3 is particularly important in antibacterial reaction. **Hereditary complement defects** are known that involve individual components of complement: C3 deficiency of Brittany spaniels, C4 deficiency of guinea pigs, C5 deficiency of mice, and C1-inactivator deficiency of humans. In most of these patients there is little or no increased susceptibility to disease, probably because other antimicrobial systems compensate for the deficit.

Incompetent cells of the immune system

Any significant functional deficit in cells of the lymphoid system, or in the cytokines or secretions that they produce, has serious consequences for the host. Plasma cells and lymphocytes operate by highly specific mechanisms that are critical for recovery and prevention of disease on second exposure to the same agent (Fig. 6.2). The actions of these cells and their products are commonly called "immune" mechanisms because they have two striking characteristics: they are **specific** (reacting antibodies and lymphocytes are specifically designed for a particular antigen), and they have **memory** (that is, they are able to be recalled on second exposure to a microorganism, and further encounter produces a more rapid and stronger immunologic response).

Plasma cells

Plasma cells are large plump cells that secrete antibodies. They develop from precursor B cells (Fig. 6.3) and are found not only in the vascular channels of lymph nodes and spleen but also at sites of infection throughout the animal. Plasmacytes have a characteristic "cartwheel" nucleus (large clumps

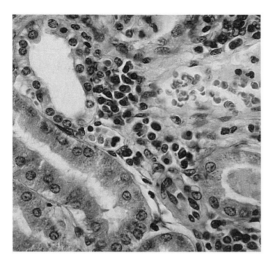

FIGURE 6.3. Plasmacytes in interstitial spaces of kidney, dog with leptospirosis.

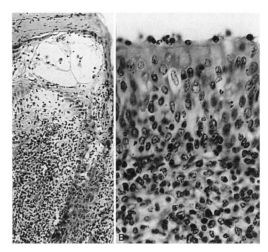

FIGURE 6.4. Lymphocytes, skin, cow with malignant catarrhal fever. A. Lymphocytes throughout dermis and in a microvesicle in epidermis. B. Small lymphocytes below, within, and above epidermis.

of chromatin at the periphery with a large central nucleolus), and their cytoplasm is filled with the machinery of protein synthesis. Globulins that plasmacytes produce are called **immunoglobulins (Ig)** because they have antibody activity (Ig and antibody are physical and functional descriptions of the same entity). Antibodies persist for long periods in serum and extracellular spaces and are the major humoral mechanism of immunity.

As immunoglobulins are secreted from plasmacytes into tissue spaces, they are drained into lymph and transported to the bloodstream. Immunoglobulins persist in circulating blood until the infectious process is resolved, and on reinfection they appear more rapidly in blood. Although antibody production occurs at sites of infection, most antibodies are released in lymph nodes and spleen.

Circulating antibody is especially efficient in preventing spread of infection. It prevents both dissemination of microorganisms through the vascular system and bacterial colonization at sites distant from the primary infection. In some viral infections, plasmablasts attach to the surface of infected cells and secrete antibody directly into the cytoplasm.

Lymphocytes

Lymphocytes play major roles in recovery and immunity by directly attacking microorganisms and by secreting cytokines that enhance many other aspects of immunity. In some infectious diseases, especially viral infections, the cellular aggregates in lesions contain not plasmablasts but a collection of small lymphocytes (Fig. 6.4). The lymphocytes in direct attack on the microorganism or target cell. Called **cell-mediated immunity** (CMI), these reactions are in contrast with the humoral immunity of antibodies. CMI is of primary importance in recovery from some viral infections, in graft rejection, and in many of the hypersensitivity diseases, including poison ivy dermatitis.

Lymphocytes secrete **cytokines** that act via autocrine and paracrine mechanisms to initiate and promote both humoral and cellular immune responses. The contact of lymphocyte with microbe causes the cell to secrete a cytokine that causes other lymphocytes to proliferate and then to attack the microbe. Bacteria that replicate intracellularly are especially prominent in their capacity to induce T cell–mediated immunity, and this reactivity is the most significant reaction in recovery in tuberculosis, brucellosis, salmonellosis, and some of the fungal infections.

Macrophages

Macrophages present antigens to T cells by special mechanisms. **Antigen presentation** involves the taking up of antigen by the macrophage, intracellular processing, and subsequent interaction of T_H cells (helper T cells). These effector T cells will recognize processed antigen only if it is presented with histocompatibility antigens. Macrophages, endothelial cells, B cells, and dendritic cells all have the capacity to present antigens to T cells. Other special antigen-presenting cells include the following:

- **Skin**—Langerhans cells (phagocytic cells within the dermis)
- **Lymph node**—follicular dendritic cells (interdigitating cells)
- **Gut**—M cells (in Peyer's patches)
- **Bone marrow**—reticular cells (lining bone marrow sinusoids)
- **Liver**—Kupffer cells (lining hepatic sinusoids)
- **Lung**—intravascular macrophages (inside alveolar capillaries)
- **Brain**—microglia

Dendritic cells

Dendritic cells (DCs) are a heterogeneous, stellate-shaped subpopulation of the monocyte-macrophage series. They ingest and display antigens on their surfaces to interact with and increase the effectiveness of other lymphocytes. Dendritic cells form a network of sentinel cells to monitor the antigenic environment. Stimulation of dendritic cells initiates their migration across endothelium into the lymphatic vessels and from there into the regional lymph nodes, where the maturing dendritic cell presents antigens to other T lymphocytes.

Blood monocytes have a capacity to differentiate into macrophages or dendritic cells, and the pathway taken is driven by cytokines. From studies in vitro, we know that one cytokine, macrophage colony-stimulating factor (M-CSF), drives monocytes into macrophages, whereas another cytokine, granulocyte-macrophage colony-stimulating factor (GM-CSF), induces dendritic cell formation. Further exposure to TNF-α irreversibly locks these cells into a maturing dendritic cell pathway. Cell signals, released during the processes of phagocytosis and migration across endothelial cells, guide and regulate the development of the mature dendritic cells. For example, differentiation is markedly enhanced during phagocytosis and passage through the vascular wall. In addition to cytokines, certain adhesion molecules are also known to divert monocytes from macrophage lineages into dendritic cell differentiation.

Lymph node and spleen

When foreign antigens first gain entrance past epithelial and inflammatory tissue barriers, they enter lymphatic vessels, drain into regional lymph, and circulate in the blood. The **lymph node** is an important barrier to the spread of infectious agents. As microorganisms arrive in afferent lymph vessels on the cortical surface of the node, they begin to percolate through the reticular cell-macrophage meshwork of the subcapsular sinuses. Long dendritic tentacles on reticular cells avidly trap bacteria. As

bacteria are phagocytized and destroyed, chemotactic factors and pyrogens are released that initiate the local acute inflammatory response and the systemic signs of bacterial infection.

As antigens pass through the cortical zones bearing germinal centers, they are trapped on dendritic webs of **follicular dendritic cells**, whose long dendrites form a network for trapping and transporting foreign proteins. During the immune response, vascular structures of the node expand in association with lymphoid proliferation, and the medullary cords become filled with proliferating plasmablasts.

Passing into the meshwork of the lymph node medulla, bacteria are surrounded not only by macrophages but also by columns of plasmacytes in the medullary cords. This is a plasmacyte-filled end of the funnel of reticular cell meshworks. In immune animals, it is here that bacterial survival is prevented. Antibodies released by plasmacytes in the cords opsonize bacteria in the sinus lymph and present the bacterial clumps to activated macrophages.

If the bactericidal processes within the lymph node sinuses are insufficient to kill virulent bacteria, multiplication of bacteria begins to dominate the balance between host defense and bacterial survival. Replication increases logarithmically within the milieu of exuding plasma proteins, degranulating neutrophils, and activated macrophages. Virulent bacteria are released into the efferent lymph to circulate via the thoracic duct into the bloodstream.

Antigens also must pass the elaborate biologic filters of the spleen. Located in the bloodstream, the **spleen** is ideally suited to trap circulating antigens. Macrophages near reticular sheaths take up and transport antigens to germinal centers in white pulp. In these areas, macrophages have a close association with B cells, the plasmacyte precursors destined to produce antibodies. Antigens are first localized on cytoplasmic extensions of dendritic cells and are then taken into the cell and rapidly degraded.

Congenital immunologic defects

Defective development of the B and T cells responsible for immunologic reactions may result in functional immunologic deficits. In some cases the B and T cell deficits are distinct (Table 6.1). **Thymic hypoplasia**, characterized by absence of thymic tissue and hypoplasia of regions in lymphoid tissues normally populated in the neonate by T lymphocytes, leads to defective cell-mediated immunity (with normal antibody production). In **agammaglobulinemia**, antibody production is depressed, but cell-mediated immunity is normal. The most common and severe defects in animals are com-

TABLE 6.1. Immunodeficiency syndromes

Primary
    Humoral: agammaglobulinemia
    Cellular: thymic aplasia (*nu/nu* mouse)
    Combined: CID of Arabian foals
    Specific Ig deficiency: IgA deficiency
Secondary
    Postviral: hog cholera, feline panleukopenia, bovine
        viral diarrhea
    Neoplasm-associated: plasmacytoma, thymoma,
        lymphosarcoma
    Aging
    Malnutrition
    Drug-induced
    Chemotherapy and radiation treatment

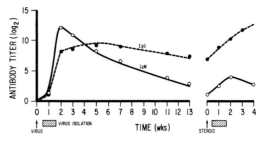

FIGURE 6.5. Corticosteroid-induced disease: viral isolation and serum antibodies in a calf given infectious bovine rhinotracheitis virus. Cortisone treatment caused exacerbation of viral excretion and a rise in antibody titer. (Data: Potgieter et al., *Am J Vet Res* 46:893, 1985)

bined **immunodeficiencies** in which both B and T cell populations are defective and in which antibody production and cell-mediated immunity are both depressed.

Combined immunodeficiency

Severe combined immunodeficiency (SCID) diseases have been reported in horses, dogs, mice, and humans. Canine SCID occurs in basset hounds, Cardigan Welsh corgis, and Jack Russell terriers; SCID in the first two breeds is an X-linked recessive trait affecting only male puppies, whereas in the last it is non-X-linked. Affected pups have generalized lymphoid atrophy, are lymphopenic with reductions in the percentage of T lymphocytes, especially CD8+ subsets, and have low levels of IgG and IgA.

A fatal, genetic combined B and T lymphocyte immunodeficiency occurs in Arabian foals. The clinical diagnosis is based on lymphopenia (less than $1000/mm^3$), hypoplasia of the thymus, absence of germinal centers and lymphoid sheaths in the spleen, and absence of one or more serum Ig class. Laboratory tests for T lymphocytes show markedly diminished function of T cells, and skin graft rejection is prolonged. Foals with combined immunodeficiency are highly susceptible to respiratory disease and usually die from pneumonia. Mortality often occurs from adenoviruses or *Pneumocystis carinii*, neither of which are clinically important in normal immunocompetent horses.

Acquired defects in immunity

Chemical immunosuppression

Immunosuppression can be induced therapeutically by many different mechanisms. These are used clinically to prolong the survival of tissue grafts, to suppress immunologic components of acute inflammation, and to kill neoplastic cells.

Many immunosuppressive agents have nonselective effects. Cortisone has profound effects on both humoral and cell-mediated immune systems (Fig. 6.5). Some agents, however, cause selective destruction of cellular mechanisms. Methotrexate is a powerful inhibitor of dihydrofolate reductase and thereby depresses DNA synthesis by suppressing thymidylate formation. Alkylating agents produce profound suppressive effects by direct toxicity to lymphocytes. They alkylate nucleic acids by forming cross-links with nucleoside bases, thereby interfering with DNA biosynthesis.

Failure of passive transfer of immunoglobulins. Failure of transfer of colostral immunoglobulins in neonates is the leading cause of acquired immunosuppression. Calves are agammaglobulinemic at birth and absorb IgG from colostrum for only 24–36 hours after birth. Any delay in suckling has a marked effect on enhancement of bacterial infection. Calves with less than 10 mg IgG_1/ml are considered hypogammaglobulinemic; values below 5 mg IgG_1/ml are evidence of passive transfer failure.

Animals with failure of Ig transfer are often treated with antibiotics and corticosteroid during the neonatal period. This extends the immune defect by permitting fungal overgrowth and by suppressing host defense mechanisms. Foals with passive transfer failure are prone to develop bacterial septicemia and, if treated with antibiotics, may develop systemic and oral fungal infections such as candidiasis.

Starvation causes immunosuppression

Atrophy of lymphoid tissue is common in cachexia and starvation, especially in young animals. **Thymic atrophy** (or congenital hypoplasia) is most prominent, and the thymus has long been considered a "barometer of nutrition." Thymic regression

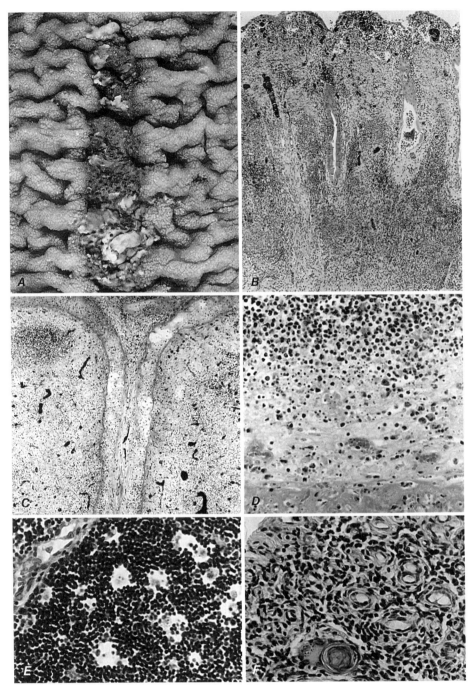

FIGURE 6.6. Depletion of lymphoid tissues in viral disease. A–B. Submucosal lymphoid tissue, jejunum, bovine viral diarrhea. A. Exudate and necrotic debris on surface of Peyer's patch. B. Histology: lymphoid tissue is atrophic, and intestinal villi are fused. C–D. Bronchial lymph node, infectious bovine rhinotracheitis (herpesvirus). C. Marked depletion of lymphoid tissue of cortex with destruction of cortical germinal centers. D. Necrotic lymphocytes. E–F. Thymus, hog cholera. E. Early phase of thymic involution: pale foci are macrophages filled with debris of necrotic lymphocytes. F. Late stage, chronic infection: lymphoid tissues are depleted, and thymic reticulum has collapsed around thymic corpuscles.

occurs in pituitary deficiencies, but the connection of growth hormone with thymic size is not known.

Immunodeficiency syndromes and retroviruses

Acquired immunodeficiency syndromes (AIDS) are progressive wasting diseases in which opportunistic microorganisms kill a host severely immunodepressed by a retrovirus. Feline immunosuppressive viruses cause feline AIDS. In nonhuman primates, several suspect viruses have been isolated, and some produce AIDS as quickly as 2–4 weeks after experimental inoculation. Monkeys given the causal retrovirus develop swollen lymph nodes characterized by marked follicular hyperplasia and reduced paracortical areas (which contain mostly T_S lymphocytes, i.e., suppressor T lymphocytes). Pathogens isolated from tissue lesions include cytomegaloviruses, papovavirus SV40, *Cryptosporidium* spp., *Candida albicans,* and various septicemia-causing bacteria.

Leukemia viruses silently cause immunosuppression

Most **leukemia viruses** produce a phase of immunosuppression soon after infection. No overt clinical disease results, but affected animals develop infections and serious diseases from agents to which that species of animal is not normally susceptible. In cats, a major result of infection with feline leukemia virus (FeLV) is loss of normal immune function. More FeLV-infected cats die from conse-quences of immunosuppression than from leukemia. Young kittens infected with feline leukemia virus often develop hemobartonellosis and other opportunistic infections.

The immunosuppression caused by leukemia viruses is part of a widespread effect on host bone marrow. **Anemia** also occurs in early stages of infection, and although often not clinically important, it is clearly revealed by hematocrit determinations at various intervals. Lymphoid leukosis virus of chickens, which replicates first in the cloacal bursa (a central lymphoid organ for antibody production), will induce an immunosuppressive phase.

Acute cytolytic viruses cause immunosuppression

Many of the viruses that cause severe systemic disease are known to produce transient immunosuppression by virtue of replication in the lymphoid and reticuloendothelial systems. Bovine viral diarrhea, canine distemper, feline panleukopenia, feline infectious peritonitis, hog cholera (swine fever), and Newcastle disease of chickens are some of the more important diseases in which immunosuppression plays a role in viral persistence (Fig. 6.6). The immune system of the host usually loses the race with a particularly virulent strain of virus during the incubation period. Immunosuppression is caused by direct virus-induced **destruction of lymphoid cells** and by several alterations in cell signal molecules that induce **programmed cell death**, or **apoptosis** (e.g., prostaglandin release, phospholi-

---

FOCUS

Feline Immunodeficiency Virus in Fetal Development

FELINE IMMUNODEFICIENCY VIRUS (FIV) is a lentivirus that induces degenerative and immunodeficiency disorders by a selective and progressive depletion of CD4+ lymphocytes. Replication of FIV in the thymus leads to marked thymic atrophy with reduced CD4$^+$/CD8$^+$ thymocytes and the production of cells that bear surface IgG. Maternal-offspring transmission can occur during intrauterine development, and a variety of maternal and viral factors control the incidence of vertical transmission in utero, during parturition, and during neonatal growth. The thymus of kittens infected with FIV as fetuses is particularly affected by atrophy but can regenerate postnatally. Despite recovery in thymus weight and architecture, thymic regeneration does not completely restore the normal phenotypic distribution of thymocytes and continues to support FIV replication.

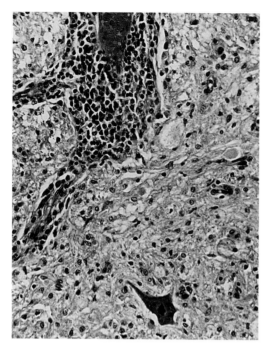

FIGURE 6.7. Postvaccinal encephalitis, rabies, dog. Large collections of lymphoid cells occur around veins and venules.

pase activation, interferon production, and activation of acute phase proteins of inflammation). A variety of chronic diseases follows acute infection by these viruses because of lymphoid destruction and immunosuppression.

Adrenal corticoids cause immunosuppression

The **adrenal cortex** plays a protective role against infection: a normal pituitary-adrenal response is necessary for survival of an animal with severe bacterial infection and septicemia. In an experiment with adrenalectomized mice maintained on graded doses of cortisone and inoculated with pneumococci, survival was greatest in groups whose maintenance cortisol most closely resembled the normal. Mortality was progressively increased toward the extremes of hypoadrenocorticism and hyperadrenocorticism.

Chronic treatment with corticosteroids renders an animal increasingly susceptible to bacterial and fungal infection. Glucocorticoids particularly cause lysis of lymphocytes and apoptotic depletion of cells in central peripheral lymphoid organs. A retrospective study of 16 cases of equine nocardiosis in California (1965–1983) showed that only 2 horses had local lesions associated with wound infection, 14 horses had disseminated

infection, and all were immunosuppressed. Eight were Arabian foals with combined immunodeficiency, 3 had ACTH-secreting pituitary tumors with secondary hyperadrenocorticism, and 3 had systemic disease also known to be associated with immunosuppression.

Can mental stress cause immunosuppression?

Mental anxiety in humans can reduce immune responses and may play a role in animals. In a study of medical students after final exams, T_H cells were reduced, and there was diminished natural killer cell activity. These results can be correlated with activation of herpes simplex and development of "cold sores." Pituitary secretion of ACTH (adrenocorticotropic hormone) and adrenal corticosteroid release are surely involved in this phenomenon.

Rabies in immunodeficient dogs and cats

Live, attenuated rabies vaccines are used to provide preexposure prophylaxis in dogs and cats and less often in cattle. Although **vaccine reactions** do occur in these animals, they are rare. Under appropriate conditions of immunosuppression, disease can be produced by vaccine strains of virus. In cats given the high-egg-passage vaccine, a syndrome of posterior paralysis has been reported. Paralysis began in one hind limb and rapidly spread to the other and then to the forelimbs. Later signs of cranial nerve paralysis occurred. In the brain, inflammatory lesions resembling those of natural rabies were seen. Immunofluorescent tests showed that viral antigens were present in brain tissue; the rabies virus was isolated and shown to be a specific vaccine strain.

In dogs, the same pattern of ascending paralysis has been seen, usually occurring 12–14 days after vaccination with chick embryo origin, the low-egg-passage Flury strain of rabies virus. More serious problems may arise when these vaccines are used in wild foxes, raccoons, and laboratory animals.

Nerve tissue: postvaccinal encephalitis

The centenary of Pasteur's first successful rabies immunization in humans was in 1985. These early vaccines, which were composed of nervous tissue, produced a variety of local and systemic reactions. Although severe local cutaneous reactions and systemic anaphylaxis were major problems, the serious cause of mortality was postvaccinal encephalomyelitis. The patients died of an immune-mediated reaction against their own nerve tissue. It was not until 1928 that it was suggested that nervous tissue in the vaccine was responsible.

Canine postvaccinal allergic encephalomyelitis is a rare complication of repeated immunization using rabies virus grown in brain tissue. Clinical signs of paralysis and disorientation are a result of lymphocyte cuffing and demyelination in the white matter of the brain and spinal cord (Fig. 6.7).

Experimental allergic encephalomyelitis, produced by injecting a laboratory animal with brain tissue extracts, is a widely studied model of immunologic central nervous system disease. The encephalitogenic antigen is a protein in myelin. The lesions are mediated by T lymphocytes and are foci of demyelination surrounded by perivascular lymphocytic infiltrates. Antibodies are present in these animals but do not play a primary role in the disease.

Canine distemper

Dogs treated with immunosuppressive drugs may die of vaccine virus–induced encephalomyelitis. Canine distemper may occur 2 weeks or more after vaccination and is characterized by diarrhea, followed by respiratory signs and then central nervous system signs: myoclonus, trembling, decreased muscle coordination, and convulsions. These signs are due to necrosis of spinal cord funiculi and dorsal horns of gray matter. Eosinophilic nuclear inclusions occur in glia that stain with immunofluorescent stains. Interstitial pneumonitis and severe respiratory disease are characteristic.

Progressive poxvirus infections

Vaccinia virus is a laboratory strain (with origins in cowpox virus) that was used for 200 years as a vaccine for smallpox. It is also used against monkeypox in several species of nonhuman primates. In normal monkeys the vaccine is scarified into the skin and gives rise in a few days to a series of changes: erythema, macule, papule, vesicle, and pustule. The pustule in the scarified dermis heals within a week or so.

In immunosuppressed monkeys, as in humans, **progressive vaccinia** produces chronic tissue damage and death. Viral growth begins to produce satellite lesions around the original site of scarification (Fig. 6.8), and these progress to produce massive necrosis and often death. In very young animals **generalized vaccinia** (the systemic spread of virus) may occur with foci of necrosis in spleen, liver, and other viscera.

Chickens and turkeys are vaccinated against fowlpox and turkeypox by scarifying these viruses into the featherless skin on the wing (the "wing-

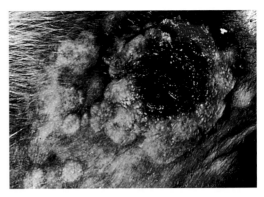

FIGURE 6.8. Progressive vaccinia, lesion that developed after vaccination of monkey with vaccinia virus to protect against monkeypox.

progressive fowlpox can also spread in immunodeficient birds to produce massive vaccine reactions.

Canine parvovirus vaccine may be immunosuppressive

Some parvovirus vaccines cause **lymphopenia** 5–7 days after vaccination, a manifestation of transient immunosuppression that can increase susceptibility to other infectious agents, including canine distemper vaccine viruses. Vaccination of dogs with mixed vaccines of canine distemper 5 days before inoculation of parvovirus enhanced the severity of canine parvovirus enteritis; vaccinated dogs became clinically ill, whereas unvaccinated dogs did not. Lymphopenia occurs after canine distemper vaccination, and parvoviruses may replicate during the rebound stage when lymphocyte proliferation is stimulated.

Gammopathy

Gammopathy is any Ig abnormality. Most gammopathies are neoplastic diseases and are associated with increased plasma immunoglobulins. The Ig arises from neoplastic B lymphocytes or plasmacytes. Systemic plasmacytomas (also called myelomas) are tumors of malignant plasmacytes and are characterized by massive production of light chains of the antibody molecules and defective assembly with the heavy chain components (light chains accumulate in the bloodstream and, because of their low molecular weight, spill over into the urine as Bence Jones proteins).

If only one specific Ig is produced, the gammopathy is called **monoclonal** (e.g., IgA monoclonal gammopathy). Monoclonal components may also be IgG, IgM, or an Ig subunit such as kappa or lambda chains. If different immunoglobulins are present in plasma, the disease is called **polyclonal**,

TABLE 6.2. Categories of hypersensitivity disease

Type	Mechanism	Disease
I	IgE-mediated disease	Anaphylactic shock Food allergy enteritis, dermatitis Postvaccination wheal-and-flare reactions Insect envenomation reactions
II	Cytotoxic disease	Blood transfusion reactions Hemolytic disease of the newborn Hemolytic reactions to drugs
III	Immune complex disease	Serum sickness Arthus reaction Anaphylaxis
IV	Cell-mediated disease	Contact hypersensitivity (poison ivy) Graft rejection syndromes Tuberculin reaction (diagnostic test)

having arisen from more than one clone of Ig-producing cells.

Clinical signs in these gammopathies result from the remarkable elevations in plasma globulins. The **hyperviscosity syndrome** of dogs, characterized by weakness, congestive heart failure, distended retinal veins, and bleeding tendencies, is due to greatly thickened plasma with excess immunoglobulins.

HYPERSENSITIVITY DISEASE

The production of antibody and lymphocytes against microbes is usually associated with **immunity**, and clinical disease does not develop when an animal is reexposed to a specific pathogenic microorganism. In certain situations, however, an excessive reaction to antibody, lymphocytes, or both results in **hypersensitivity** (allergy), which is an exaggerated reaction to antigen.

Hypersensitivity diseases arise from several mechanisms (Table 6.2). Many naturally occurring hypersensitivity diseases are a mixture of these mechanisms, and the reaction that dominates must be differentiated in each individual disease. This section deals only with diseases that are solely due to mechanisms of hypersensitivity. There are many other clinical syndromes in which hypersensitivity reactions play a minor role. For example, the chronic phases of many infectious diseases are complicated by a hypersensitivity component that aggravates the clinical situation but does not significantly affect the outcome of the disease.

IgE-mediated mast cell reactions (type I hypersensitivity)

Type I hypersensitivity (referred to as **anaphylactic hypersensitivity**) arises from interaction of an antigen with antibodies bound to mast cells or basophils in an animal that has been previously sensitized to the antigen. The reaction occurs rapidly, within minutes after antigen-antibody contact. Mast cell release reactions due to non-IgE mechanisms are sometimes called **anaphylactoid reactions** and can arise from other mast cell secretagogues such as interleukin-8, melittin of bee venom, and physical agents such as ultraviolet light, heat, and cold.

Explosive IgE-mediated mast cell reactions of anaphylaxis occur only during a second exposure to certain types of antigens. The antigen must contact cytophilic antibodies bound to the surfaces of mast cells or basophils. IgE is involved in most reactions: receptors on surfaces of mast cells and basophils combine with the Fc part of the IgE molecule during the immune response and are held there in wait for contact with antigen. In subsequent exposure, antigen forms bridges between antibody molecules to trigger the rapid release of inflammatory mediators.

On contact with antigen, sensitized mast cells release their granules, which contain pharmacologically active agents that produce the clinical signs. Histamine, heparin, eosinophil chemotactic factor, and neutrophil chemotactic factor are the primary mediators of mast cell damage. Secondary factors arise from products released from plasma membrane breakdown, all of which induce acute inflammatory reactions. Platelet-activating factor (PAF) causes platelets to aggregate at the sites of reaction. Leukotrienes (LTs) C_4 and D_4 are more potent than histamine in producing vascular permeability and smooth muscle contraction (e.g., bronchoconstriction in the lungs). LTB_4 is chemoattractive for eosinophils, neutrophils, and monocytes. The flow of the reaction is as follows:

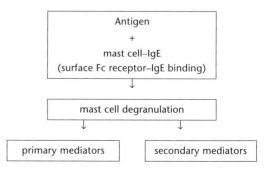

Antigen
+
mast cell–IgE
(surface Fc receptor–IgE binding)
↓
mast cell degranulation
↓   ↓
primary mediators   secondary mediators

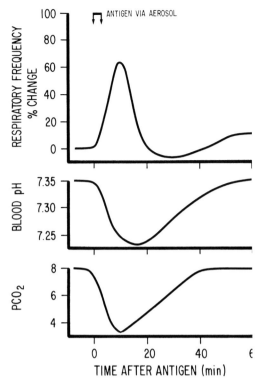

FIGURE 6.9. Anaphylaxis: changes in respiratory rate, blood pH, and oxygen.

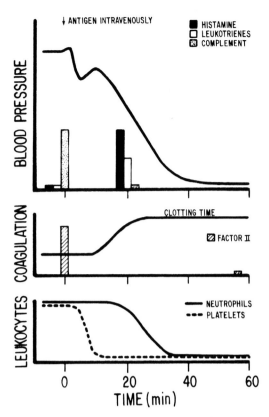

FIGURE 6.10. Changes in blood pressure and blood during anaphylactic shock (aggregate anaphylaxis).

Systemic anaphylaxis

Rapid systemic distribution of antigen is a requirement for systemic anaphylaxis, and the severe form of this disorder, **anaphylactic shock**, usually follows an intravenous injection. As antigens combine with antibodies on mast cell surfaces and granules are released, there are precipitous decreases in blood pressure accompanied by smooth muscle contraction, capillary dilatation, and edema—all systemic effects of mast cell granule release. Accumulation of edema fluid is particularly severe in the upper respiratory tract (especially if that is the site of antigen entry), and affected animals may die from laryngeal obstruction and asphyxia. If the animal survives for several hours, platelets and neutrophils may be trapped in lungs and lead to intravascular coagulation.

Early signs involve lung; death is due to shock. Anaphylaxis is an unusual or exaggerated allergic reaction. It is most common after parenteral administration of drugs or vaccines but also can occur after inhalation or oral exposure. The signs of anaphylaxis are respiratory distress, a precipitous decrease in blood pressure, leukopenia, and decreased amounts of fibrinogen and complement in plasma (Fig. 6.9). All these clinical signs can occur, or any one of them may appear as an isolated manifestation. Horses are prone to die of respiratory problems and cardiovascular collapse during anaphylaxis and show tachypnea, harsh wheezing sounds, increased heart rate, weak thready pulse, cyanotic mucous membranes, and prolonged capillary refill times.

Different species show differing reactions in anaphylactic shock. In dogs and horses, the intestine may be an important "shock organ," especially if the antigenic challenge is prolonged. Increased peristalsis leads to diarrhea and hemorrhagic lesions in the intestine. Cattle, sheep, and swine may react similarly. In dogs, the liver is also an important shock organ. Severe congestion is followed by ischemic necrosis of hepatocytes, largely due to vasoconstriction's causing blood to pool in liver and intestine, which leads to hypotension and shock (Fig. 6.10).

Local anaphylaxis

Focal, pruritic, edematous cutaneous lesions characterized histologically by mast cell degranulation and vascular hyperpermeability are referred to as **wheals**. Assumed to be IgE-dependent, these lesions are transient and respond to drugs that suppress acute inflammation.

In dogs and cats, flea bites are seasonally recurring dermatitides with unusual dorsal body distribution and intense pruritus. Flea allergy is the most common small animal hypersensitivity skin disease. It probably results from a hypersensitivity reaction to insect saliva similar to that occurring in horses associated with repeated bites by *Culicoides* spp. Cats with ear infections of *Otodectes cynotis* have precipitins to mite antigens and develop wheal-and-flare reactions at sites of reinfection. In Australia, Queensland itch is an allergic dermatitis caused by hypersensitivity of horses to biting midges (*Culicoides robertsi*). Papules form and are followed by pruritus, alopecia, and crusting.

The term **atopy** implies a familial association with localized anaphylaxis. Atopic reactions are immediate and involve such organs as skin (urticaria), upper respiratory tract (rhinitis, or hay fever), and bronchioles (asthma). Antigens can, in some cases, be demonstrated to be bound to mast cells.

Allergic inhalant dermatitis

Only in dogs has IgE-mediated atopic disease been adequately studied. Skin is the target organ and pruritus the primary sign; it is an "itch that rashes rather than a rash that itches." Like humans, most atopic dogs are multisensitive and allergic to many allergens. Curiously, there is no significant difference in amounts of serum IgE between normal and atopic dogs.

The cause of **allergic dermatitis** in dogs is usually pollen allergy, most often ragweed pollen, and many pollens are unreactive in atopic dogs (e.g., nettle pollen). Clinical associations include age (most frequently 1–3 years), season (spring and summer), and intercurrent skin disease (flea infestation). In some areas, nearly one-third of dogs admitted for dermatologic examination are atopic, and there is some breed predisposition. Of 29 atopic dogs in a California study, 38% were golden retrievers; 56% were born during pollen seasons, suggesting that sensitization during the first month of life is important. Viral infections appear to predispose to allergy in atopic dogs. Pups vaccinated for canine distemper before being given pollen extract had greater IgE antibodies in serum than did unvaccinated pups.

Food allergy enteritis-dermatitis

Intestinal mucosal immune responses to food antigens may be due to atopic allergy. For example, atrophy of intestinal villi and lymphocytic infiltration into the lamina propria have been seen in calves and piglets fed soy proteins. Although atopic reaction may be responsible for malabsorption in neonates, cell-mediated immunopathic enteritis usually is the source of the problem in adults.

Cytotoxic disease (type II hypersensitivity)

Cytotoxic diseases are initiated when circulating antibodies (either IgG or IgM) attach to antigens on cell surfaces. Cell lysis is caused when circulating complement attaches to the cell-bound antibodies, and neutrophils then bind to the Fc portion of antibodies. The attack sequence of complement components is responsible for the actual lysis of cells.

Complement-induced cytolysis

Clinical disease resulting from cytotoxic reactions involves predominantly blood cells. Although the most severe clinical reactions occur against erythrocytes (to cause anemia), cytotoxic diseases also develop from antibody-mediated, complement-induced attack on leukocytes (causing granulocytopenia) and platelets (causing thrombocytopenia). In all of these diseases, antibodies bound to the cell surface attract complement, the attack sequence of which causes 100-nm holes to appear in the plasma membrane. Lysis results from loss of potassium ions and from entry of sodium and calcium ions and water into the cell.

Naturally occurring cytotoxic diseases are complex and may also involve cell-mediated mechanisms, that is, the direct action of sensitized lymphocytes on cell surface antigens. Recent studies indicate that some lymphocytes (those with natural killer and T cell cytotoxicity activities) produce tiny membranous vesicles called **perforans** that are released on contact with target cells. Perforans attach to the cell surface of the target cells and induce holes similar to those produced by complement.

Transfusion reactions

Isoantibodies are formed against antigenic cell proteins (isoantigens), which differ among individuals of the same species. Generally, isoantibodies are important in relation to cellular antigens, such as those on erythrocyte surfaces. In normal baby pig sera, isoantibodies may develop against globulins that have crossed the maternal-fetal barrier.

In 1900, Karl Landsteiner discovered the isoantigens A and B (and consequently the blood groups A, B, AB, and O) in human red blood cells. These form the strict limitations of human red blood cell transplantation. "Blood type" is based on differences in sugar moieties of glycoprotein isoantigens of the erythrocyte's plasma membrane: type A contains an enzyme that transfers acetylgalactosamine to the core protein, type B an enzyme that transfers galactose, and type O lacks both enzymes.

Similar antigenic differences exist in animals. Although some of these are termed A, B, and so on, they are unrelated serologically to human isoantigens or to each other. Isoantigens are not confined to red blood cells but are present on surfaces of endothelial and epithelial cells of the epidermis, thymic corpuscles, and intestines.

Transfusion reactions result when blood with erythrocyte **isoantigens** of one type is transfused to individuals with circulating **isoantibodies** against it—for example, blood with A isoantigen given to an individual with type B blood (and A isoantibodies). Clumping and lysis of the donor erythrocytes in the vascular system of the recipient result in embolization, pulmonary vascular blockade, and death. Because of the rapid dilution of donor antibodies, the opposite reaction of clumping of recipient erythrocytes by donor isoantibodies does not cause clinical disease.

Hemolytic disease of the newborn

Hemolytic disease occurs in newborn horses, mules, calves, and swine. The fetus, by virtue of inheritance from the sire, develops erythrocyte antigens not present in the mother. When these cells gain access to the mother's bloodstream, they induce antibody formation. If these antibodies are returned to the newborn via colostrum, severe hemolytic anemia is induced. Absorption of antibodies occurs via milk in horses and swine, but in humans, transplacental transfer of antibody occurs, resulting in a similar disease called erythroblastosis fetalis. Thrombocytopenia caused by a similar mechanism has been reported in piglets and puppies with platelet deficiency and hemorrhages.

Hemolytic anemia caused by antibodies to erythrocytes can occur when the mother has been injected with blood or blood products; for example, antierythrocyte immunoglobulins appear in serum and colostrum of cows vaccinated against anaplasmosis with vaccines containing blood cells.

Hemolytic reactions to drugs

Hemolytic anemia during prolonged drug therapy, particularly with penicillin, occurs in some animals. The most common mechanism involves the formation by the drug of a hapten on the erythrocyte surface that then binds antihapten antibodies to cause erythrocyte lysis.

In cats, propylthiouracil is used for treatment for hyperthyroidism and may cause a hemolytic reaction. Clinical signs, which appear in 20–35 days, include lethargy, weakness, anorexia, and bleeding. Severe anemia is accompanied by thrombocytopenia. The direct antiglobulin (Coombs') test is positive, and serum antinuclear antibody titers exceed 1:10. Cessation of treatment is accompanied by disappearance of anemia.

Anemia has been reported in response to sulfadiazine in Doberman pinschers. The dominant sign was lymphocytic polyarthritis, and the dogs also had lymphadenopathy, myositis, and skin rashes.

Immune complex disease (type III hypersensitivity)

Immune complex diseases are due to the damage induced in tissues by antigen-antibody-complement complexes that produce an inflammatory response. They occur in two ways: (1) when antigen-antibody complexes form in the bloodstream and circulate to lodge in delicate vascular channels such as the renal glomerulus, choroid plexus, or vascular channels of synovia; and (2) when circulating antibody attaches to antigens in tissue sites, with production of a damaging inflammatory reaction directly in the tissue.

The size and character of the antibody are often more important than the nature of the antigen. Small complexes remain in circulation and are not trapped in blood vessels. Large complexes are insoluble and are quickly removed by the reticuloendothelial system. Medium-sized complexes remain in circulation, fix complement, and are trapped in small capillaries.

In situ deposition of immune complexes

Arthus reaction. The classic **Arthus reaction** is produced in rabbits by two intradermal injections of the same antigen at the same site at an interval of greater than 24 hours. Antibody produced locally after the sensitizing injection reacts with the antigen injected on the second, challenge dose. Antigen-antibody-complement complexes form directly within vascular walls and lead to acute vasculitis with hemorrhage, infiltration by neutrophilic leukocytes, and necrosis of the blood vessel wall (Fig. 6.11). Complement is strongly chemotactic for neutrophils, which rapidly degrade antigens. However, lysis of neutrophils also occurs, and release of enzymes from neutrophil granules causes the disastrous tissue injury.

Arthus reactions are common, subtle components of parenteral immunization procedures. Antigens in the vaccine localize in the vascular wall, complex with antibody (produced during previous immunizations), and combine with complement. Most of these reactions are transient and subclinical. Although occasional bothersome dermal lesions occur after immunization, they are more likely to involve acute reactions induced by reaginic antibodies and histamine release.

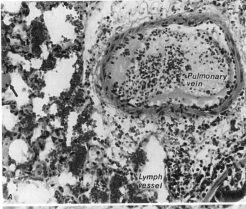

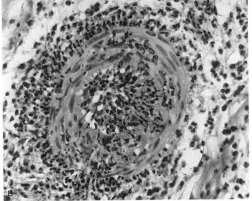

FIGURE 6.11. *Top,* anaphylaxis, lung: dilatation of the pulmonary vein, capillaries of alveolar septa, and lymph vessel. Fibrin thrombi *(arrow)* block some capillaries. Erythrocytes are present in interstitial spaces (hemorrhage). Part of a bronchiole is at lower right corner. *Bottom,* Arthus reaction, skin, rabbit. Heterophils (rabbit neutrophils) have infiltrated and destroyed the wall of an artery.

Arthus-type reactions occur in the recovery stages of some infectious diseases, for example, the ocular lesions following acute infectious canine hepatitis. Partial resolution of the acute, primary, virus-induced iridocyclitis occurs, with viral antigens persisting in the anterior uvea. Antibody produced locally by plasmacytes in the iris and limbus reacts with cell-associated antigen, triggering a hypersensitivity reaction that appears clinically as corneal opacity, or "blue eye" (Fig. 6.12).

Focal edematous lesions of skin that appear as exacerbations of acute infectious disease may be due to the interaction of systemic antibody with persisting dermal antigens. A subacute dermatitis caused by *Sarcoptes scabiei* heals and disappears, and a generalized pruritus with erythematous skin lesions may appear several weeks after infection.

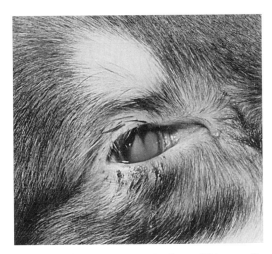

FIGURE 6.12. Corneal edema ("blue eye"), sequel to vaccination for infectious canine hepatitis.

Allergic alveolitis

An immunologic reaction, largely of the Arthus type, is induced on the alveolar wall of sensitized animals by large aerosols of extrinsic particulate antigens. Lesions in the lung include infiltration of the alveolar wall with lymphocytes, macrophages, and plasmacytes. In severe cases, epithelioid granulomas that obliterate bronchioles occur, probably because of a complicating cell-mediated type of hypersensitivity.

Allergic alveolitis occurs in cattle and horses exposed to spores of *Micropolyspora faeni,* which are common in old, moist hay. *Thermoactinomyces* spp. are also responsible for pulmonary allergies in animals, especially *T. viridis,* one cause of "fog fever" of cattle. The large number of allergic pneumonitides that occur in humans are named according to the occupational hazard involved: for example, "farmer's lung" (due to *M. faeni*), "cheese washer's lung" (due to *Aspergillus clavatus* and *Penicillium casei*), "wood pulp worker's lung" (*Alternaria* spp.), and "paprika slicer's lung" (*Mucor* spp.). The lesions in these diseases are usually a chronic Arthus reaction, for there are multiple exposures of the lung to antigen. Lung biopsies reveal extensive fibrosis, vascular reactions, and perivenular lymphocyte accumulations. This suggests the participation of cellular hypersensitivity, which is often the case in these complex reactions.

Immunologic reactions of the respiratory system to organic dusts depend on the distribution pattern of antigens and on host reactivity. Atopic dogs and humans have bronchial asthmatic reactions, which are mediated by nonprecipitating reaginic antibodies. Nonatopic individuals react to dust antigens predominantly with precipitating antibodies, which induce alveolitis typical of an Arthus-type reaction.

Glomerulonephritis

Immunologic injury to the renal glomerulus can result from the direct deposition of circulating immune complexes, from attachment of circulating immune complexes, or from attachment of circulating antibodies to exogenous antigens trapped in the glomerular filtration barrier. In the rare autoimmune glomerulonephritides, antibodies that cross-react with antigens that are components of the normal glomerular basement membrane will combine in situ with that material to produce glomerular disease.

All lesions of **immune complex glomerulonephritis** involve irregular granular hyalin deposits beneath the vascular endothelium (Fig. 6.13). Immunofluorescent staining can reveal the presence of antigens, complement, and immunoglobulins within these dense deposits. Affected glomeruli are hypercellular because of infiltration of inflammatory cells. Accumulations of monocytes (with some activation to macrophages) are the most common, although neutrophils dominate in some types of immune complex reactions. The actual site of trapping in the glomerulus may be in the capillary endothelium, its basement membrane, or the slits of foot processes of the epithelium. The normal renal filtration barrier restricts molecules greater than 4.5-nm in diameter. Trapping in the glomerulus is influenced by the size of the immune complex (large complexes cause mesangiopathic glomerulonephritis, whereas smaller complexes lead to membranous glomerulonephritis) and the charge of the complex (highly cationic complexes are trapped most avidly). Systemic factors that influence trapping include (1) drugs (corticosteroid hormones and amine antagonists); (2) liver disease (failure of the liver to trap circulating immune complexes, especially IgA); and (3) thrombosis-enhancing factors. Furthermore, excess circulating antigen may cause release of complexes in glomeruli by conversions of large latticed deposits to smaller complexes.

Chronic infection is the major cause of **immune-mediated glomerulonephritis**. Membranous glomerulonephritis is especially common in **bacterial sepsis**, especially chronic infections involving *Escherichia coli* (e.g., colisepticemia, coliform mastitis, and cystic endometritis of dogs). Local bacterial lesions have massive infiltration of plasma cells and produce large amounts of immunoglobulins, which form complexes with antigen that in some way become trapped in the renal glomerulus to cause basement membrane thickening and expansion of the glomerular mesangium.

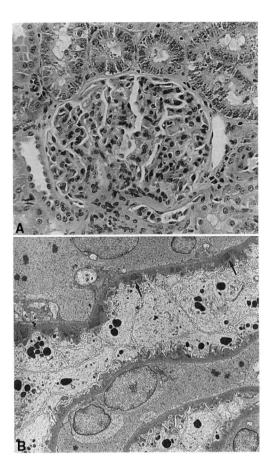

FIGURE 6.13. Immune complex membranous glomerulopathy. A. Dog with dirofilariasis. Capillaries in the glomerulus have markedly thickened basement membranes. B. Ultrastructure of electron-dense granular deposits in the basement membrane of the capillary *(arrows)*.

Some **chronic viral infections** characteristically induce immune complex glomerulonephritis: bovine viral diarrhea, hog cholera, and equine infectious anemia. Malignant lymphoma in cats, mice, and humans due to leukemia viruses induces renal glomerular deposits stainable for immunoglobulins and viral antigens (glycoproteins from the viral envelope). Renal lesions develop in feline infectious peritonitis, a lethal disease involving ascites, and diffuse fibrinous peritonitis has a major immunologic component; kittens with antibody in their serum develop more serious disease than do kittens that have not been exposed to the virus.

Aleutian disease, a major problem of commercial mink ranching, is caused by a parvovirus that replicates in macrophages and persists in high tier in blood, spleen, and lymphoid tissues. Viral replication is not associated with overt tissue lesions but induces an extreme immune response to viral antigens. Disease results from deposition of virus-antibody complexes and plasmacytes in tissues. Like many of the viral glomerulopathies, intravascular coagulation often contributes to the glomerular lesions.

In canine Lyme borreliosis, a unique glomerulonephritis involving diffuse tubular necrosis and progressive interstitial nephritis, 10% of affected dogs develop membranous glomerulonephritis with subendothelial deposits of IgG, IgM, and C3.

Serum sickness

Serum sickness was a disease of animals and humans in preantibiotic days when large amounts of horse serum were injected intramuscularly to produce passive immunity to infectious diseases. Lesions begin when antibody forms and appears in serum before the injected antigen has been removed. Antigen-antibody complexes develop in the bloodstream and are deposited in joints, kidney, and sites of serum injection. The renal glomerulus is the significant site of injury. Deposits of antigen, antibody, and complement below the capillary endothelium block the passage of glomerular filtrate. With immunofluorescent techniques applied to sections of the kidney, the antigens, host immunoglobulin, and complement can be detected in the granular deposits along the capillary basement membrane.

FOCUS

Anaphylactic Shock

SERUM SICKNESS WAS COMMON in animals used in serum laboratories in the 1890s. It was also known that some horses repeatedly immunized with tetanus or diphtheria antigens to produce antiserum suddenly collapsed and died when given a second or third injection. In 1894, Simon Flexner reported that dogs immunized to proteins died abruptly after a second exposure to the same protein. Human deaths were brought to light after a notorious case of the daughter of the renowned pathologist Paul Langerhans; she was taken to a clinic for preventative treatment for diphtheria and died within 5 minutes after receipt of antiserum.

These syndromes occur through complex mechanisms but are grouped together as **anaphylaxis**, a term coined in 1902 to describe the dichotomous response to immune serum; the immunizing, or "prophylactic," response occurred when serum was given initially, and the hypersensitizing, or "anaphylactic," response occurred after repeated inoculation.

Anaphylactic shock, an immediate life-threatening reaction, arises from two mechanisms: (1) IgE-mediated mast cell degranulation (type I hypersensitivity) and (2) deposition of immune complexes, which induces coagulation in the pulmonary capillary bed. This "aggregate anaphylaxis" occurs when large amounts of antigen are given intravenously. Antigens combine with IgG, and the resulting antigen-antibody complexes bind complement. Complement causes the complexes to stick to endothelium and to attract leukocytes. In the binding to complement, fragments of complement are released that induce blood coagulation and leukocyte degranulation.

Aggregate anaphylaxis killed Flexner's dogs. The animals died because the pulmonary circulation was irreversibly blocked by clots of fibrin, platelets, and neutrophils that were trapped in the pulmonary vascular bed.

Cell-mediated hypersensitivity (type IV hypersensitivity)

Cell-mediated hypersensitivity arises from specific, sensitized T cell–induced damage; B cells and antibody are not required. This pattern of diseases involves **recognition** of antigen of T lymphocytes (T_{dh} subset), secretion of **cytokines** by the activated T cell, and **attraction of effector cells**, chiefly monocytes activated by the process and transformed into macrophages. Effector cells produce tissue injury by secreting lymphotoxins or by directly attacking target cells. Histologically, the typical cell-mediated hypersensitivity lesion is composed of aggregates of lymphocytes and monocytes. With time, the lesion transforms into accumulations of activated macrophages.

T cell–mediated cytotoxicity is an important component of many infectious diseases. It often complicates exudative and necrotic processes that are induced by antibodies and affects clinical signs and pathologic evidence of tissue injury. Because of its powerful activating effect on macrophages, the cytokine interferon-γ (IFN-γ) is very important in cell-mediated reactions. IFN-γ increases the capacity of macrophages to kill bacteria, viruses, and fungi.

Contact hypersensitivity

Cell-mediated mechanisms are the most prominent in skin, largely because the sensitizing agent must diffuse through the skin barrier and can avoid stimulating antibody production, which would complicate the disease process. Drugs and toxins act as haptens by combining with protein in the skin epithelium. The conjugate is then carried to the regional lymph node, where it stimulates an immune response by lymphocytes. On the second exposure, the antigen is trapped in the epithelium by specialized macrophages (epidermal Langerhans cells). They have Fc and immunoglobulin receptors and antigens of the major histocompatibility complex on their surface. They play a key role in taking up and presenting antigens to lymphocytes during induction of delayed hypersensitivity in skin.

Contact hypersensitivity is common. Dermatitis caused by proteins in poison ivy, cosmetics, or drugs is a frequent type of human contact hypersensitivity. One of the most common contact hypersensitivities is "cement eczema," caused by allergy to hexavalent chromium salts present in cement. In animals, hypersensitivities to protein components in vaccines are probably the most common. Cell-mediated reactivity as a **component** of other syndromes can be proved by testing on the skin using a dermal patch. Filter paper soaked in dilute sensitizing antigen is placed on the skin, cov-

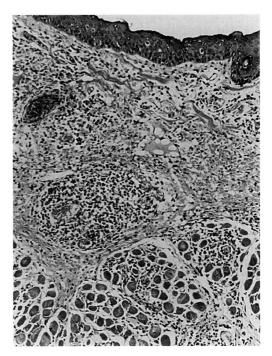

FIGURE 6.14. Tuberculin reaction, eyelid, rhesus monkey. The dermis is expanded by edema fluid. Large aggregates of small lymphocytes occur in the dermis around venules.

ered with tape, and examined after 12 hours. Swelling peaks at 24–48 hours and is taken as a positive sign of cell-mediated reactivity.

Delayed hypersensitivity

The **tuberculin reaction** is a diagnostic test produced by a delayed hypersensitivity response. Tuberculin (purified protein derivative, or PPD) is a relatively nonantigenic extract of soluble mycobacterial proteins. When injected intradermally into a tuberculous animal, it incites an inflammatory reaction characterized by increased vascular permeability to fluid and neutrophils and perivascular accumulation of lymphocytes and macrophages (Fig. 6.14). The character of the lesion is determined by the purity of the tuberculin and the severity of tuberculosis.

Although a vigorous tuberculin reaction develops in the early stages of tuberculosis, **anergy** occurs in the terminal stages. Anergic animals do not respond to tuberculin, probably because of extensive dissemination of bacillary antigens throughout the host that depletes lymphoid tissue and renders remaining host lymphocytes and macrophages unresponsive.

Hypersensitivities of this delayed type can be elicited in skin in most infectious diseases, but only in tuberculosis and some fungal diseases are they used clinically as diagnostic aids.

Graft rejection

If the technical aspects of skin grafting are correct (e.g., proper surgical alignment and absence of infection), skin transplants between **syngeneic** (genetically identical) animals vascularize and become accepted as host tissue. Grafts between **allogeneic** animals (not identical but of the same species) become necrotic and slough in 10–14 days. Rejection of grafted skin is preceded by infiltration of the dermis by small lymphocytes and monocytes, largely in a perivenous location. Vascular damage occurs and induces ischemia, which in turn causes death of the graft.

A second skin transfer and graft from the same donor will result in a more rapid rejection by the recipient. This rapid "second set" reaction is specific for the original donor skin and has other characteristics of a specific immune reaction; that is, rejection is inhibited by immunosuppressant drugs and can be transferred with lymphocytes but not with serum. In dogs given bone marrow grafts, two graft-versus-host syndromes occur. **Acute** rejections (median onset, 13 days; median survival, 29.5 days) are characterized by skin erythema, jaundice, diarrhea, and gram-negative bacterial infections. **Chronic** rejections (median onset, 124 days; median survival, 150 days) include skin ulceration, ascites, cirrhosis, gram-positive infections, and epidermal atrophy.

Histocompatibility antigens cause rejection. The immunologic basis of rejection of grafted tissue is a direct expression of genetic differences between donor and recipient. Rejection occurs against **histocompatibility antigens**, which are proteins inserted in the membranes of the cell surface of the grafted cells. The nature of these histocompatibility antigens has been well defined. In all cases these antigens make immune reactions highly specific.

Lymphocytes directly attack graft tissue. The majority of grafted organs in nonimmunosuppressed recipients are rejected within 4 weeks by mechanisms of cell-mediated immunity. Contact between sensitized lymphocytes and foreign cells destroys the latter. How the small lymphocytes mediate graft rejection is not precisely known. It is theorized that sensitized cell–antigen interaction releases a factor involving nonsensitized monocytes. The monocytes dominate in the graft, and release of lysosomal enzymes is responsible for tissue damage.

Tissue grafts are rejected by complex mechanisms. Human organ transplantation has revealed complex mechanisms of tissue rejection.

For example, kidney allografts may be rejected at three time periods after grafting, each representing a different dominant mechanism. (1) **Peracute rejection** begins immediately and is mediated through activation of complement; platelets and neutrophils are prominent in the lesions and accumulate in glomerular and peritubular capillaries. (2) **Acute rejection** begins in a few days and is caused by the cellular immunologic processes described above; small lymphocytes accumulate around intertubular capillaries in the grafted kidney and destroy it. (3) **Chronic rejection** may occur after many months; it is related to vascular degeneration.

Graft-versus-host reaction

The **graft-versus-host reaction** is an immunologic response that occurs when lymphocytes are transplanted and proliferate to attack the recipient animal, because they react against histocompatibility antigens of the host. The recipient of immunologically active lymphocytes is destroyed by the attack of these cells on its tissue.

There are three requirements for graft-versus-host reactions. First, the donor and recipient must have different strong histocompatibility genes. Second, the recipient must be incapable of an efficient immune response to reject the graft, so neonatal animals are the best candidates. Third, donor cells must be immunocompetent; adult lymphocytes are best, and the reaction is accelerated with cells from a preimmunized donor. Grafts such as epithelium cannot mount an immune response and so are incapable of initiating this reaction.

Clinical signs of graft-versus-host reactions are growth failure (often called runt disease), diarrhea, and emaciation. At necropsy, lymphoid depletion and hepatosplenomegaly are seen. Myocardium, intestinal mucosa, liver, and other organs contain accumulations of macrophages. In animals, graft-versus-host reactions are a complication of bone marrow grafting used in the treatment of immunodeficient or stem cell–deficient animals. In combined immunodeficiency of Arabian foals, injection of thymic cells has been followed by widespread infiltration of tissues with lymphocytes and death of the recipient.

AUTOIMMUNE DISEASE

In **autoimmune disease**, the animal's own tissue acts as an endogenous antigen to incite production of antibodies or sensitized lymphocytes. The normal **state of tolerance** is broken. That is, an autoimmune disease results from breakdown of the tolerant state for self-proteins, and this leads to the production of autoantibodies and sensitized lymphocytes.

In the normal animal, the mechanisms that prevent autoimmune responses to self-antigens include central tolerance, peripheral tolerance, and clonal avoidance. **Central tolerance** depends upon the death of developing T and B lymphocytes as they encounter self-antigens in the thymus and bone marrow. Sometimes called clonal deletion, this mechanism involves the removal and elimination of T cells that begin to express self-antigens during development. **Peripheral tolerance** depends on lymphocyte destruction when these cells encounter self-antigens in peripheral tissues, outside the thymus or bone marrow. Peripheral tolerance depends on a continuous monitoring of lymphoid cells for reactivity to self-antigens, and their removal from the body by some form of cell death. **Clonal avoidance** depends on the sequestration of self-antigens from immunocompetent lymphocytes, either by anatomic isolation or by defective presentation of self-antigens to lymphocytes (in the absence of co-signals that are required for an effective immune response). Antigen recognition by lymphocytes without second signals may lead to this state of functional unresponsiveness, also called clonal anergy.

Programmed cell death of self-reacting lymphocytes is brought about by several mechanisms, and mutations in genes that control death processes can lead to induction of autoimmunity. One of the major mechanisms that triggers induction of programmed cell death is the interaction of that cell surface protein and its receptor, Fas–Fas ligand (FasL). Fas–FasL interactions on the lymphocyte surface are responsible for activation of programmed cell death of developing and mature T lymphocytes. Mutations in the Fas or FasL gene are associated with autoimmune syndromes of lymphoproliferation. Other single-gene defects that appear to be causal in autoimmunity include the interleukin-2–IL-2 receptor interaction.

Autoimmune disease typically develops without any clearly established predisposing disease process, and the mechanisms by which self-tolerance is reduced in specific autoimmune diseases is not always clear. Whatever the case, the **tolerance of CD4+ T_H cells** is critical in preventing autoimmunity. Breaking of T_H cell tolerance is triggered by exposure or modification of previously masked self-antigens, and a subsequent reaction of these antigens with nontolerant T_H cells.

Two important mechanisms for breaking T_H tolerance are (1) **autoantigen modification** through complexing of self-antigens with drugs or microorganisms (e.g., some autoimmune hemolytic anemias appear to arise from drug-induced alteration of the erythrocyte surface); and (2) **partial degradation of autoantigens** that exposes new antigenic determinants (e.g., the partial enzymatic degradation of collagen appears to make this molecule more antigenic than normal collagen).

In some diseases, new antigens generated by molecular change can trigger autoimmunity—by exposure of new epitopes on normal proteins. Rheumatoid factors, a group of human antibodies directed against γ-globulin, are among the most common autoantibodies of humans. They are present in very low amounts in normal individuals and in higher concentrations in patients with immunologic disease, especially those with rheumatoid arthritis and lupus erythematosus.

The frequent association between infections and autoimmunity is thought to be due to activation of anergic, self-reaction lymphocytes by neighboring cells that are reacting to microbial antigens. For example, viral infections are thought to trigger some autoimmune diseases, but the causal association in most cases is tenuous. A genetic component is often involved, and many autoimmune diseases tend to have a familial pattern of development.

Tissue-specific autoimmune disease

Autoimmune thyroiditis

Lymphocytic thyroiditis with signs of thyroxin deficiency occurs naturally in dogs, rats, chickens, and humans. Thyroiditis may be caused either by autoantibodies or by lymphocyte-mediated mechanisms. Most affected animals have antithyroid antibodies in serum, but the precise mechanism of pathogenesis seems to involve T lymphocytes. In most species, there is a genetic predisposition to disease. In dogs, Dobermans have a high incidence and are predisposed to develop thyroiditis as pups.

Biopsy of affected thyroids reveals infiltrates of lymphocytes and plasma cells, often in large interstitial masses with germinal centers. T cells attack surfaces of thyroid follicular epithelial cells and cause the dog to be hypothyroid. Thus, the clinical signs of dogs with autoimmune thyroiditis include obesity, lethargy, hair loss, hyperlipidosis, and pyoderma. Circulating antibodies to thyroid hormone are present in about 50% of hypothyroid dogs and circulating antigen-antibody complexes in about 20%. In early cases, dogs are symptomatic (or until three-fourths of the thyroid is nonfunctional).

Thyroiditis in a strain of white Leghorn chickens is used as a model of B lymphocyte–mediated thyroiditis. Adults have excess body fat, small skeletons, silky feathers, poor laying records, and sensitivity to low environmental temperature—all changes associated with hypothyroidism. Plasmacytes and even germinal centers develop in the thyroid and circulating autoantibodies to thyroglobulin are present in serum.

Autoimmune hemolytic anemia of dogs

Autoimmune hemolytic anemia of dogs is characterized by severe hemolytic anemia and thrombocytopenia. The anemia is usually regenerative; thus high reticulocyte counts are common, and increased erythroid activity is demonstrable in bone marrow smears. Antibodies attached to the surface membranes of erythrocytes induce hemolysis or promote removal of the cells by macrophages in the spleen. The spleen becomes filled with degenerate and dead erythrocytes.

Clinical laboratory tests corroborating the diagnosis of autoimmune hemolytic anemia include a positive direct antiglobulin (Coombs') test and low hemoglobin with spherocytosis of erythrocytes. The positive Coombs' test indicates that the dog has antibody or complement on erythrocyte surfaces (but it does not establish that antibody is specifically directed toward the erythrocyte); false positive results may occur in drug toxicity and parasitemia.

Thrombocytopenia usually accompanies autoimmune anemia. In the first major study of 19 cases of canine autoimmune hemolytic anemia, 14 dogs had thrombocytopenia, and 6 of these had purpura. Glomerulonephritis with wire-loop lesions (thick basement membranes encircling capillaries of the glomerulus) were seen in some cases. These phenomena must be differentiated from idiopathic thrombocytopenia (where only antiplatelet antibodies are present) and lupus erythematosus.

Autoimmune anemia may be acute or chronic. The pathogenesis of autoimmune anemia is complex because of the variation in types of antibodies involved. Affected dogs may have the following categories of autoagglutinins: (1) saline-reacting antibody, which causes erythrocyte clumping visible on drawing blood into saline solution (disease in these dogs is usually sudden with a poor prognosis); (2) in vivo hemolysin, which causes massive intravascular erythrocyte destruction accompanied by sudden onset of icterus; (3) incomplete antibody, in which erythrocytes are coated but not lysed and are removed by the spleen (onset tends to be gradual); and (4) cold hemagglutinin, in which the autoantibody is not fully active at body temperature (hemoglobinuria may occur, and skin lesions develop caused by ischemia from intravascular agglutination; Coombs' tests are negative at 37°C but positive at 4°C).

Cold hemagglutinin disease occurs in dogs and horses. Cold hemagglutinin disease, also called cryopathic autoimmune hemolytic anemia, is a subtle syndrome. IgM-class autoantibodies are present in large amounts in serum. Anemia is much less evident than in "warm" anemia, except when animals are exposed to cold. Skin lesions arise from capillary stasis because of erythrocyte agglutination and lysis. In dogs, they involve the nose, ears, and extremities.

Immune complex conjunctivitis

Bilateral conjunctivitis and recurrent vaginitis have been reported in poodles associated with immune complex deposition. Severe keratitis and corneal ulceration often develop. In the human form (Sjögren's syndrome), plasmacytic aggregates develop in conjunctivae and lacrimal glands, and autoantibodies against nictitating membrane epithelium (a tear-forming organ) are present. Parenchymal destruction of salivary and lacrimal glands by invading lymphocytes leads to decreased secretion and fibrosis.

Immune complex orchitis

Rare cases of autoimmune orchitis have been reported in several species. Normally, sperm is isolated and not exposed to immune process, but under conditions poorly understood, an immune response is directed toward spermatozoa. A naturally occurring infertility in black mink males is associated with autoimmune orchitis. Affected mink have antisperm antibodies in serum, aspermatogenesis, and monocytic orchitis. Autoimmune orchitis is characterized by decreased size of epithelial cells, increased thickness of basement membranes, and deposition of dense deposits of immune complexes.

Immune complexes develop in the testes after vasectomy, which confines sperm to the epididymis and proximal vas deferens, where they degenerate and are engulfed by macrophages. During this process, sperm antigens leak into the circulation and, in some animals, stimulate formation of autoantibodies.

Idiopathic polyneuritis

Idiopathic polyneuritis of dogs ("coonhound paralysis") is a postinfectious autoimmune disease. Progressive paralysis begins 7–14 days after the dog has been bitten or scratched by a raccoon. Affected dogs are afebrile and alert, and signs of disease vary from weakness to flaccid symmetric quadriplegia. The ventral nerve roots of the spinal cord and some peripheral nerves have lesions of segmental demyelination and perivenular lymphoid infiltrates.

Experimental allergic neuritis of dogs (produced by injecting ground nerve tissue) has similar lesions. Neutrophil infiltration, both perivascular and in foci, occurs early, followed by nerve degeneration and demyelination, especially in lumbar and sacral spinal roots.

Neuritis of the cauda equina, a disease of equine spinal nerves, resembles the Guillain-Barré syndrome. The clinical signs of paralysis of the tail and urinary and intestinal sphincters are due to disintegration of myelin and infiltration of monocytes and macrophages into the sacral intradural rootlets.

Idiopathic polyneuritis (Guillain-Barré syndrome), a postinfectious paralytic disease of humans, resembles canine polyneuritis. Guillain-Barré syndrome is usually transient and follows upper respiratory infections such as influenza. An autoimmune mechanism is involved in the segmental demyelinating lesions in the spinal nerve roots and peripheral nerves that cause the clinical signs.

Myasthenia gravis

Progressive muscular weakness and low tolerance to exercise, the clinical signs of **myasthenia gravis**, result from autoantibodies that bind to and block acetylcholine receptors at motor endplates. Affected endplates become short, with wide, attenuated secondary synaptic clefts (their terminal axon remains normal). In late stages, lymphoid cells invade synaptic clefts, diminishing the total area of the postsynaptic membrane and the release of acetylcholine.

Dogs affected with myasthenia gravis suffer from muscle weakness that responds to anticholinesterase therapy. Alterations have been demonstrated in the presynaptic and postsynaptic elements of the junctional regions of the motor endplate by electron microscopy. A **congenital form** of myasthenia gravis in Jack Russell and smooth fox terriers has reduced acetylcholine receptors in muscle without any demonstrable autoantibodies to receptors in serum.

Pemphigus

Pemphigus is a group of diseases of dogs and humans characterized by bullous lesions of the skin and mucous membranes. In canine pemphigus, which arises as an autoimmune disease of oral mucous membranes, bullae develop because of loss of coherence of epithelial cells and development of acantholysis. Autoantibodies in serum are directed against glycoproteins of epithelial cells.

Pemphigus foliaceous is a variant of pemphigus in which bullae occur on the face and ears. It is a painful skin disease manifest by pus-filled blisters (pustules) and crusts and is the most common autoimmune skin disease of domestic animals. Bullae form under the stratum corneum rather than just above the basal layer. They progress to scabs and alopecia. Footpad lesions develop in most dogs. Bearded collies, Akitas, schipperkes, and Newfoundlands have an increased risk for pemphigus foliaceous.

Autoimmune **pemphigoid** is a similar disease, but autoantibodies are directed against the epithelial basement membranes and to antigens in the glycocalyx of keratinocytes.

Eosinophilic granuloma complex of cats

The **eosinophilic granuloma complex** of cats may be an autoimmune lesion. In a retrospective study of sera of 29 cats with this complex, 68% of the cats had circulating antibodies to components of normal cat epithelium. These autoantibodies may be secondary, however; that is, the granuloma may release altered self-antigens to which the cat's immune system responds.

Systemic autoimmune diseases

Lupus erythematosus

Lupus erythematosus (LE) is a rare disease of dogs and humans, characterized by arthritis, anemia, lymphadenopathy, and nephritis. Widespread vascular lesions are induced by circulating antigen-antibody complexes. Thus the clinical and pathologic manifestations resemble those of serum sickness more than those of autoimmune "organ" diseases such as thyroiditis. Serologic abnormalities include autoantibodies against IgG, nucleoprotein, DNA, RNA, thyroglobulin, and erythrocyte membrane antigens.

In general, flare-ups of disease correlate with drops in complement levels, and antigen-antibody-complement complexes can be demonstrated directly in vascular and renal lesions. Deposition of immune complexes in the renal glomeruli produces alterations in renal function that can lead to uremia. In skin, dogs develop lymphocytic infiltrates around dermal blood vessels. Complexes also occur in other vascular organs such as choroid plexus, myocardium, skin, and gonads.

Autoantibodies to host proteins develop. Autoantibodies to chromatin (DNA-protein complexes) produce dense, extracellular "hematoxylin bodies" (remnants of nuclear debris) in tissue. Other autoantibodies react with erythrocyte surfaces to cause mild hemolytic anemia. Anti-DNA antibodies are the basis of the LE test, in which suspect serum is added to leukocyte suspensions. Nuclei of susceptible cells undergo dissolution with release of nuclear chromatin, which is then phagocytized by other leukocytes. These appear as LE cells, large cells with hematoxylin-staining inclusions.

Canine lupus erythematosus. The complex disorder of **canine lupus erythematosus** leads to progressive hemolytic anemia, thrombocytopenic purpura, proteinuria, and polyarthritis. Renal failure, due to irregular, spotty, chronic membranous glomerulonephritis with accumulations of plasmacytes, is a frequent cause of death. Lymphoid follicles develop in medullary areas of the thymus.

Anemia occurs as acute, severe hemolytic crises, during which there is a strong, direct, positive antiglobulin (Coombs') test. Eluates from affected erythrocytes sensitize normal canine erythrocytes to an indirect antiglobulin test (confirming that autoantibodies are responsible for the hemolysis).

Thrombocytopenia purpura, which occurs because of platelet destruction, is manifest as hematuria, epistaxis, and petechiae or ecchymoses in the skin and mucous membranes. Autoantibodies to platelets have been demonstrated. Circulating antigen-antibody complexes (unrelated to platelets) may also exert a cytotoxic effect.

ADDITIONAL READING

Aleksandersen M, et al. 1995. Scarcity of γΔ T cells in intestinal epithelia containing coccidia despite general increase of epithelial lymphocytes. *Vet Pathol* 32:504.

Dambach DM, et al. 1997. Morphologic, immunohistochemical, and ultrastructural characterization of a distinctive renal lesion in dogs putatively associated with *Borrelia burgdorferi* infection: 49 cases (1987–1992). *Vet Pathol* 34:85.

Foley JE, et al. 1999. Outbreak of fatal salmonellosis in cats following use of a high-titer modified-live panleukopenia virus vaccine. *J Am Vet Med Assoc* 214:67.

Holmberg CA, et al. 1985. Immunologic abnormality in a group of *Macaca arctoides* with high mortality due to atypical mycobacterial and other disease processes. *Am J Vet Res* 46:1192.

Hurvitz AI. 1980. Canine pemphigus vulgaris. *Am J Pathol* 98:861.

Ihrke PJ, et al. 1985. Pemphigus foliaceus in dogs. *J Am Vet Med Assoc* 186:59.

Iwasaki T, et al. 1995. Canine bullous pemphigoid (BP): identification of the 180-kd canine BP antigen by circulating autoantibodies. *Vet Pathol* 32:387.

Johnson CM, et al. 1998. Biphasic thymus response by kittens inoculated with feline immunodeficiency virus during fetal development. *Vet Pathol* 35:191.

King NW. 1986. Simian models of acquired immunodeficiency syndrome (AIDS): a review. *Vet Pathol* 23:345.

Kuhl KA, et al. 1994. Comparative histopathology of pemphigus foliaceous and superficial folliculitis in the dog. *Vet Pathol* 31:19.

Parijs LV, Abbas AK. 1998. Homeostasis and self-tolerance in the immune system: turning lymphocytes off. *Science* 280:243.

Pertile TL, et al. 1996. Immunohistochemical detection of lymphocyte subpopulations in the tarsal joints of chickens with experimental viral arthritis. *Vet Pathol* 33:303.

Ploegh HL. 1998. Viral strategies of immune evasion. *Science* 280:248.

Quimby FW, et al. 1979. A disorder of dogs resembling Sjögren's syndrome. *Clin Immunopathol* 12:471.

Randolph GJ, et al. 1998. Differentiation of monocytes into dendritic cells in a model of trans-endothelial trafficking. *Science* 282:480.

Reiser H, Stadecker MJ. 1996. Costimulatory B7 molecules in the pathogenesis of infectious and autoimmune diseases. *New Engl J Med* 335:1369.

Roosje PJ, et al. 1998. Increased numbers of CD4+ and CD8+ T cells in lesional skin of cats with allergic dermatitis. *Vet Pathol* 35:268.

Roth JA, Kaeberle ML. 1983. Suppression of neutrophil and lymphocyte function induced by a vaccinal strain of bovine viral diarrhea virus with and without the administration of ACTH. *Am J Vet Res* 44:2366.

Winkelstine JA, et al. 1981. Genetically determined deficiency of the third component of complement in the dog. *Science* 212:1169.

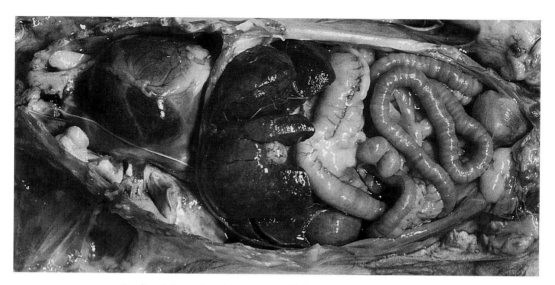

Cardiac failure, dog. Late stage, with heart stopped in diastole. Massive enlargement of heart with blood-filled right atrium and vena cava. Liver markedly enlarged, mottled, and granular.

PART 3

Circulatory Disorders

IN PART 3 WE DEAL WITH different pathologic changes that are connected by their development in the vascular system and their interrelatedness in terms of clinical effects in the animal. On the opposite page, we see the effects of long-standing cardiac failure in a dog. Diminished cardiac function leads to serious consequences throughout the body, especially in the liver.

Your understanding of how fluids pass from tissue into the vascular system and back again affects how well you understand disease and its treatment. Changes in blood vessels are associated with most serious diseases. Edema, heart failure, shock, thrombosis, and inflammation are life-threatening processes, and all are caused by or lead to alterations in endothelium and the vascular wall.

The capillary bed has the capacity to expand under the influences of the nervous system, humoral substances, and vasodilatory drugs. Endothelial cells constantly secrete glycoproteins that blanket the luminal surfaces of endothelium. Exposed to flowing blood, these glycoproteins inhibit clotting and protect the delicate junctions between endothelial cells. When endothelium is injured, the synthesis and release of surface glycoproteins are diminished, causing defects in hemostasis and fluid transport. Just as injured epidermis fails to protect underlying subcutis, injured endothelium does not permit normal transport of needed substances into and out of tissue.

In capillaries, substances are transported across the endothelial cell in three ways: (1) **direct diffusion** (e.g., ions, water, and very small molecules passively diffuse across the vessel wall); (2) **active transport**, which occurs via special ion pumps embedded in the plasma membranes at the cell surface (i.e., charged particles cannot pass the cell's plasma membrane and must be moved into and out of cells via membrane proteins that function as active pumps); and (3) **endocytosis and exocytosis**, in which tiny vesicles on the luminal surface of the endothelium take up materials, pinch off from the surface, and carry materials across the cytoplasm to exit at the basal surface.

Arterioles and venules regulate blood flow through the capillary bed. **Precapillary arterioles** contain small myocyte sheaths that are innervated and that contract to control blood flow entering the capillary bed. Pharmacologic manipulation of these arterioles is important in indirectly controlling the exudation of fluids in the vascular bed. **Postcapillary venules** are extraordinarily susceptible to some toxins and, along with capillaries, are sites of fluid exudation.

Regional differences in capillary permeability depend on structural variation in the vascular wall. Studies on transport kinetics show that permeability to macromolecules varies in limbs, intestine, liver sinusoids, and brain. Restricted transport in capillaries of the brain, the **blood-brain barrier**, is due to very tight intercellular junctions reinforced by covering of the capillaries by astrocyte foot processes. In contrast, the bone marrow sinusoidal endothelium is exceptionally open to passage of both soluble and particulate material.

Cyclic changes occur in vessels of some endocrinologically controlled organs. For example, endo-thelium of capillaries of the uterine mucosa is flattened and relatively structureless in sexually inactive females. They become markedly enlarged and filled with ribosomes upon stimulation with progesterone during the mating season.

Blood pressure exerts an effect on passage rates of low-molecular-weight proteins. When hypertension is induced experimentally, there is evidence that protein tracer molecules pass into tissue in massive amounts. This implies a loss of barrier function in endothelium under high pressure.

FOCUS

Dirofilariasis: A Cause of Cardiac Hypertrophy in Dogs

MECHANICAL OBSTRUCTION of the right ventricle and pulmonary artery by the heartworm *Dirofilaria immitis* leads to marked enlargement of the heart. Dirofilariasis is an insect-borne disease. Microfilariae sucked from the blood of infected dogs by mosquitoes are transmitted as larvae to other dogs, where they develop to adult worms within the right ventricle and pulmonary artery.

Clinical signs in affected dogs (weakness, anorexia, and respiratory difficulty) are progressive. Clinical pathologic examination in early stages reveals microfilariae in the blood. Radiologic examination shows a markedly enlarged heart with dense areas distributed throughout the lungs. At necropsy, myocardial walls are thickened and chambers are enlarged. Lungs are large, pale, and meaty and do not collapse. Fluid is usually present in the abdominal and thoracic cavities.

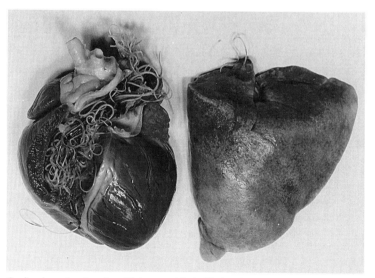

Cardiac hypertrophy, dog. Right ventricle is filled with masses of adult *Dirofilaria immitis*. Lung is solid with nematodes in bronchi.

▶

Pathologic diagnoses include (1) **cardiac hypertrophy**, with obstruction of the right ventricle and pulmonary artery; (2) **chronic multifocal granulomatous pneumonitis** due to embolization of adult parasites and microfilaria in the capillary bed of the lung; (3) **bronchiectasis** with mucous hyperplasia of bronchial epithelium; and (4) **centrolobular fatty degeneration** of the liver with foci of necrosis and fibrosis.

In canine heartworm disease, disastrous increases of workload on the right ventricle occur by several mechanisms. First, adult parasites mechanically obstruct blood flow. Second, pulmonary arterial vascular lesions develop and shed thromboemboli into the pulmonary capillary bed. This leads to chronic inflammatory disease of the lung, with hemosiderosis, alveolar wall fibrosis, and focal granulomatous lesions. Last, live microfilariae are shed into the pulmonary capillary bed. These factors, when combined, initiate the cycle of pulmonary edema–heart failure. Fluid accumulates in the alveolar wall, and fibrosis and emphysema develop. These, in turn, increase the heart workload. The failing right ventricle cannot pump sufficient blood to the lung. Death may occur during cardiac hypertrophy because of sudden embolization of microfilariae and thrombi, or it may not occur until cardiac failure and severe dilatation have developed.

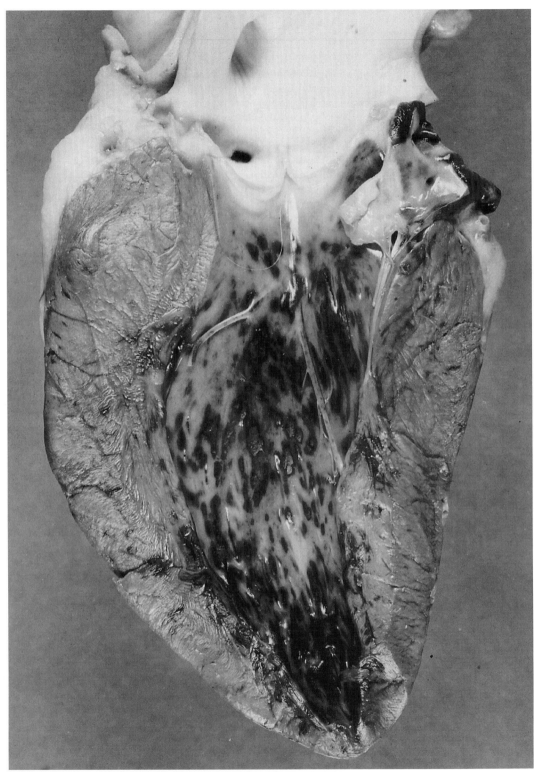

FIGURE 7.1. Ecchymotic hemorrhages, endocardium, heart, horse given endotoxin of *Escherichia coli*.

CHAPTER 7

Fluid Balance and Blood Volume Disorders

HEMORRHAGE

Hemorrhage is commonly due to trauma. The blood vessel is torn, and whole blood escapes. Hemorrhage may be external or internal and in either case may deprive the animal of blood (**exsanguination**). Accumulation of blood in the thoracic cavity, pericardial space, or peritoneal space (abdominal cavity) are called **hemothorax, hemopericardium**, or **hemoperitoneum**, respectively.

When blood escapes into tissue (rather than through broken surfaces), it accumulates as a blood-filled space, or **hematoma**. In dogs, hematomas are common on the concave surfaces of the pinna; they are a consequence of trauma, commonly due to violent head shaking and scratching from aural pain and usually develop in clefts formed by trauma in the ear cartilages.

Hemorrhage from surfaces may occur in abnormal tissue masses that protrude into lumens or onto surfaces in such a way that trauma easily causes already fragile blood vessels to rupture. Neoplasms of skin, spleen, and intestine are prone to this kind of hemorrhage. Genital hemorrhage occurs in mares with varicose (enlarged and tortuous) veins of the vaginal wall; these varices probably arise during the physical impairment of venous return from the vagina during pressure from a gravid uterus.

Very tiny hemorrhages into the skin, mucous membranes, and serosal surfaces are designated as **petechiae**. Their presence often indicates a severe generalized process. Petechiae are commonly seen in septicemia, where endothelium is destroyed by bacterial toxins, and in viral infections, in which the virus replicates in vascular endothelium. The viral diseases hog cholera, equine viral arteritis, Newcastle disease of birds, and epidemic hemorrhagic disease of deer are all characterized by multiple petechiation caused in part by necrosis of endothelial cells.

Hemorrhages slightly larger than petechiae, a condition called **purpura**, are associated most commonly with disturbances of the clotting mechanisms that allow more extensive escape of blood because of failure of blockage of the injured vessel. **Ecchymoses** are large hemorrhages (greater than 1 cm in diameter); large bruises are ecchymoses (Fig. 7.1).

Hemorrhages are rapidly resorbed. Bleeding into the skin produces a red ecchymotic blotch that gradually becomes darker and then purple, fading to brown-yellow and disappearing in 2–3 weeks. In the process of repair, erythrocytes are lysed or are phagocytized by macrophages (erythrophagocytosis). Hemoglobin is released and is degraded into bilirubin and hemosiderin, which impart their characteristic yellow brown colors to the tissue. Bilirubin may form yellow crystals called hematoidin.

The significance of lost blood depends on the acute or chronic nature of the hemorrhage and how much blood has been lost. The consequence of acute blood loss may be hypovolemic shock; the consequence of chronic loss, anemia.

EDEMA

Edema (Gr. *oidema,* swelling) is the abnormal accumulation of excess fluid in interstitial tissue spaces or in body cavities. Edematous tissue, when examined grossly, is wet, gelatinous, and heavy. In several species, fluids are slightly yellow, especially if proteins have exuded. Microscopically, tissue spaces are distended by eosinophilic proteinaceous fluids. Hyperemia is often obvious, and lymph vessels are always dilated. **Local edema** is usually due to lymphatic blockage, and evidence of lesions in efferent lymphatics should be sought. **Generalized**

TABLE 7.1. Causes of edema

Mechanism	Clinical example
Inflammatory	
Increased endothelial permeability	Burns
	Trauma
	Surgery
	Infection
Noninflammatory, systemic	
Increased hydrostatic pressure	Congestive heart disease
	Pericarditis/myocarditis
	Severe liver disease
Reduced oncotic pressure of plasma	Malnutrition
	Gastroenteritis
	Glomerulonephropathy
Increased osmotic pressure of interstitial fluid related to sodium retention	Reduced renal perfusion
	Increased tubular resorption
Noninflammatory, local	
Lymphatic obstruction	Neoplasia
	Inflammatory scarring
	Congenital malformations
Lymphatics	
Impaired venous drainage	Trauma

edema, on the other hand, results either from increased hydrostatic pressure of blood (as in the venous system of heart failure) or from decreased colloid osmotic pressure of plasma proteins. In heart failure, pressure in the veins rises and is transmitted to the capillary bed, where fluid exudes. Massive accumulation of edema fluid in the body tissues is referred to as **anasarca**.

Accumulation of edema fluid in the major body cavities is termed **hydroperitoneum**, **hydrothorax**, or **hydropericardium**, depending on the cavity involved. Hydroperitoneum (also called **ascites**) is the accumulation of fluid in the abdominal cavity. It is common in chronic heart failure, in which it is caused by a rise in intrahepatic portal venous pressure. **Pulmonary edema**, seen as frothy, pale, massive lungs, leads to suspicion either of circulatory problems or of sudden diffuse and direct damage to the capillary bed of the lungs. **Effusion** (L. *effusio*, a pouring out) is the escape of fluid into tissue. The term is used by some clinicians to distinguish fluid escaping from serous surfaces (e.g., pleural effusion).

There are two major types of edema: inflammatory and noninflammatory (Table 7.1). This section concerns noninflammatory edema, in which fluids move into tissue spaces because of colloidal osmotic and hydrostatic pressure changes. Edema fluid closely resembles lymph. In this type of edema, the fluid is "protein poor," characterized as a **transudate**; that is, it has a low protein content, a specific gravity below 1.012, and low cellularity. In the sec-

FOCUS

End-stage Heart Disease

CONGESTIVE HEART FAILURE is the clinical syndrome resulting from the inability of cardiac output to keep pace with venous return. It is the final common pathway for several types of heart disease. Retention of water and sodium ions (from decreased renal blood flow and adrenal cortical mechanisms) may result in overhydration with increased blood volume. This distends the venous bed so that the heart chambers cannot keep up with the amount of blood delivered. The venous bed is distended further, and fluid begins to accumulate in the tissues.

Signs of congestive heart failure are due to the secondary effects of stasis and congestion. Lesions are extensive in the lungs and liver. They are rare in kidneys, brain, and subcutis, although lesions of anoxia and fluid exudation occur in these organs.

▶

ond major type of edema, inflammatory edema, endothelial damage leads to increased capillary permeability. The transudate is rapidly converted to an **exudate** that is high in protein and specific gravity and contains increased numbers of leukocytes. The massive edema of the subcutis in severe burns and trauma are characterized by exudation of large amounts of albumin and fibrinogen.

Edema results when the forces that move fluid from the vascular lumen to the interstitium are augmented over those producing the reverse effect. Starling's law states that hydrostatic pressure in the vascular system (aided slightly by perivascular os-

motic pressure) moves fluid out of the system (Fig. 7.2). The forces holding the fluid within the blood are osmotic pressure of the plasma proteins and, to a lesser extent, tissue pressure around blood vessels.

Total body water consists of fluids of plasma, interstitial tissue spaces, and intracellular spaces. The distribution of water among these compartments is a carefully controlled homeostatic mechanism, and deviations from normal have profound effects on the body. Plasma fluid can be manipulated directly by intravenous fluid therapy, and thus both interstitial and intracellular fluids can be indirectly controlled.

Blood backs up in **lungs** of dogs with cardiac failure, and the increased pressure in the pulmonary veins is transmitted to the capillaries. Fluid accumulates in the alveolar wall and overflows into alveoli, causing pulmonary edema. Lesions seen postmortem include capillary dilatation (hyperemia), hemorrhage into scattered alveoli, and eosinophilic granular debris in alveoli. In long-standing heart failure, alveolar walls are thickened from fibrosis (collagen fibers are deposited in the interstitium). Alveoli contain edema fluid and iron-laden macrophages called **heart failure cells**, which arise from enhanced erythrophagocytosis that is due to stasis of blood flow in the pulmonary capillary bed.

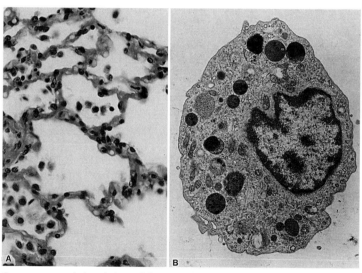

Consequences of chronic heart failure. A. Alveolar walls of the lung are thickened. Note the capillaries projecting into the alveoli. B. Macrophages in the alveoli (heart failure cells) contain iron pigments.

In chronic heart failure, the centrolobular areas of the liver slowly become fibrotic. These lesions are called **cardiac sclerosis,** or cardiac cirrhosis. Abnormalities of portal system congestion are also responsible for **ascites.**

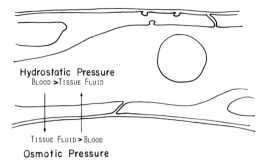

Hydrostatic Pressure
BLOOD >TISSUE FLUID

TISSUE FLUID > BLOOD
Osmotic Pressure

FIGURE 7.2. Forces that move fluid out of and into the capillary.

Interstitial fluid is the intermediary through which all metabolic products pass to enter or leave the cells. It is in constant exchange both with plasma and with cellular fluids. Maintenance of its normal volume is the sum of two sets of forces having contrasting action:

1. Forces promoting passage of fluid from intravascular plasma into the interstitium
   a. Hydrostatic pressure of the blood
   b. Osmotic pressure of interstitial fluid

2. Forces promoting passage of fluid in the opposite direction, from interstitium to plasma
   a. Osmotic pressure of blood
   b. Hydrostatic pressure of tissue fluids

These forces operate normally only when blood vessels and lymphatics are intact. Endothelium, along with its underlying basement membrane, permits free passage of water and ions but opposes passage of plasma proteins. It is the most vital element in the maintenance of blood volume.

In **healthy mammals** the hydrostatic pressure at the arteriolar end of the capillary bed is about 35 mm Hg. At the venular end it is 12–15 mm Hg. The colloidal osmotic pressure of the plasma is approximately 20–25 mm Hg (rising slightly at the venular end as fluid escapes in the arteriolar end and returns in the venular end). In **edema** there is expansion of interstitial fluid or accumulation of fluid in body cavities (e.g., the pleural and peritoneal cavities).

Local edema

Edema may be general or local. Local noninflammatory edema is nearly always due to **lymphatic blockade** or **impaired venous drainage**. The normal flow of interstitial fluid into lymphatics is prevented, and edema fluid accumulates locally. This type of edema is associated with lymphatics damaged by surgery, neoplasms, and intravascular para-

sites. Causes of generalized edema, such as chronic cardiac failure or reduced osmotic pressure of plasma, do not cause local edema.

Rare hereditary malformations of the lymphatic vessels occur in dogs, calves, and pigs. Because of blockade in the lymph vessels, the diseases are manifested as local subcutaneous edema of the limbs.

Generalized edema

Generalized edema occurs most often in one of two basic mechanisms: **increased hydrostatic pressure of blood** or **decreased colloid osmotic pressure of plasma proteins**. Decreased levels of plasma proteins are seen in chronic blood-loss anemia, in chronic renal disease (with loss of albumin in the urine), and in starvation. When protein levels in plasma fall below 5%, the potential for edema is present. Fluid is usually found in the subcutis of the cervical areas and around the legs. In large animals, several liters of fluid may accumulate in interstitial tissue spaces before edema is obvious clinically.

The sites of edema are important factors in both diagnosis and prognosis. In most tissues, fluid does not have immediate clinical significance to the patient. In lungs and brain, however, edema may rapidly produce severe disease and even death. Fluid in locations that relate to severe clinical affection often have special designations: **anasarca**, swelling of the subcutis due to severe generalized edema; **hydrothorax**, fluid in the thoracic cavity; **hydropericardium**, fluid in the sac around the heart; and **hydroperitoneum**, fluid in the peritoneal cavity.

Anasarca occurs in cardiac failure

When edema is severe and generalized and causes diffuse swelling of all tissues, it is called **anasarca**. Anasarca is especially prominent in the subcutis of some species. In progressive cardiac failure, generalized edema is nearly always present. Fluid seeps into the body cavities and subcutaneous tissues, particularly in the limbs. Because the heart cannot pump the amount of blood received from the veins, venous pressure rises and is transmitted to the capillary bed, where fluid exudes, resulting in fluid stasis and pooling.

Endothelial cells of capillaries and veins involved in stasis are swollen, and cell organelles are disoriented. Fluid and protein precipitates disrupt the basement membranes and pericapillary spaces. In the end stage of cardiac failure, capillaries of the myocardium are involved in edema. In these final stages of cardiac failure, other secondary problems are superimposed on the capillaries. Retention of chlorides by the kidney aggravates the already existing edema. The continued escape of protein low-ers the osmotic pressure of blood and raises that of tissue, enhancing fluid exudation.

Ascites

The intraperitoneal accumulation of fluid, known as **ascites**, involves retention of sodium ions and water, hypoalbuminemia, and decreased colloid osmotic pressure. Ascites is not mediated solely by increased hydrostatic pressure in all species (e.g., surgical ligation of the portal vein in dogs does not cause remarkable accumulation of fluid in the peritoneal cavity).

Pulmonary edema

Pulmonary edema is the accumulation of edema fluid in alveoli of the lungs. It is brought about by excessive amounts of plasma exuding into alveoli

from the capillary bed of the lung. In the lungs, the balance of hydrostatic and osmotic pressure between intravascular and extravascular compartments is influenced by air pressure, lymphatic drainage, and surface tension of alveolar walls. In the earliest phases, fluid accumulates in the interstitium of the alveolar wall, where it disrupts the basement membranes of the endothelial cells and pneumocytes. The first histologic evidence of edema appears perivascularly in the alveolar wall. Fluid is rapidly drained along connective tissue fibers to perivascular cuffs leading to lymph vessels.

Two major mechanisms are involved in the causation of pulmonary edema: (1) **circulatory failure–induced changes in pulmonary hemodynamics**, which result in a slow exudation of fluid into alveoli; and (2) any sudden diffuse and direct

---

FOCUS

Plasma Proteins and Edema

THE INDIVIDUAL NET CHARGES of plasma proteins are used to separate them by **electrophoretic migration**. In the electrophoresis unit, a small sample of plasma is placed on paper wetted with buffer, and migration is induced by opposing electrical charges at the ends of the paper strip. Proteins on the paper are then stained, and the pattern is transposed to graphic form, the **electrophoretogram**, by a densitometer. The percentage of each plasma protein can be determined by partitioning the peaks on the electrophoretogram and calculating the various percentages from the total plasma protein concentration. For practical purposes, the protein most affected in edema and hypoproteinemia is albumin.

The albumin molecule, at 69,000 MW, is the smallest of the major plasma proteins. It regulates the exchange of water between blood and tissue and is a major factor in maintaining osmotic regulation; each gram percent of serum albumin exerts osmotic pressure of 5.5 mm Hg. Albumin also acts as a buffer because it is amphoteric and can combine with both acids and bases.

Albumin levels in blood do not rise above normal except during hemoconcentration or dehydration. Hypoalbuminemia is a common finding in edema and in other acute diseases such as glomerulonephritis and protein–losing diarrhea, in which the albumin molecules escape from the vascular system. Reduced plasma protein concentration is reflected in the lower peak of albumin in the electrophoretogram.

Albumin is synthesized in the liver and can be detected in hepatocytes by a specific fluorescent antialbumin antibody stain. Developed in late gestation, albumin production by hepatocytes peaks soon after birth. With growth, albumin production declines, but in plasma protein-losing diseases such as cirrhosis and nephritis, all hepatocytes again convert to albumin production.

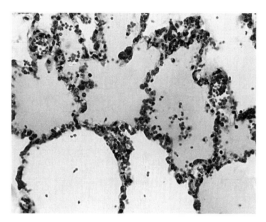

FIGURE 7.3. Pulmonary edema, dog with dirofilariasis *(Dirofilaria immitis).* Precipitates of albumen are in the alveolus.

damage to pulmonary capillary endothelium. The latter is usually a peracute stage of inflammation and, if the animal survives, is followed by pneumonitis. Both of the above conditions are associated with marked capillary dilation; the distinction between extreme hyperemia and pulmonary edema is often arbitrary.

Pulmonary edema associated with cardiac failure is inevitably chronic. Lymph flow increases, lymphatics enlarge, and the alveolar walls become thickened. Hyperplasia of granular pneumocytes is common, and these cells may line the alveoli. In long-standing pulmonary edema, collagen is deposited in the alveolar walls, diminishing the resiliency of the respiratory lobules (Fig. 7.3).

Edema of the brain

Edema of the brain is seen in trauma to the calvaria, obstruction of venous outflow, and intracranial infections (meningitis, brain abscess, and encephalitis). At necropsy, the brain is heavier than normal. Sulci are narrowed, and gyri are swollen and become flattened by contact with the skull. On section, white matter is gelatinous and appears softer than normal. The external layer of the gray matter is widened. Histologically, there is expansion of the perivascular (Virchow-Robin) spaces, which are seen as clear halos in the neuropil around blood vessels (Fig. 7.4).

SHOCK

Shock is the syndrome resulting from a disproportion between **blood volume** and **volume of the circulatory system** that needs to be filled, that is, an acute generalized failure of the capillary bed. The fundamental disturbance is that blood volume is too small to fill the vascular system. The accom-

panying cell damage is due to **inadequate perfusion of tissue**, which directly causes **hypoxia.**

Shock is most often due to one of three events: blood loss, reduced cardiac output, or loss of peripheral vasomotor control. Death may occur at any phase of shock; its attendant damage is due to circulatory failure in the central nervous system, myocardium, and other organs.

Loss of blood pressure is a common finding in shock. Arterial blood pressure is maintained normally by a proper amount of blood in the system, by adequate cardiac output, and by total vascular resistance. Shock may follow marked depression of any of these mechanisms. It is an ominous sign, often terminating in death, despite treatment.

Animals in shock are lethargic and unresponsive to external stimuli. Muscle weakness is a prominent sign. Body temperature is apt to be subnormal (because of lowered metabolism), and there is pallor and coolness of the skin. Heart rate is increased in most types of shock but may be slow and irregular. Depression of renal function and urine production often occurs.

Because shock can be caused by diverse types of injury, the clinical appearances cannot be rigidly defined. Factors such as pain, cold, general anesthesia, hypoproteinemia, dehydration, and exhaustion do not cause shock directly but do augment the mechanisms that cause circulatory collapse. Trauma impairs thermoregulation, and in the presence of a cold environment, body temperature and oxygen consumption both fall, suppressing mechanisms that operate to overcome the shock state.

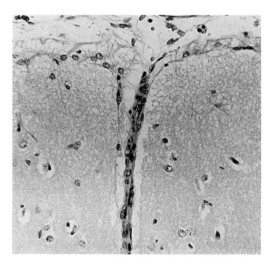

FIGURE 7.4. Acute swelling and edema, brain, dog with acute encephalitis caused by *Escherichia coli.* Water accumulated in the neuropil makes the tissue section pale and causes spaces around blood vessels to expand.

Cytopathology

Tissue lesions of shock are a result of **hypoxia**. As a consequence of inadequate peripheral circulation, there is decreased oxygen delivery. Hypoxia leads to decreased oxidative phosphorylation and ATP production in cells, and mitochondria degenerate. Pyruvate cannot enter the citric acid cycle; as a result, cells are forced to obtain energy by anaerobic glycolysis. Lactate accumulates and leads to metabolic acidosis. Thus, in the terminal stages of shock, a metabolic disease accompanies the circulatory deficiency. Although hyperglycemia is characteristic of early shock (related to catecholamine release), hypoglycemia occurs in the later stages because of depletion of liver glycogen and hyperinsulinemia. During shock there is a prolongation of insulin half-life because of reduced peripheral utilization.

Pathogenesis

The brain and heart are highly susceptible to hypoxia generated by a fall in blood pressure; foci of necrosis and hemorrhage develop in these organs in most species. Tissues vary in the amount of oxygen removed during blood flow. Although the average is approximately 25%, myocardium removes 75% of the oxygen of blood flowing through the capillaries of the heart. When cardiac output is diminished by one-fourth and blood oxygenation is reduced, as happens in shock, the total oxygen transported to the heart cannot meet the requirement of myocardial metabolism (Table 7.2).

Counterregulatory mechanisms are activated during shock regardless of its cause; they are evoked by low blood pressure and diminished cardiac output (via pressure receptors). These mechanisms stimulate the sympathetic nervous system to produce **peripheral vasoconstriction** and **tachycardia**. Hemodynamic alterations of the pulmonary circulation reduce the active ventilatory surface, resulting in hypoxic stimulation of respiratory centers in the brain. Catecholamine output, stimulation of the renin-angiotensin system, and activation of the sympathetic nervous system maintain blood flow to critical organs. Flow is increased to heart, brain, kidney, and lungs at the expense of reduced flow to peripheral tissues such as skeletal muscle and skin.

Progressive deterioration of the circulatory system occurs in massive burns and blood loss, despite these compensatory mechanisms. The designation **irreversible shock** implies the refractory state of circulatory failure with inability to control the disease clinically. When blood is removed from a dog in sufficient quantity to produce shock and is not replaced for 4 hours, the dog will enter a shock state that cannot be reversed despite total restoration of blood volume. The infused fluid or blood seems to be sequestered in the peripheral capillary beds, suggesting vasomotor paralysis of the microcirculation, caused in part by hypoxia.

Hypovolemic shock

Hypovolemic shock is shock due to loss of blood volume. A common cause is massive loss of whole blood during hemorrhage, called **hemorrhagic shock**. Loss of blood volume can also occur deceptively when large amounts of plasma exude into tissue, as happens in severe burns and crush injuries.

Extensive blood loss is required before animals develop hypovolemic shock. Healthy animals may lose one-fourth of their blood volume without showing immediate clinical signs, and loss of one-

TABLE 7.2. Lesions of shock in dogs

Organ	Gross appearance	Microscopic lesions	Mechanisms
Liver	Congested Swollen	Hyperemia of sinusoids Serous exudation (in spaces of Disse)	Constriction of myocytes of hepatic vein and increase in portal venous pressure
Intestine	Hyperemia Hemorrhage (blood in feces)	Hyperemia of villi Subepithelial edema Necrosis and sloughing of villous tips	Elevated portal venous pressure
Stomach	Hyperemia	Mucosal erosions	Hypoxia; back diffusion of H^+
Heart	Hyperemia Subendocardial hemorrhage	Focal necrosis of cardiac myocytes	Hypoxia (also medial necrosis of aorta); inadequate coronary artery blood flow
Lung	Hyperemia Edema (rare)	Hyalin thrombi in capillaries	Vascular stasis; intravascular platelet aggregation or coagulation
Adrenal	Hyperemia Hemorrhage (rare)	Foci of necrosis and hemorrhage	?
Muscle	Pale	Foci of necrosis	Vasoconstriction; hypoxia

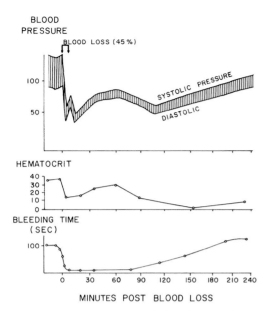

FIGURE 7.5. Hematologic changes during acute hemorrhage.

half the blood volume may be required to produce death. When much blood is lost, the arterial blood pressure drops, and venous return to the heart decreases. The heart rate may increase, but stroke volume and cardiac output are diminished.

Vasoconstriction: rapid response to hypotension

Arterial **vasoconstriction** produces increased peripheral resistance, which shunts blood from the skin and viscera to the heart and brain. The interacting mechanisms that enhance vasoconstriction include (1) **lessened stimulation of baroceptors** in the aortic arch and carotid sinus, which decreases the afferent vasodilatory and cardioinhibitory neural discharges; (2) **vagal and vasomotor discharge** from the medulla oblongata; and (3) **release of catecholamines** from the adrenal medulla. Norepinephrine constricts peripheral vascular beds; epinephrine also constricts most of these and dilates the coronary arteries. Vasoconstriction initiated by the early outpouring of catecholamines is maintained by the renin-angiotensin system.

If arterial blood pressure is measured during and after extensive blood loss, two plateaus in the pressure curve occur (Fig. 7.5). The first, which begins during blood loss, is due to **pressoreceptor reflexes**. These produce strong sympathetic stimulation (and parasympathetic inhibition) to blood vessels when the arterial pressure begins to fall. The response is vasoconstriction and contraction of the spleen, spewing erythrocytes and platelets into the

blood. General anesthesia blocks these compensatory mechanisms; animals whose reflexes have been so removed lose arterial pressure from the onset of blood loss. Another later and more powerful plateau is the central nervous system **ischemic reflex**. This reflex is activated when arterial pressure drops enough to cause brain ischemia.

Blood

Hemorrhagic shock causes slow capillary blood flow, which depletes oxygen and favors aggregation and sludging of erythrocytes. Slow flow instantly affects tissue pH, which may fall below 7.0 (even though lungs blow off CO_2 and tend to produce an early transient alkalosis). Severe capillary acidosis with endothelial injury and release of clotting factors may lead to immediate and striking **hypercoagulability**.

Platelet surfaces become sticky in shock, so platelets tend to aggregate. Platelet-leukocyte microemboli are found in blood removed from dogs with hypovolemic shock. Although hemorrhagic shock produces hypercoagulable blood, intravascular coagulation does not occur unless clot-initiating factors are released. These factors are more common in shock involving bacterial toxins and the massive thromboplastin release in trauma and burns.

As blood is lost, tests on blood for the packed cell volume (**hematocrit**) show decreased values. As blood cells are sequestered in the expanded pulmonary capillaries, there are also decreases in circulating leukocytes (**leukopenia**) and platelets (**thrombocytopenia**). Cell damage in hypoxic tissues is reflected in increased amounts of certain cellular enzymes in plasma; that is, creatine phosphokinase and other enzymes seep out of damaged cells into the circulation. There is a positive correlation of amounts of these enzymes with the severity of shock.

Lung

The lungs of dogs in hypovolemic shock are wet, solid, and frothy, usually with tiny hemorrhages near the surface. Pulmonary edema and increased pulmonary vascular resistance occur because of trapping of platelets and leukocytes in the capillary bed (if trauma with extensive tissue injury has occurred, megakaryocytes may also be found in capillaries of the lungs). As capillaries of the alveolar walls are obstructed, vascular endothelium swells and enhances the edema.

As platelets disintegrate within the pulmonary capillaries, they release vasoactive factors and chemoattractants. Neutrophils are attracted and degranulate at these sites to release lysosomal enzymes that damage tissue. **Platelet-leukocyte em-**

boli may detach from the capillary walls and be released into the circulation. Fibrin is not a major component of the emboli, probably because of mast cell histamine release and the intense activation of the pulmonary fibrinolytic system that occur in shock.

Liver

The liver is a prominent organ affected in shock of the dog. Constriction of veins within the liver raises the **portal venous pressure** and causes **stasis** in both the liver and intestine. Because of the hypoxia associated with stasis, hepatocytes degenerate, resulting in failure of effective detoxification. Kupffer cells fail to remove macromolecules. Bacteria, endotoxins, and split products of fibrinolysis, which arrive in the liver from the portal vein, are allowed to pass into the general circulation.

In shock, liver cells must adapt to hypoxia associated with decreased blood flow. The first few hours of massive blood loss are characterized by hyperglycemia, increased blood lactate, and decreased blood pyruvate, all evidence of the switch to anaerobic glycolysis by the hepatocyte. **Mitochondrial degeneration**, a result of hypoxia, is an early hepatocellular lesion of shock.

Kidney

The effects of extensive loss of blood volume produce profound changes in the kidney. Renal vasoconstriction reduces perfusion and causes the juxtaglomerular cells to degranulate. Plasma renin concentration rises and activates the angiotensin system. **Angiotensin** tends to raise the falling blood pressure by causing peripheral vasoconstriction. It also stimulates the secretion of **antidiuretic hormone** (ADH, or vasopressin) by the pituitary, which acts to conserve water normally lost from the lower nephron. **Aldosterone** secretion by the adrenal cortex is augmented, leading to increased resorption of salt and water by the renal tubule. All these mechanisms conserve fluid and support blood volume.

Small amounts of dilute urine are produced in hypovolemic shock. The decreased glomerular filtration and oliguria (reduced urine output) are consequences of increased renal vasoconstriction. Loss of urine-concentrating ability is related to the decreased medullary sodium osmotic gradient.

Heart

Myocardial damage in hemorrhage shock consists of two types of lesions: **subendocardial hemorrhage and necrosis** due to hypoxia (which mimics lesions produced by exogenous catecholamines) and **zonal lesions** deep in the myocardium caused

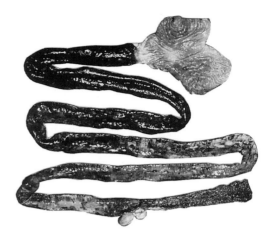

FIGURE 7.6. Lesions of postsurgical shock, intestine, dog. Marked hyperemia and hemorrhage of the duodenum.

not by hypoxia but by the heart's beating strongly and rapidly at very low ventricular volumes. Zonal lesions of necrosis, unique to hypovolemic shock, are foci of supercontracted areas within myocytes that involve several sarcomeres, located adjacent to intercalated disks. Foci of myocardial necrosis are common in dogs with shock due to pooling of blood in the intestinal tract. Experiments in dogs have shown that zonal lesions are produced only in a hypovolemic situation with low end-diastolic volume, intense sympathetic stimulation, and increased force and rate of the heartbeat.

Adrenal gland

Adrenal glands are markedly hyperemic. As blood loss becomes severe, **epinephrine** rises promptly in circulating blood. Degranulation of adrenaline-producing cells of the adrenal medulla occurs within a few minutes and progresses to total degranulation with vacuolar degeneration as hypotension becomes critical (norepinephrine-producing cells are little changed). If endothelial damage is superimposed on shock (as in septic or toxic shock), adrenal glands become hemorrhagic with foci of necrosis.

Gastrointestinal tract

Hyperemia and mucosal erosions occur throughout the gastrointestinal tract in hemorrhagic shock (Fig. 7.6). As the intestine becomes hypoxic, it releases vasoactive serotonin into the portal circulation, which enhances alterations in blood vessels. Mucin biosynthesis is diminished by hypoxia, and loss of the mucosal barrier exposes the mucosa to proteases that initiate erosions.

In severe shock, tips of intestinal villi may become necrotic because the villous countercurrent mechanism is bypassed; oxygen is shunted from the large central capillary of the villus directly to the descending peripheral capillaries and does not reach the villous tips. Although blood flow to the villi is not markedly changed, the villous tips become ischemic.

Skeletal muscle

Peripheral vasoconstriction induced by catecholamines such as adrenaline quickly leads to **pale muscle**. In prolonged hemorrhagic hypotension, vasodilation may occur in skeletal muscles, chiefly because hydrogen and potassium ions, which stimulate capillary dilation, are released into surrounding interstitial spaces after mild hypoxia.

Shock caused by pooling of blood

Expansion of the capillary bed beyond the capacity of blood to fill it results in shock. **Vasodilation** is a potent mechanism for reducing arterial blood pressure. When the splanchnic blood vessels are fully dilated, they have the capacity to accommodate nearly the total blood volume. If this occurred, blood pressure would drop to zero. Normally, continual vasoconstriction of the terminal arterioles prevents this from happening. However, toxins and other substances that cause peripheral vasodilation may lead to the shock state. This type of shock, common in animals, is seen particularly in septic conditions.

Toxic shock

Toxic shock is mediated by toxins released from damaged tissue, venoms, and microbial endotoxins that cause vascular paralysis. It commonly accompanies severe burns and intestinal gangrene. The mechanism is decreased cardiac output and arterial pressure secondary to sequestration of venous blood in the hepatosplanchnic bed. Severe injuries may be accompanied by release of hepatic lysosomal hydrolytic enzymes in a free, active form; elevation of acid phosphatase may accelerate the appearance of shock.

Major effects of **burn shock** occur in kidneys and lead to oliguria and dilute urine. As blood flow to the kidney is reduced, both glomerular filtration and tubular function are suppressed. This suppression occurs within minutes after burn injury (before hypovolemia develops), initiated by nervous system control of renal function.

Gangrene of the gastrointestinal tract promptly leads to shock. In dogs, an important cause is gastric dilatation and volvulus. Release of vasoactive factors into the circulation from necrosis of the gastric mucosa initiates pooling of blood and hypo-

tension. Shock is enhanced by subsequent compression of the posterior vena cava and portal vein by the engorged stomach and by acidosis.

"**Tourniquet ischemia**" shock is an example of a generalized vascular response to marked local tissue destruction. Products from large areas of ischemic tissue enter the circulation and cause circulatory collapse. Widespread vascular damage with release of kinins, prostaglandins, and histamine dilates blood vessels throughout the body.

Shock in bacterial disease

Lysis of gram-negative bacteria releases potent cytotoxic lipopolysaccharides of the bacterial cell wall called **endotoxins**. Endotoxins adsorb to surfaces of endothelium, erythrocytes, leukocytes, platelets, and mast cells. They induce plasma membrane defects that cause both cell degeneration and release of biologically active substances that produce the clinical signs of endotoxic shock. In addition to vasodilation and circulatory collapse, these signs include fever, coagulation, thrombocytopenia, and leukopenia. In contrast to hypovolemic shock, **endotoxic shock** is manifest by intense activation of the coagulation, fibrinolytic, kinin, and complement systems. The critical organ is the lung; lesions involve microthrombi and vascular leakage in both alveolar capillaries and bronchial veins. After experimental intravenous injection of endotoxin, there is a precipitous decline in arterial blood pressure, with simultaneous elevation in portal venous return and cardiac output. Examination of the splanchnic veins 1 hour later reveals marked congestion and dilatation. Venous pooling plays a highly significant role in endotoxic shock. In dogs, pooling in the hepatoportal system is responsible for a significant decrease in venous return of blood to the heart.

Slow capillary flow and release of thromboplastic substances from damaged endothelium trigger intravascular coagulation, and fibrin is deposited throughout the vascular system. The fibrinolytic system is activated, degrading fibrin into split products, which may prevent serious coagulation problems. However, if endotoxemia is severe and sustained, **disseminated intravascular coagulation** may develop. This disastrous condition has two important effects: depletion of coagulation factors, or consumption coagulopathy; and multifocal infarction caused by microthrombi in vessels of kidney, heart, and liver.

Platelet aggregation has immediate and disastrous effects in the lung. Platelet-leukocyte-fibrin thrombi obstruct the capillary bed and induce hypovolemic shock. Endotoxin-induced leakage of bronchial veins augments the already serious interstitial edema. Acute death in shock of gram-negative septicemia is usually due to respiratory failure. In clinical cases treated with anticoagulant therapy, fibrin may not be deposited in large amounts, because of the combined effects of heparin and naturally occurring fibrinolysis.

Pathologic changes in other organs may also lead to death. In **kidney**, the combined effects of hypotension and capillary injury may lead to necrosis. Peritubular capillaries are particularly damaged and show acute tubular necrosis in the renal cortex. Endothelium of capillaries and venules of the **brain** often show severe extravasation. Early serious effects on the **heart** are complicated by edema of the heart valves.

In **liver**, sludged erythrocytes and microthrombi occlude and damage sinusoidal endothelium. Because sinusoids are further blocked by swollen Kupffer cells and endothelium, flow of blood may be reversed from the hepatic artery into the portal vein. Parenchymal cells of all these organs are affected by the metabolic defect in shock. After the initial period of hyperglycemia, the progressively developing hypoglycemia and hypoinsulinemia of canine endotoxic shock are associated with impending death.

It may be important to distinguish two pathways in which endotoxin produces injury: (1) **gram-negative bacteremia**, in which both circulating and phagocytized bacteria are killed, releasing cell wall fragments; and (2) **endotoxemia**, in which endotoxin, generated by intestinal bacteria, penetrates the mucosa to enter the portal venous system, producing an initial effect on the liver. (Because endotoxin is difficult to assay, this second mechanism is still hypothetical.)

Septic shock (exotoxic shock) occurs in any overwhelming infection caused by cocci and other gram-positive bacteria. These bacteria lack endotoxin but induce shock through release of other toxins. It is therefore essential that blood pressure be maintained in severe systemic infections. Increased blood viscosity is a factor that may reduce blood flow to the capillary bed.

Shock in severe systemic viral disease

Viruses that replicate in endothelial cells tend to be associated with severe, often fatal, systemic disease, and most of these viral diseases terminate in shock (e.g., simian hemorrhagic fever, epizootic hemorrhagic disease of deer, and equine viral arteritis). The collapse and death that characterize terminal stages of equine viral arteritis are due to a fatal sequence of events: capillary necrosis, increased vascular permeability, loss of intravascular plasma volume, hemoconcentration, and finally hypotension.

Other factors such as thrombocytopenia, decreased prothrombin levels, adrenal necrosis, and lymphocyte depletion play roles in the process, but the hypovolemic shock is the most important factor in mortality.

Other types of shock

In addition to the two principal patterns of shock, there are less important ways in which shock syndromes occur. The varying adjectives applied to shock indicate the complexity of reactions leading to the final common pathway.

Neurogenic shock

Neurogenic shock occurs in animals with severe fright, pain, and trauma (without hemorrhage). It is commonly seen in restrained wild birds and mammals, especially in cold weather. Animals enter a shock state mediated by the nervous system—that is, nervous stimulation induces peripheral vasodilation, which leads to loss of effective circulating blood volume.

Shock accompanying severe crush injury involves neurogenic shock. If tourniquets are applied to limbs crushed experimentally, external fluid loss is prevented but not circulatory collapse (if nerves remain intact). In contrast, sectioning of the nerves, even without the tourniquet, prevents shock. Neurogenic shock is true circulatory collapse and should not be confused with fainting.

Cardiac shock

Cardiac shock occurs due to the precipitous decrease in cardiac output that accompanies sudden extensive damage to the heart. Most animals succumb directly to myocardial inadequacy. In those rare animals that do not, shock may ensue because of pooling of the blood in capillary beds.

Anaphylactic shock

Anaphylactic shock is circulatory collapse accompanying the binding of antigens to cell-bound antibodies. It is mediated through the massive intravascular release of histamine, which induces increased arteriolar and venous dilation. Clinical signs are great reductions in arterial pressure and venous return of blood to the heart. The syndrome may be complicated by immune complex–induced platelet aggregation, trapping of aggregates in the lung, and increased pulmonary vascular resistance.

INFARCTION

Infarction is a local area of ischemic necrosis in a tissue caused by occlusion of the arterial supply or venous drainage. Infarcts are classified on the basis

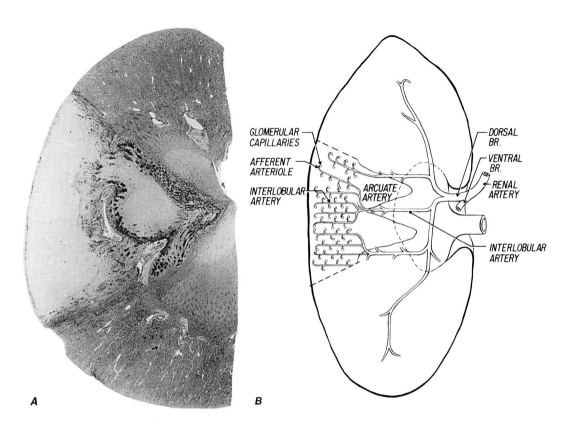

GLOMERULAR
CAPILLARIES

AFFERENT
ARTERIOLE

INTERLOBULAR
ARTERY

ARCUATE
ARTERY

DORSAL
BR.

VENTRAL
BR.

RENAL
ARTERY

INTERLOBULAR
ARTERY

A   B

FIGURE 7.7. Infarction, kidney, pig. A. Pale infarct with hemorrhagic borders, infarct
due to blockade of interlobular artery. B. Site of block in artery.

of color (white or red) and bacterial contamination (bland or septic). **White infarcts** lack blood (they are also called anemic); in contrast, **red infarcts** are filled with blood and usually contain hemorrhages. The amount of blood that escapes into the oxygen-deprived area is determined by age of the infarct, type of injury, and type of tissue. Most infarcts are hemorrhagic initially but become pale in a very short period. White infarcts usually have a red zone at the periphery, because capillaries at the border of the infarct undergo dissolution and blood seeps into the area of necrosis.

Most infarcts result from thrombosis or embolism. Viruses that produce endothelial damage commonly cause thrombi, which expand to block arterioles and to cause infarction in organs with end arteries (kidney, heart, and spleen). Multiple causes are often involved; for example, an artery whose endothelium is injured by viral disease is more prone to be blocked by emboli arising from distant sources.

Infarcts tend to be wedge-shaped; the base of the wedge is at the periphery, with the occluded vessel at the apex (Fig. 7.7). The margins of the infarct may be irregular, a reflection of the vascular supply

from adjacent, nonaffected tissue. Initially, infarcts are ill defined and hyperemic (hemorrhage occurs in organs with loose parenchyma). By 48 hours, most infarcts become progressively paler. At necropsy, infarcts of the kidney are usually white (ischemic). In contrast, lungs usually develop red (hemorrhagic) infarcts.

Within the infarct, the parenchyma undergoes ischemic coagulation necrosis, providing that the animal survives for several hours. In myocardial infarction, the affected area of necrosis is sharply demarcated from normal tissue (Fig. 7.8). All tissues are affected, including blood vessels, mesenchymal cells, and nerves; there is no regeneration. If the infarcts arise from septic emboli, the infarcted area may be converted into an abscess (which may not even be recognized as an infarct at necropsy). Ultimately, infarcts are replaced by scar tissue, which forms an indentation over the surface of the organ.

The consequences of a block in a muscular artery depend on a combination of several factors; that is, the combined factors determine whether infarction occurs and how serious that infarct will be for the host. The most important factor is the **degree of injury to the vascular supply**—whether a large ar-

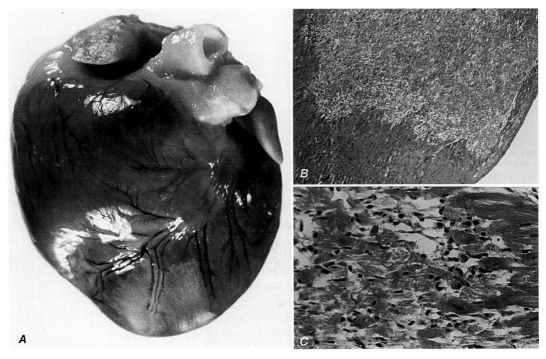

FIGURE 7.8. Infarction, heart. A. Pale infarct at tip of left ventricle. B and C. Histology of infarcted area.

tery is affected, whether the artery is totally blocked, and whether blood vessels surrounding the affected area can expand to supply the tissue. Other factors that affect infarction include the **rate of development** of the infarct, the **vulnerability of the cell types** involved, and the **oxygen-carrying capacity of the blood** at the time of infarction. Infarcts are larger in anemic animals than in normal animals.

Damage in infarcted tissue results from a combination of ischemic necrosis of parenchymal cells, ischemic necrosis of vascular endothelium, and the indirect effect of neutrophil-mediated tissue death that occurs at the margins of the infarct and in the parenchyma if reflow of blood is established. Reflow injury results from damage induced by neutrophils that attach to injured vascular endothelium. It has special clinical significance because it can be reduced by certain therapies. The selectins mediate the attachment of neutrophils in vasculature of ischemic tissue, and blockade of selectin ligands by oligosaccharides has markedly reduced reflow injury in myocardial infarction.

Systemic infections are associated with infarction

Any disease that causes widespread damage to endothelium predisposes to infarction. Many bacterial diseases produce disseminated infection and sep-

ticemia in which vascular endothelium is damaged; thrombi obstruct the vascular system and tissue necrosis ensues (Fig. 7.9). In classic cases of hog cholera (swine fever), virus replicates in endothelial cells to produce marked vascular injury. Thrombi form at sites of viral injury in the arteries and arterioles and lead to occlusion of the blood vessel and infarction. Infarcts in hog cholera commonly occur in the spleen and intestine.

Obstruction of veins

Obstruction of veins is not apt to produce infarction but may cause slowly developing stasis, with engorgement of the tributary venous system. The most serious effects result when the anterior or posterior vena cava is obstructed. The **vertebral vein system** is an alternate route for return of blood from body to heart, via anastomoses with anterior systemic veins and azygos veins that bypass the caval systems.

EMBOLISM

Embolism is the sudden blocking of an artery or vein by an obstruction that has arrived in the bloodstream. The consequence of an embolus is infarction. Emboli can be composed of many materials, although the most frequent sources of emboli are thrombi. Many of the causes of thromboemboli

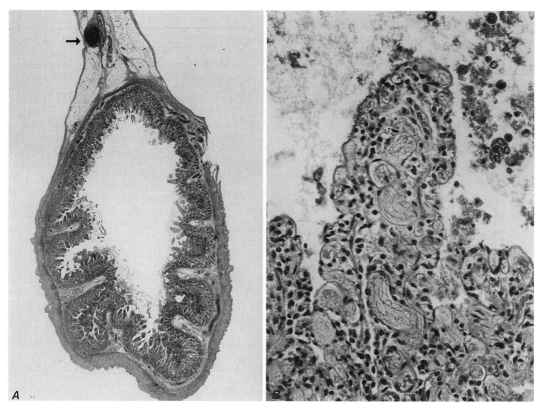

FIGURE 7.9. Infarction, intestine, cow with *Corynebacterium equi* infection. A. Thrombus *(arrow)* in mesenteric vein and necrosis of intestinal mucosa. B. Necrosis of intestinal villi with deposition of fibrin in capillaries. Epithelial cells have sloughed from the villous surface, leaving the capillaries of the tunica propria exposed.

and infarction are systemic infections in which endothelium has been injured; thrombi then form, and thromboemboli are discharged into flowing blood.

Thromboembolism

Thromboembolism can be lethal. Thromboemboli arising in the venous system are transported through the heart to be trapped in the lungs. Pulmonary thromboemboli cause sudden death by blocking respiration; they are associated with vascular infectious processes, disseminated intravascular coagulation, and extensive neoplastic disease. In dogs, thromboemboli occur in dirofilariasis and as a complication of hypothyroidism, hyperadrenocorticism, renal amyloidosis, and pancreatitis.

Thromboemboli that arise in the left side of the heart or in the major arteries and are released then travel to the smaller vessels of the arterial system. Arterial thrombi cause disease by blocking the arterial supply, and the common clinical result is infarction. In cats, thromboemboli arising from valvular endocarditis lodge at the aortic bifurcation and in the origins of the iliac arteries. Emboli that lodge in and straddle the iliac arteries are called **saddle emboli**. Clinical signs in cats with aortic emboli or saddle emboli of the iliac arteries are cool, edematous limbs and lack of femoral pulse. If complete block of the arteries occurs, paralysis and shock are inevitable.

Parasite emboli commonly cause infarction

Live and dead parasites that enter the bloodstream can cause infarction of the **lung**. Emboli of live, adult *Dirofilaria immitis*, which reside in the right heart and pulmonary artery of the dog, can cause large infarcts in the lungs. Pulmonary emboli that occur in canine dirofilariasis may also be due to dead adult parasites, groups of microfilariae, or thrombi that originate from parasite-induced erosions in the wall of the pulmonary artery. Ascarid larvae and other nematodes may lodge in the **brain** to produce foci of necrosis that end as abscesses containing dead parasites.

Infarction of the **intestine** is common in horses that are infected with larvae of *Strongylus* spp. These larvae invade, disrupt, and produce thrombi in

Atherosclerosis

ATHEROSCLEROSIS IS THE ACCUMULATION of lipids in larger arteries in the form of elevated, lipid-filled plaques called **atheromas**. Necrosis and fibrosis follow the deposition of lipid and result in progressively enlarging lesions that expand the arterial wall. The consequences of severe atherosclerosis are often fatal. **Ischemia** and **infarction** develop in affected organs because of the encroachment of the vascular lumen. Less commonly, **aneurysms** develop from weakening of the arterial wall. **Rupture** of the artery with hemorrhage into surrounding tissue can be fatal.

Canine atherosclerosis is uncommon. In 21 cases in a 14-year period at the Animal Medical Center in New York City, 8 were males, and there was a preponderance of miniature schnauzers, Doberman pinschers, and Labrador retrievers. Severe systemic atherosclerosis is most often seen in dogs with **hypothyroidism**, which leads to hypercholesterolemia and indirectly to atherosclerosis. Lesions are prominent in the media as well as intima of large muscular arteries of the heart, kidney, intestine, bladder, and other organs. Lipids fill the cytoplasm of myocytes, and lipid-laden **foam cells** distort the media of the vessel wall.

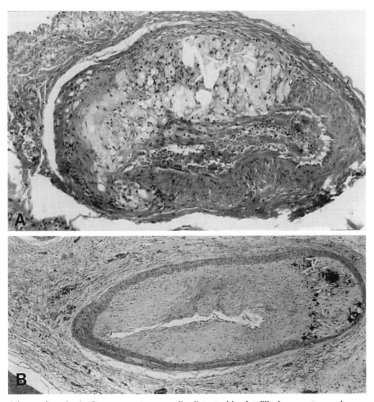

Atherosclerosis. A. Coronary artery, media distorted by fat-filled myocytes and macrophages, dog with hypothyroidism. B. Coronary artery, vessel wall containing evidence of acute and chronic changes, human female with diabetes mellitus.

▶

▶

As constructed from serial examination of naturally occurring lesions, this involves (1) endothelial injury, (2) seepage of plasma lipids and lipoproteins into the intima, (3) invasion of the intima by circulating monocytes that transform into macrophages and then phagocytize lipids, (4) myocyte migration through fenestrae of the inner elastic membrane, (5) proliferation of myocytes in foci within the intima, and (6) accumulation of lipids within the cytoplasm of the vascular smooth muscle cell.

Macrophages contain the very low density lipoproteins (VLDLs) that characterize atherosclerosis and play a critical role in the development of atherosclerosis in dogs. Glutathione peroxidase, which has been detected immunohistochemically in the large foamy macrophages of atherosclerotic lesions, appears to oxidize LDLs in ways that may promote atherogenesis.

Reference
Kagawa Y, et al. 1998. Immunohistochemical localization of apolipoprotein B-100 and expression of glutathione peroxidase (GSH-PO) in canine atherosclerotic lesions. *Vet Pathol* 35:227.

endothelium of the mesenteric artery and its branches. Thrombi are the most common in the ileocecocolic branch of the cranial mesenteric artery; emboli arising from this site may be thrombi or emboli of parasitic larvae. Thromboemboli also lodge in the peripheral vasculature within the intestinal wall. Aortic verminous thrombotic lesions may give rise to parasite emboli that lodge in blood vessels of the brain to produce **cerebral infarction**.

Fibrocartilaginous emboli cause spinal cord infarcts

Infarction of the spinal cord caused by emboli of fibrocartilaginous material from ruptured intervertebral disks occurs in dogs, cats, horses, and pigs. Emboli lodged in arteries or veins of the leptomeninges and spinal cord cause a pattern of infarction and necrosis called **necrotizing myelopathy**. Material from the nucleus pulposus may herniate directly into venous sinuses or enter smaller arteries and pass back through the arterial system.

Fat emboli lodge in highly vascular tissue

Fat emboli arise as a complication of bone fractures, prolonged surgery, or osteomyelitis. They seldom cause infarction. Although gross lesions are usually not obvious, capillaries in the lungs contain small masses of fat. Retrograde embolism of fat may occur at slaughter during the agonal period; when the

jugular vein is opened for exsanguination, fatty tissue can be sucked from the wound into the right atrium, inferior vena cava, and hepatic veins.

Fat emboli also lodge in the renal glomerulus, and in dogs, "lipid glomerulopathy" is a rare but fatal complication of trauma to fat tissue.

COLLATERAL AND COMPENSATORY CIRCULATION

Sudden total blockage of most any artery will produce infarction. If the block is incomplete, slowly progressive, or in an organ with anastomosing capillaries, however, collateral circulation will develop. When one **femoral artery** of the dog is experimentally ligated, transient lameness and edema may develop in the limb, but anastomosing vessels will enlarge and new channels will form to bypass the ligated artery. When the kidney is made ischemic by blocking the arcuate arterial system (intraarterial injection of latex beads is a common experimental model), new arterial channels develop from several neighboring vascular sources.

The greater the blood supply, the more rapidly that collateral circulation develops. If the **right mammary** and **right external pudic arteries** are ligated in a young calf, circulation will be totally restored by adulthood. The vascular supply to gland tissue is completely supplied by surrounding vessels. At lactation, milk production in the right mammary glands will be identical to that in the left, as the caudal branch of the left mammary artery fully restores the blood vessels of the right mammary gland.

Where alternative pathways of circulation exist, vascular blockage results in compensatory enlargement of what was a previously minor flow route. Bilateral blockage of the **common carotid arteries** of the dog shunts blood through vertebral arteries and also incites development of anastomotic connections of the internal carotid to the maxillary and ascending pharyngeal arteries.

Blockage of the pulmonary artery

Obstruction of the pulmonary artery can accompany pneumonia, congenital heart disease, bronchiectasis, and parasite infestations. The pulmonary artery is commonly blocked in dogs with dirofilariasis when dead worms lodge in the arterial wall, causing proliferative changes. In walls of affected pulmonary arteries, vasa vasorum are dilated proximal to and at sites of obstruction. As compensation, anastomoses develop between pulmonary artery and bronchial arteries (the bronchial arteries originate from the first to fourth intercostal arteries and supply the hilar lymph nodes, vasa vasorum of the pulmonary arteries and veins, and bronchioles). In severe dirofilariasis, the dilated tortuous bronchial arteries around the bronchial tree can be seen to terminate in branches in the periphery of lung lobes; this collateral circulation occurs most often in the right diaphragmatic lobe.

Blockage of the portal vein

Blockage of the portal vein leads to infarction of the intestine. Animals with this condition rarely survive. In dogs, **gastric torsion** leads to striking obstruction of the portal venous system. Twisting at the pyloric and cardiac areas of the stomach blocks tributaries of the portal vein. Occlusion of the portal vein leads to severe venous congestion. Vascular stasis of the intestine causes ischemia, loss of endothelial integrity, and tiny hemorrhages along the veins at the mesenteric attachments of the gut wall (Fig. 7.10). Sudden complete block of the portal veins leads rapidly to shock.

Blockage of the posterior vena cava

When the posterior vena cava is blocked, blood is shunted into the azygos vein. In the dog, the single azygos vein begins at the third lumbar vertebra by confluence of intervertebral veins and has an anastomotic branch with the posterior vena cava (Fig. 7.11). It joins the precava at its termination in the right atrium opposite the third intercostal space. Although obstruction may cause edema of the limbs and engorged veins, many animals with extensive blockage of the posterior vena cava are asymptomatic. Enlargement of preexisting pathways gradually permits these vessels to compensate and normal tissue perfusion to occur.

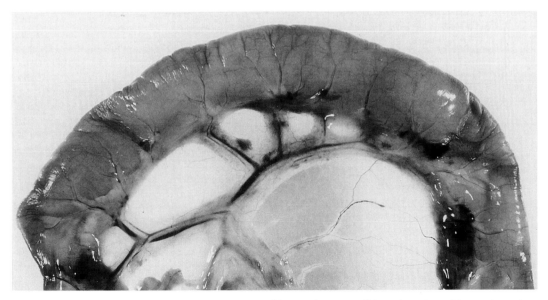

FIGURE 7.10. Congestion and hemorrhage, small intestine, dog with gastric torsion. Intestine has hemorrhages along mesenteric border. Marked congestion of capillaries and venules of intestinal walls.

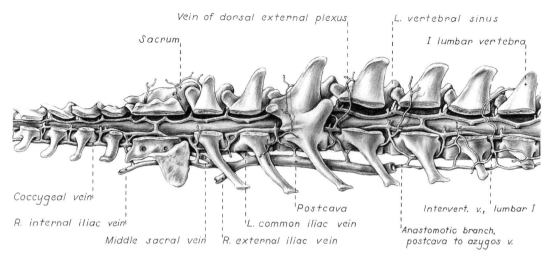

FIGURE 7.11. Anastomotic branch of postcava to azygos vein, which markedly enlarges to permit survival in blockade of posterior vena cava. (Drawing: Karl Reinhard)

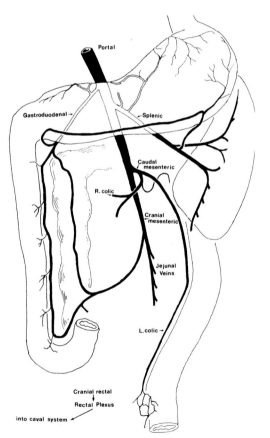

FIGURE 7.12. Arterial supply to viscera affected by gastric torsion.

Gastric torsion

Torsion of the canine stomach leads to striking obstruction of the portal venous system by twisting at the pyloric and cardiac areas, resulting in blockage of tributaries of the portal vein (Fig. 7.12). At the cardia, torsion of 180–360° occurs in a clockwise direction; the degree of torsion determines the extent of vascular obstruction. Although veins are obstructed, arteries often remain intact, leading to engorgement and stasis of the portal and vena caval systems.

Gastric torsion is most common in Great Danes and other giant breeds (especially the males). It develops in the following progression: overeating → gastric dilatation → torsion of gastroesophageal junction → accumulation of fluid and gas. Early, the greater curvature moves ventrally (especially in deep-chested dogs), the gastrohepatic ligament becomes lax, and the pylorus is freed to move dorsally, cranially, and to the right—all preludes to **volvulus**. Gas accumulates largely from bacterial fermentation (stomach contents usually have the sweet odor of silage), although aerophagia and the action of HCl and H_2CO_3 also contribute.

Distension of the stomach has important secondary effects. (1) There is direct pressure necrosis of **gastric mucosa** due to vascular stasis, especially at the greater curvature of the fundus, where small vessels anastomose with the left epigastric artery. The mucosa shows hyperemia, hemorrhages, edema, and necrosis (gangrene), probably due to histamine release and increased capillary permeability. (2) **Portal venous stasis** leads to hypoperfusion of viscera, causing release of prostaglandins and phospholipases. (3) Pressure on the thorax may precipitate **lung** dysfunction. (4) The **duodenum** is compressed. (5) The **spleen** is engorged from venous occlusion as it twists on its long axis.

Pressure on the **posterior vena cava** shunts blood through the vertebral veins, ventral vertebral sinuses, and azygos veins. Signs at this stage are extreme abdominal pain. Blockade of the gastroesophageal junction causes belching, retching (without vomiting), decreased venous return to the heart, and decreased cardiac output—a "slow-flow syndrome" that can precipitate intravascular coagulation.

VASCULAR SHUNTS AND FISTULAE

Portosystemic venous anomalies

Anomalous shunts between the portal vein and the posterior vena cava are most commonly reported in dogs. When severe, the clinically important changes are central nervous system signs, small liver, and high blood ammonia levels. Excretion of tracer dyes by the liver is delayed, and bile acids are increased in serum.

Canine congenital venous anomalies, in which portal blood bypasses the liver in its return to the right atrium, include (1) persistent patency of the fetal ductus venosus; (2) atresia of the portal vein, usually with functional collateral portosystemic shunts; (3) anomalous connection of the portal vein to the caudal vena cava; (4) anomalous connection of the portal vein to the azygos vein; and (5) drainage of the portal vein and caudal vena cava into the azygos vein. In normal dogs the hepatic artery supplies about 25% of the blood to the liver; the remainder comes from the portal vein. In severe portosystemic venous anomalies, the total hepatic blood flow is reduced to near 50% of normal, despite a compensatory increase in hepatic arterial flow. The liver undergoes atrophy partly because of loss of hepatotropic factors (which arise from pancreatic and gastroduodenal sources) that are normally present in portal blood.

Arteriovenous malformations

Vascular malformations of skin and nervous tissue, characterized by large irregular venous channels, are found in several species. They are generally of little significance. These defects arise at various sites in the developmental pathway of blood vessel formation and may be due to mutant **growth factors**

or **growth factor receptors** for the fibroblast growth factor (FGF) or vascular endothelial growth factor (VEGF) families. Angiopoietin, secreted by mesodermal cells, binds to ligands on vascular endothelium to activate release of growth factors that control the formation of the vascular wall.

$$\text{Mesoderm} \xrightarrow{\text{FGF}} \text{angioblasts} \rightarrow$$

$$\text{endothelial cell} \xrightarrow{\text{VEGF}} \text{blood vessel}$$

Hepatic encephalopathy

The brain becomes progressively more sensitive to various exogenous and endogenous substances in chronic hepatic dysfunction. Affected animals are much more sensitive to hypoxia and electrolyte imbalance. Encephalopathy is associated with marked increases in blood ammonia, which arises in the colon. Normally, NH_3 is absorbed and carried via the portal vein to the liver, where it is incorporated into the ornithine cycle and converted into urea. In dogs with portal venous anomalies, serum NH_3 concentrations are 2–11 times higher than normal. Methionine, amino acids, and short-chain fatty acids have been reported as contributing to the CNS signs of hepatic encephalopathy.

Acquired portacaval shunts

During increased pressure in the portal venous system (portal hypertension), blood bypasses the liver and returns to the heart by various collaterals. As portal hypertension rises, blood begins to flow through channels that normally are not patent. For example, the **azygos vein** dilates and accepts blood from the portal system. Commonly, a complex of varices connecting the portal vein to the 13th intercostal vein (which drains into the azygos vein) can be seen in dogs with portal hypertension.

Varices between the cranial mesenteric vein and the caudal vena cava, and the shunting of portal venous blood into the caudal vena cava via a patent ductus venosus, can also be found in portal hypertension.

Portal hypertension arises from conditions such as carcinoma of the adrenal cortex growing into the caudal vena cava (see Fig. 12.7), tumors of the right atrium of the heart, and liver disease, both posthepatic (obstruction of the hepatic veins) and prehepatic (obstruction of the portal veins).

Intrahepatic shunts

Communications between branches of the **hepatic arteries and portal venous radicles** result in retrograde flow into the portal vein. Most arteriovenous fistulae are congenital defects (resulting from

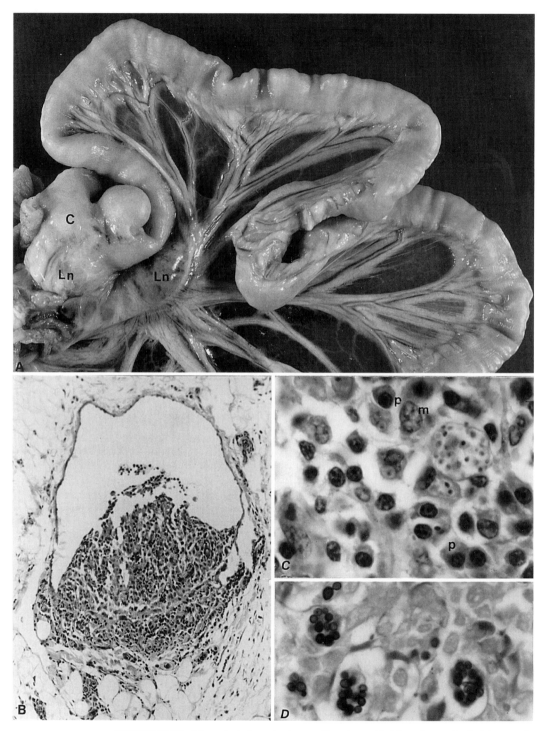

FIGURE 7.13. Mesenteric lymphadenopathy, dog with histoplasmosis. A. Mesenteric lymph nodes are enlarged and meaty but do not exude milky fluid; *C,* cecum; *Ln,* lymph node. B. Granulomatous inflammatory tissue eroding through a lymphatic vessel in lymph node. C and D. *Histoplasma capsulatum* in macrophages. Hematoxylin-eosin stain in *C;* capsule is a clear hole; *m,* macrophage; *p,* plasma cell. Silver stain in *D.*

failure of differentiation of embryologic anlagen with persistence of many vascular communications). Other causes include trauma to the abdomen, rupture of an aneurysm of the hepatic artery, and surgery or diagnostic procedures of the abdominal vasculature.

Lesions are often found during angiography or surgery and include dilated, tortuous, pulsating vessels on the surface of the liver. On cross section, large cavernous vessels are found within the liver lobes. These make the liver large despite its reduced mass of hepatocytes. Microscopically, the arterial branches have foci of intimal hyperplasia, and there is reduplication and splitting of the inner elastic membrane. Within the abnormal vessels is evidence of thrombosis and recanalization.

Dogs with arteriovenous fistulae have evidence of **portal hypertension**: ascites, enlargement of the azygous vein, and extrahepatic portacaval venous shunts. Arteriovenous fistulae between **hepatic artery** and **hepatic vein** are very rare and are associated with rapid onset of cardiac failure.

LYMPHATIC BLOCKAGE

Blockage of lymphatic vessels leads to accumulation of lymph in tissue or in body cavities. When damaged by surgery, neoplasms, and intravascular parasites, the normal flow of interstitial fluid into lymphatics is prevented, and edema fluid accumulates locally. Lymphatic vessels are enlarged, and if they are on the serosal surfaces lining body cavities, they may ooze fluid to cause ascites or hydropleura (Fig. 7.13).

Rare, hereditary malformations of lymphatic vessels in dogs, calves, and pigs are manifest as local subcutaneous edema of the limbs.

Thoracic duct obstructions

Duct rupture leads to chylothorax

Chyle, the milky fluid taken up by the lacteals from food in the intestine, is composed of lymph and triglyceride droplets. When the thoracic duct is ruptured, chyle flows into the thoracic cavity. The presence of effused chyle in the thoracic cavity is called **chylothorax** (or chylopleura). This syndrome is manifest by dyspnea and tachypnea on exertion and has been alleviated by ligation of the thoracic duct.

Chylothorax in dogs and cats is most often caused by trauma (such as surgery and the tearing that occurs in vomiting and chronic coughing). It can also accompany congenital defects, neoplasms, and granulomas such as blastomycosis and histoplasmosis. For example, *Histoplasma capsulatum* grows within lymph vessels to produce lymphangi-

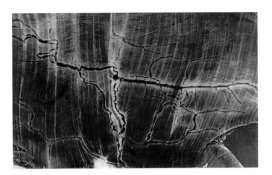

FIGURE 7.14. Lymphatic dilatation, surface of diaphragm, dog with chronic histoplasmosis. Granulomatous inflammatory lesion blocks lymph vessels.

tis, blockade of the lymph vessel lumen, and rupture of the vessel wall (Fig. 7.14).

In dogs, the thoracic duct lies on the right side of the caudal thorax and crosses to the left side at the level of T6, the 6th thoracic vertebra. In cats, the duct lies entirely on the left side of the mediastinum. There are marked individual variations in thoracic duct anatomy in normal cats and dogs.

Thoracic lymphangiectasia is a cause of chylothorax

Partial or total obstruction of the thoracic duct can cause lymphangiectasia and chylothorax. Effusion of chyle occurs because fluid oozes from dilated lymphatics (in contrast to the more rapid flow when the thoracic duct is ruptured). Many of these lesions are malformations (e.g., lymphaticovenous anastomoses) and can be diagnosed only by radiography. Oil-based contrast agents are injected into hindlimb lymphatics to outline the thoracic duct.

ISCHEMIA

In this section we consider the ischemic variety of anoxia. Ischemia is essentially a localized tissue anemia. Failure of blood to circulate through tissue leads to a progressive, cascading series of events that ends in necrosis. If there is anoxia, cells quickly die from oxygen depletion and shutdown in ATP production. Ischemia-induced pathologic processes are major causes of death in animals. They are also the major causes of death in humans, especially myocardial infarction and cerebral ischemia.

- **Hypoxia**—a reduction of oxygen below normal amounts in a tissue.
- **Ischemia**—local deficiency of blood in tissue due to obstruction or constriction of a blood vessel.
- **Hyperemia**—increased blood in tissue resulting in distension of blood vessels.

Active hyperemia is due to dilatation of blood vessels, **passive hyperemia** to hindered drainage.

- Congestion—an abnormal accumulation of fluid within the vessels of an organ. This is usually taken to mean blood, but the term occasionally is applied to mucus. Congestion is often equated with passive hyperemia but is a broader, less precise term.

Consequences of ischemia

The earliest cellular change in ischemia is swelling and disintegration of mitochondria. Loss of energy in turn leads to cell membrane damage, which permits entry of water, electrolytes, and plasma proteins into the cells. Increases in cellular calcium lead to irreversible cytopathic changes and necrosis. Cellular enzymes are liberated into the interstitial fluids as the cell dies.

Two phases of ischemic injury

Ischemic injury occurs in an **anoxic phase**, during which blood flow is shut down, and in a **postischemic phase**, as blood flow begins again. In clinical situations in which animals survive an ischemic event, much of the tissue injury occurs during this reflow period.

Superoxide radicals in postischemic injury

In ischemia, oxygen deficiency enhances production of superoxide radicals from "leaky" sites in the mitochondrial electron transport chain. A major source of superoxide in postischemic tissues is the enzyme **xanthine oxidase**, which is especially rich in intestine, lung, and liver:

$$\text{Xanthine} + H_2O + NAD \xrightarrow{\text{xanthine oxidase}}$$
$$\text{uric acid} + 2O_2 + 2H^+$$

In ischemic tissue the enzyme xanthine dehydrogenase is converted to xanthine oxidase, a reaction initiated by a drop in cell energy. The cell fails to operate its membrane pumps, which maintain ion gradients across its membranes. Ions are redistributed, especially calcium, which is elevated in the cytosol and activates a protease that converts the dehydrogenase to oxidase. ATP is depleted, and AMP accumulates and is catabolized to adenosine inosine and then to hypoxanthine. Hypoxanthine serves as an oxidizable purine substrate of xanthine:

$$\text{Xanthine (or hypoxanthine)} + O_2$$
$$\xrightarrow{\text{xanthine oxidase}} \text{uric acid} + 2O_2 + 2H^+$$

In ischemia, there is a new enzyme (xanthine oxidase), a new substrate (hypoxanthine), and oxygen.

Intestinal ischemia

Ischemia of the intestine is a major cause of mortality in animals. The intestine becomes ischemic in three situations: (1) **blockade of the portal vein**; (2) **shock**, during which blood is shunted away from the intestinal mucosa to brain and myocardium (sometimes called flow ischemia); and (3) **obstruction of a mesenteric artery**. Horses are especially liable to intestinal ischemia; it arises from malposition of the gut or from strongyle larvae–induced thrombosis of the cranial mesenteric artery. In terminal stages of many equine diseases, low cardiac output accompanying low perfusion pressure of endotoxic shock perpetuates mucosal necrosis.

Ischemia of the gut is "multifactorial"

Mucosal damage causes decreased intestinal net fluid and electrolyte absorption. Three factors are implicated in intestinal lesions of ischemia: (1) **hypoxia at the tips of villi** (extravascular short-circuiting of oxygen in the villous countercurrent exchanger underlies the hypoxia present in villous tips, while intraluminal administration of oxygen experimentally prevents the mucosal lesions of shock); (2) **superoxide radicals** released during reflow of blood (damage is ameliorated by superoxide dismutase treatment); and (3) **pancreatic proteases** acting on mucosa when the ischemic mucosa ceases to produce protective mucus—the epithelial lining becomes vulnerable to luminal enzymes, particularly trypsin and chymotrypsin (intraluminal application of protease inhibitors prevents mucosal damage).

Blood is shunted away from villous tips

In all species, intestinal ischemia induces inhibition of epithelial transport, bleeding from the mucosal capillaries into the lumen, and loss of epithelial cells from the villi. In the villi, blood is shunted from the central arteriole to peripheral capillaries. Thus blood bypasses the tips of the villi, which become hypoxic and slough into the intestinal lumen.

Bleeding is especially common in dogs, in which bloody diarrhea is a sequel to shock. The first sign of ischemic mucosal damage is subepithelial spaces at the tips of the villi. This space expands, and the epithelial layer is lifted from the lamina propria. If ischemia is prolonged, this process continues down the side of the villus, which becomes denuded of epithelial cells (see Fig. 7.9). Even with severe mucosal damage, the deep layers of the intestine are relatively normal.

Bacteria leak into lymphatics and portal vein

Ischemia results in an imbalance of gut bacterial flora and usually leads to an increase in anaerobes (*Clostridium* spp. and *Bacteroides* spp.) and a decrease in aerobic bacteria. *Clostridium* spp. and *Bacteroides* spp. increase in most species with intestinal ischemia. There is a progressive leak of bacteria into the portal vein and peritoneal lymphatics, thus creating a tendency to septicemia when intestinal ischemia occurs.

Ischemia of the small intestinal mucosa is much more often lethal than colonic ischemia. Absorption of bacterial toxins, fermentation products, luminal enzymes, and products of necrotic tissue (i.e., peptides, lysosomal enzymes, and membrane fragments) leads to irreversible shock, then to thrombosis, and finally to intestinal infarction.

Vasospastic ischemia

Vasospastic ischemia, a nonocclusive ischemia, or "abdominal angina," that arises from severe constriction of intestinal blood vessels, is comparable to nonocclusive ischemia in coronary arteries of the heart. Excessive tension in smooth muscle of arterioles, the major control sites of blood flow in the intestine, causes release of cardiotoxic factors, which circulate and predispose to shock and infarction.

Evaluation of gut ischemia during surgery

Evaluation of intestinal viability is important in resection of necrotic portions of the intestine. It is done visually during surgery. Spontaneous peristalsis is the best index of intestinal viability. Other criteria include color of the serosa, reflex motility, refill following blanching, and inspection of the mucosa via enterotomy. These criteria are not reliable, however, and some surgeons resort to special manipulations for a more precise analysis of the extent of ischemia, such as intravenous injection of sodium fluorescein. Fluorescein given intravenously is rapidly distributed to all perfused tissues. Intestine with a blood supply fluoresces under ultraviolet light; areas with reduced circulation show less or no fluorescence.

ADDITIONAL READING

Adams HR. 1997. Following up endogenous nitric oxide article. *J Am Vet Med Assoc* 210:888.

Darien BJ, et al. 1995. Morphologic changes of the ascending colon during experimental ischemia and reperfusion in ponies. *Vet Pathol* 32:280.

Davies AP, et al. 1979. Primary lymphedema in three dogs. *J Am Vet Med Assoc* 174:1316.

Fikes JD, O'Sullivan MG, Bain FT, Mayo MJ, Harber ES, Carlson CS. 1996. Gastric infarction in cynomolgus monkeys *(Macaca fascicularis)*. *Vet Pathol* 33:171.

Flynn DM, et al. 1996. A sialyl Lewis[x]-containing carbohydrate reduces infarct size: role of selections in myocardial reperfusion injury. *Am J Physiol* 271:H2086.

Folkman J, D'Amore PA. 1996. Blood vessel formation: what is its molecular basis? *Cell* 87:1153.

Harber ES, O'Sullivan MG, Mayo MJ, Carlson CS. 1996. Cerebral infarction in two cynomolgus macaques *(Macaca fascicularis)* with hypernatremia. *Vet Pathol* 33:431.

Hayes MA, et al. 1978. Acute necrotizing myelopathy from nucleus pulposus embolism in dogs with intervertebral disk degeneration. *J Am Vet Med Assoc* 173:289.

Liu S-K, et al. 1969. Pulmonary collateral circulation in canine dirofilariasis. *Am J Vet Res* 30:1723.

Moore PF, Whiting PG. 1986. Hepatic lesions associated with intrahepatic arterioportal fistulae in dogs. *Vet Pathol* 23:57.

Neu H, von Rautenfeld DB. 1996. Primary congenital lymphoedema in seven Labrador retriever puppies, one German shepherd puppy, and one Canadian wolf puppy. *Eur J Comp Anim Med* 5:52.

Nordstoga K, Aasen AO. 1979. Hepatic changes in late canine endotoxin shock. *Acta Pathol Micriobiol Scand* [A] 87:335.

Scavelli TD, et al. 1986. Portosystemic shunts in cats. *J Am Vet Med Assoc* 189:317.

Suter MM, et al. 1985. Primary intestinal lymphangiectasia in three dogs. *Vet Pathol* 22:123.

Ware WA, Fenner WR. 1988. Arterial thromboembolic disease in a dog with blastomycosis localized in a hilar lymph node. *J Am Vet Med Assoc* 193:847.F

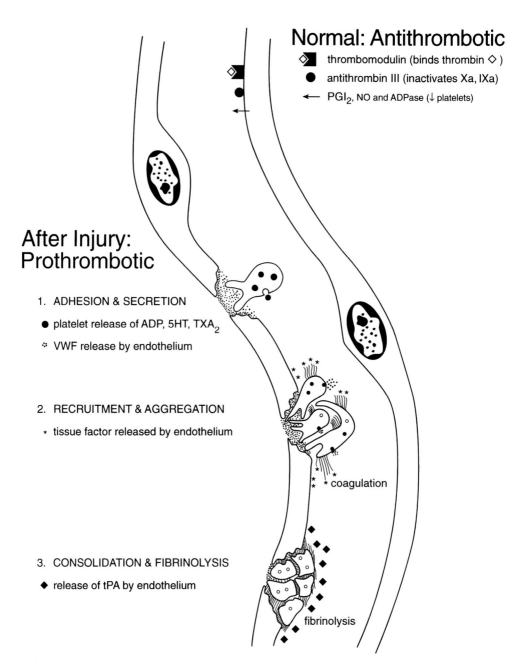

Normal: Antithrombotic

◈ thrombomodulin (binds thrombin ◇)
● antithrombin III (inactivates Xa, IXa)
← PGI$_2$, NO and ADPase (↓ platelets)

After Injury: Prothrombotic

1. ADHESION & SECRETION

● platelet release of ADP, 5HT, TXA$_2$
✢ VWF release by endothelium

2. RECRUITMENT & AGGREGATION

✳ tissue factor released by endothelium

✳ coagulation

3. CONSOLIDATION & FIBRINOLYSIS

◆ release of tPA by endothelium

fibrinolysis

FIGURE 8.1. Phases of hemostatic plug formation. 1. Adhesion and secretion. Immediate platelet adherence to basement membrane fragments and collagen (binding incorporates von Willebrand factor); release of ADP, serotonin (5-HT), and thromboxane A$_2$ (TXA$_2$)—all of which attract and activate circulating platelets; release of prostaglandins and nitric oxide, which limit thrombus expansion. 2. Aggregation. As platelets aggregate, they undergo the platelet release reaction, which is characterized by secretion of clot-promoting substances into the environment of the platelet mass. Phospholipoproteins on platelet surfaces attract thrombin, which initiates fibrin formation. 3. Consolidation. The vascular defect is impermeable. Neutrophils and erythrocytes contact and are incorporated into the developing thrombus, and the clot retracts. Fibrinolysis is initiated by release of tissue plasminogen activator (tPA) from endothelium. Thrombosis is contained by endothelial release of thrombomodulin (thrombomodulin binds thrombin, which activates protein C; protein C in turn cleaves factors Va and VIIIa) and heparin-like molecules that complex with antithrombin III to inactivate thrombin and coagulation factors Xa and IXa.

▦ CHAPTER 8

Hemostasis

Hemostasis (*hemo-* + Gr. *stasis,* halt) is the arrest of bleeding, either by clot formation, vasoconstriction, or physical means. In hemostasis, blood flow is interrupted through the vascular lumen. Bleeding must be prevented or stopped so that blood is contained within the vascular lumen and maintained in a fluid state. Bleeding, even from trivial or minor wounds in tissue, can be prevented by a combination of the following mechanisms:

- Platelet aggregation
- Coagulation
- Vasoconstriction
- Physical obstruction of the blood vessel

Vasoconstriction is an immediate, often transient, response to trauma that plays a significant role in reducing blood flow but rarely has a significant effect on extensive hemorrhage. Reduction of blood flow not only reduces blood loss through vascular defects but also slows the movement of blood past the endothelial surface and allows the enzymatic reaction of coagulation and platelet aggregation to be more effective.

The crucial reaction in stanching blood flow in wounds is the interaction of platelets and coagulation factors within the vessel lumen to form thrombi. The critical events within the vascular lumen at sites of endothelial injury are platelet aggregation (which loosely covers the endothelial defect) and coagulation, the polymerization of fibrinogen into fibrin. As hemorrhage occurs and blood increases in tissue spaces, there is increased pressure. Blood accumulating extravascularly may inhibit or prevent further extravasation.

In small wounds, the initial event in clot formation is the transformation of normal antithrombotic endothelium into prothrombotic endothelium. Activation of endothelial cells—whether by trauma, bacterial endotoxin, leukocytes, or cytokines—causes endothelium to transform to a procoagulant surface.

When endothelium is destroyed, circulating platelets are exposed to a complex milieu of subendothelial ground substances that includes collagen, fibronectin, and laminin. Von Willebrand factor, released by injured endothelial cells, plays a critical role in binding platelets to these substances. Endothelial injury leads directly to these events: (1) collagen and other thrombogenic materials are exposed at sites where endothelium is injured; (2) injured endothelial cells release **von Willebrand factor** (vWF), a large glycoprotein (which is also present in platelets and serum), into the site of injury; (3) vWF adheres to collagen and then binds circulating platelets via **platelet surface proteins** called **GpIb**, causing platelets to cover the endothelial defect; (4) **thromboplastin** is released by damaged tissue and acts directly to initiate coagulation; (5) platelets express surface receptors for fibrinogen, and because fibrinogen is present in the area of the developing clot, multiple fibrinogen bridges enhance platelet aggregation (Fig. 8.1). The **coagulation cascade** forms a large clot at the site of endothelial injury, and the clot is bound to the developing platelet mass.

As platelets aggregate to cover the vascular defect, they are stimulated to undergo the **platelet release reaction**: a marked change in platelet shape, accompanied by release of granules and activation of surface receptors and adherence molecules. Various soluble factors in platelet granules are spewed into the developing platelet plug and act to recruit new platelets to the mass, to enhance vasoconstriction, and to initiate the process of coagulation.

Surfaces of activated platelets serve as an assembly area for an enzyme cascade of coagulation factors that produce the protein-cleaving enzyme **thrombin**. The target of the protease thrombin is

fibrinogen, a large protein circulating in plasma. When contacted by platelet-bound thrombin, fibrinogen molecules undergo a remarkable polymerization, linking together to form **fibrin**, a large threadlike polymer. Fibrin forms a network in the vicinity of platelets (where thrombin is generated), giving the clot stability. The rapidity and intensity of fibrin production determine the extent of clot formation. The final stages of blood coagulation, generally referred to as the common pathway of blood coagulation, are as follows (roman numerals in parentheses indicate the official designation of the blood coagulation factor).

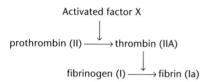

The small fibrin clot is only a transitory device, rapidly formed and soon dismantled by fibrinolysis. The **fibrinolytic system** is a distinct group of enzymes that degrade fibrin into split products. Fibrinolysis prevents excessive coagulation that might otherwise kill the host. During fibrinolysis, a circulating plasma protein is activated to form the fibrinolytic enzyme **plasmin**, which cleaves fibrin. Plasmin also operates to dismantle large clots, thus permitting the permanent repair system of **fibroplasia** and **endothelial regrowth** to return the tissue to normal gradually.

PREVENTION OF COAGULATION BY NORMAL ENDOTHELIUM

When activated within the vascular system, the combined effects of platelet aggregation and activation of the coagulation system would, if uncontrolled, lead to disastrous accumulation of fibrin thrombi within blood vessels. To prevent disseminated intravascular coagulation from following even trivial and minor wounds, three potent mechanisms of resistance to thrombosis are present:

- **Thromboresistance** of endothelial surfaces
- **Inhibition of thrombin** by antithrombin III and heparin
- **Lysis of fibrin** by the fibrinolytic system

Normal vascular patency depends on an equilibrium between coagulation and fibrinolysis. Clinically, the breakdown of these systems leads to dissem-

inated intravascular coagulation, a major cause of death in severe burns, sepsis, and other severe injuries.

Thromboresistance of endothelium

Normal endothelial cells release factors that limit the extent of coagulation, platelet activation, and fibrinolysis. Endothelial cells control the early events of the hemostasis. In contrast, activated or injured endothelium releases procoagulant factors that enhance the clotting process and override these normal anticlotting systems.

Normal endothelium is resistant to thrombosis because of several different mechanisms (Table 8.1). α_2-Macroglobulin, present in the glycocalyx that coats luminal surfaces of endothelial cells, inhibits proteases of the coagulation, fibrinolytic, and kinin systems that operate extracellularly. There are, however, two powerful surveillance systems that cooperate to prevent thrombosis during normal body functioning: thrombin inhibition and control of platelet activation.

Thrombin inhibition

Thrombomodulin, a protein on endothelial surfaces, is a specific receptor for thrombin and plays a critical role in preventing thrombus formation. When bound to thrombin, thrombomodulin converts it from a procoagulant to an anticoagulant function, thereby decreasing its ability to catalyze clot formation. This action occurs indirectly; the thrombomodulin-thrombin complex activates protein C, which then decreases clotting by proteolytically cleaving factors Va and VIIIa.

Protein C, a zymogen of a serine protease, is a potent anticoagulant that selectively inactivates blood coagulation factors Va and VIIIa. Produced in

TABLE 8.1. Characteristics that prevent and promote thrombosis on endothelial surfaces

Mechanism	Antithrombotic	Prothrombotic
Platelet aggregation	PGI$_2$ NO ADPase	Von Willebrand factor Platelet activating factor
Coagulation	Thrombomodulin α_2-Macroglobulin Antithrombin III Proteins C and S	Thromboplastin Binding factors IXa, Xa Factor Va
Fibrinolysis	Tissue plasminogen activator (tPA)	tPA inhibitor

Note: Normal endothelium is anticoagulant. Activated endothelial cells are converted to procoagulant states.

the liver, it is activated at endothelial surfaces by thrombin. Protein C also stimulates fibrinolysis. **Protein S**, a cofactor for protein C, is also synthesized and released by endothelial cells. Anticoagulant effects are also produced by a membrane-associated heparin-like molecule that is secreted by endothelium and catalyzes the anticoagulant protein antithrombin III.

Control of platelet activation

Prostaglandins (particularly PGI_2 and PGE_1) are formed from endoperoxides by enzymes within endothelial cells. Antiplatelet effects on endothelial surfaces are mediated through the secretion of **prostaglandin I_2** and **nitric oxide**, substances that not only are potent vasodilators but also strongly inhibit the aggregation of platelets. PGI_2 (prostacyclin) inhibits platelet functions in all species of animals, including secretion of granules, release of arachidonic acid metabolites, and expression of fibrinogen receptors on platelet surfaces.

Thrombin inhibition by antithrombin III and heparin

Activated clotting factors are short-lived because they are diluted by blood, removed by the monocyte-macrophage system, degraded by proteases, and inactivated by specific inhibitors. Thrombin, the major player in the final fibrinogen-to-fibrin conversion, is inhibited by several circulating proteins. Referred to as **serpins** (serine protease inhibitors), these proteins include the following:

- Antithrombin III
- α_2-Macroglobulin
- Heparin cofactor II
- α_1-Proteinase inhibitor

Antithrombin III, the major physiologic anticoagulant, is a plasma protein that inactivates thrombin by irreversibly complexing with it (it also inhibits other clotting factors). The thrombin-inhibiting action of antithrombin III is enhanced by heparin. **Heparin** achieves its anticoagulant effect by increasing the formation of irreversible complexes between thrombin and antithrombin III. The antithrombin III molecule has two critical domains: one that binds thrombin, and one that binds heparin (and other glycosaminoglycans). Binding of both domains markedly accelerates thrombin inactivation. Heparin is a potent anticoagulant widely used in the laboratory to prevent coagulation of blood and in clinical treatment to inhibit coagulation. Treatment of an animal with heparin suppresses coagulation and induces a prolonged activated partial thromboplastin time (aPTT).

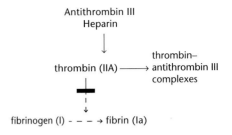

Fibrinolysis

Once a platelet-fibrin clot forms over a wound, endothelial cells bordering the wounded area release materials that activate fibrinolysis. **Fibrinolysis** begins when a circulating plasma protein is activated to form the fibrinolytic enzyme **plasmin** (sometimes called fibrinolysin).

Fibrin, the end product of coagulation, is the substrate for plasmin; that is, plasmin degrades fibrin and releases fibrin breakdown products into the circulation. The fibrinolytic system is the biologic converse of the coagulation mechanism. It includes **plasminogen**, a proenzyme that is converted by **plasminogen activators** to the active enzyme **plasmin**, which in turn digests fibrin into split products.

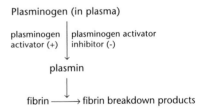

Plasmin

Plasmin is a broad-acting, trypsinlike enzyme that is formed by the action of **plasminogen activator** on the inactive proenzyme, **plasminogen**, a β-globulin present in normal plasma. Binding of plasminogen to plasminogen activator converts plasminogen to plasmin chiefly on the surfaces of thrombi, although conversion also occurs in circulating blood.

Plasmin is a relatively nonspecific serine protease. It degrades not only fibrin but also, to a lesser degree, several circulating proteins, including fibrinogen and other coagulation factors. Plasmin also enhances breakdown of the extracellular matrix by activating procollagenases to collagenases that degrade collagens (invasive growth in conditions from embryogenesis to neoplasia is associated with increased plasmin production). Breakdown of fibrinogen produces fibrinogen fragments that are also anticoagulant.

The detection of plasmin is not clinically meaningful in animal blood, because the stress of collection tends to give faulty data and because the immense amount of antiplasmin in plasma makes plasmin detection in plasma difficult. Therefore, knowledge of how plasmin functions in disease is limited.

Plasminogen activator

Plasminogen activator is synthesized by endothelial cells and macrophages. Fibrinolytic activity is most prominently associated with vascular endothelium but also occurs around leukocytes and some epithelial cells. Macrophages that enter inflammatory sites produce large amounts of plasminogen activator, for example, and the secretion of this enzyme enables them to transect fibrin barriers encountered during migration. In severe, acute bacterial infections, increased amounts of activa-

tors of plasminogen can be detected in plasma. An increase in plasminogen activators also occurs in plasma during ischemia, shock, and disseminated neoplastic disease. Some neoplastic cells produce large amounts of plasminogen activators, which may promote tumor invasion.

The two types of plasminogen activators are (1) **tissue plasminogen activator** (tPA), which is strongly stimulated by fibrin that binds to both plasminogen and tPA; and (2) **urokinase-type plasminogen activator** (uPA) which involves binding of plasminogen and uPA to cell surfaces (especially in embryogenesis and programmed cell death). Both have the same end point: plasmin formation.

Plasminogen activator circulating in plasma is slightly different from that found in tissue. The tissue plasminogen activator (tPA), which can be purchased commercially, is more specific than most plasminogen activators; it has a low affinity for circulating plasminogen and has been called clot specific. Used experimentally as a thrombolytic agent

---

FOCUS

Physiologic Control of Vasoconstriction

ENDOTHELINS, THE MOST POTENT physiologic vasoconstrictors known, arise from large peptides (proendothelins) that are converted to active form by endothelin-converting enzymes. Endothelin synthesis is stimulated by a wide variety of vasoactive substances including thrombin, bradykinin, TNF-α, IL-1, and vasopressin. The genes that encode endothelin, endothelin-converting enzymes, and endothelin receptors are known for many mammals.

Endothelin 1, which is found only in endothelial cells, was discovered in supernatants of cultured porcine aortic endothelial cells. Isopeptides (endothelins 2 and 3) are found in many other tissues. Intravenous injection of endothelin 1 causes (in addition to vasoconstriction) bronchoconstriction, aldosterone secretion, and contraction of uterine smooth muscle. Endothelins activate calcium channels in smooth muscle to initiate contraction. Their biochemical structure and activity are closely related to those of sarafotoxins, a family of peptides isolated from venom of the poisonous snake *Atractaspis engaddensis*.

All of the endothelins interact with inflammatory cytokines and play important roles in inflammation, particularly in sepsis, endotoxemia, and other causes of the systemic inflammatory response syndrome. Plasma levels of endothelin are high in endotoxic shock; endothelin appears to arise from endothelial damage in this syndrome and to partially underlie the severe vasoconstriction of the peripheral vascular bed.

to study removal of clots injected intravenously into animals, tPA is also used in human medicine to remove intravascular thromboemboli.

Exogenous activators of plasminogen include the bacterial products **streptokinase** and **staphylokinase**. Vampire bat saliva is a potent source of fibrinolytic activity, enabling these predators to feed on the blood of cattle and other mammals. Injections of histamine and adrenaline also induce enhanced fibrinolysis in dogs.

Thrombolysis

Pharmacologic dissolution of blood clots is the basis for thrombolytic therapy for thromboembolic disease. Inhibition of the fibrinolytic system can be induced by blocking plasminogen activators with **plasminogen activator inhibitor–1** or by blocking plasmin with α_2-antiplasmin. Thrombolytic agents that have been used in patients include streptokinase, urokinase, and recombinant tissue-type plasminogen activator (and its derivatives).

Fibrinolysis in vivo involves specific molecular interaction between tPA, plasminogen, and fibrin: plasminogen is preferentially activated at fibrin surfaces (plasmin so generated efficiently degrades fibrin because it is protected from rapid inhibition by α_2-antiplasmin). Exogenous non-fibrin-selective agents such as streptokinase (used in therapeutic thrombolysis) activate both systemic and fibrin-bound plasminogen indiscriminately and are less efficient for clot dissolution because they cause systemic generation of plasma with depletion of α_2-antiplasmin and coagulation factors. There is marked species variation in fibrinolytic responses; e.g., dogs have high sensitivity, but cattle and rats low sensitivity to staphylokinase.

PLATELET AGGREGATION

Circulating platelets, or **thrombocytes**, are necessary for maintenance of normal vascular integrity. As endothelial cells age and detach, platelets extend long pseudopods that attach to subendothelial collagen and cover the defect. After attachment, platelets release soluble factors that induce them to aggregate with other platelets. When mammalian blood is devoid of platelets, capillaries and postcapillary venules develop fenestrations and are extraordinarily susceptible to hemorrhage.

Mammalian platelets originate from bone marrow megakaryocytes. Platelet formation occurs as invaginations of the megakaryocyte surface spread inward to dissect the cell, using endoplasmic reticulum as guidelines. Disintegration results in production of 3,000–4,000 platelets per megakaryocyte. When platelets are decreased in circulating blood,

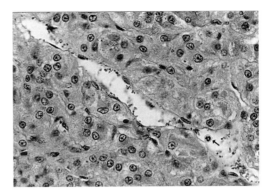

FIGURE 8.2. Platelets adhering to veins in the adrenal medulla, sheep, endothelial injury associated with hemorrhagic shock. Neutrophil *(arrow)* in the venous lumen.

megakaryocytes undergo hypertrophy; they may be prematurely spewed into the circulation and can be detected in blood or lung tissue.

Platelet surfaces are highly reactive. An amorphous layer of carbohydrate-rich glycoproteins covers the surface, making it highly reactive and negatively charged. This **glycocalyx** is made of glycoprotein molecules embedded in the plasma membrane. These molecules either circulate in the bloodstream or are produced by the platelet. By receptor-mediated attachments, platelets readily absorb clotting factors and fibrinogen, giving the platelets an extreme tendency to aggregate when in contact with rough surfaces (Fig. 8.2).

The surface membranes of activated platelets exhibit large amounts of a fibrinogen receptor, the glycoprotein molecule $\alpha_{IIB}\beta_3$ (this receptor is also known as GpIIb-IIIa, but here we use the integrin nomenclature). Fibrinogen, by binding to $\alpha_{IIB}\beta_3$, acts as a cofactor in platelet aggregation. During platelet activation, the molecular transformation of $\alpha_{IIB}\beta_3$ from its resting, closed form to an active, or open, form is a major change in the clotting process. When activated, the outer portions of the $\alpha_{IIB}\beta_3$ molecule open and spread to accommodate the ligand epitopes of fibrinogen that have clustered on the platelet surfaces. Binding causes many receptors to cluster together and causes their transmembrane signal to pass to the platelet cytoskeleton to be translated into platelet shape change, movement, and the platelet release reaction. New antiplatelet drugs used in the prevention of clot formation include drugs that block this receptor.

The role for $\alpha_{IIB}\beta_3$ given above is oversimplified, and the natural phenomenon of platelet aggregation involves multiple, complex interplatelet adhesion molecules. $\alpha_{IIB}\beta_3$ is promiscuous and also functions as a ligand for von Willebrand factor,

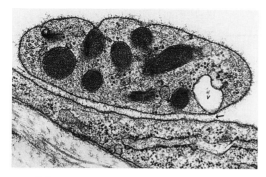

FIGURE 8.3. Ultrastructure of platelet adhered to endothelium. Adhesion of glycocalyx of platelet to glycocalyx of endothelium *(arrow).* Platelet α-granules are large and dense; *v,* vacuole.

fibronectin, and other connective tissue molecules. In addition, prothrombin is an activation-independent ligand of $\alpha_{IIB}\beta_3$ and bound prothrombin is efficiently activated to thrombin.

In response to interactions with thrombin and subendothelial collagen, platelets release **prostaglandins** (PGs), which mediate many actions of platelets. The first step in PG synthesis is the release of arachidonic acids from degradation of phospholipids within the plasma membrane by phospholipases. The freed arachidonic acid is used to form specific PGs that constrict vascular smooth muscle and induce platelet aggregation: thromboxane A_2, PGG_2 and PGH_2. In the normal blood vessel, the balance between two dominant eicosanoids, PGI_2 and TXA_2, maintains blood flow:

- Endothelial cell-derived PGI_2 is a vasodilator and inhibits platelet aggregation.
- Platelet-derived TXA_2 is a vasoconstrictor and activates platelet aggregation.

After endothelial injury and platelet activation, this balance is tipped in favor of platelet aggregation.

Platelet storage granules contain potent aggregation factors and procoagulants. Mammalian platelets contain two types of granules that are important in thrombosis: α-granules and variable-sized granules often called dense granules. **Dense granules** contain surface reactants, most of which are absorbed and taken into the platelet from plasma. These include amines (serotonin, or 5-hydroxy-tryptamine), calcium, and a metabolically inactive nucleotide, ADP. When released, ADP induces rapid aggregation of other platelets.

α-Granules contain a variety of proteins that are synthesized in the megakaryocyte, including **thrombospondin, platelet factor 4** (which coun-

teracts the anticoagulant effect of heparin), and **platelet-derived growth factor** (a potent mitogenic stimulant). α-Granules also contain fibrinogen, fibronectin, and cationic proteins that mimic those of neutrophils (although with much less effect) in attracting granulocytes from the circulation and increasing vascular permeability.

Platelet release reaction

The process whereby platelets transform from tranquil, discoid bodies to spiked, sticky aggregates that discharge their granules is called the **platelet release reaction**. The reaction is initiated when platelets contact collagen and other thrombogenic substances that surround the damaged endothelium. Adhesion is mediated by formation of an enzyme-substrate complex between galactosyl hydroxylysine groups of collagen and transferases located in the platelet surface.

Receipt of these coagulation signals at the platelet surface induces several events in the plasma membrane that are translated into striking surface changes. Some of the molecular events include loss of normal asymmetry of membrane phospholipids, movement of surface proteins, exposure of fibrinogen receptors and anionic lipids, activation of membrane-bound enzymes (such as phospholipases), and alteration of subsurface cytoskeletal fibrils, all of which lead to movement of the platelet surface. Influx of Ca^{2+} during platelet activation disturbs the enzyme aminophospholipid transferase, which maintains the normal asymmetry of membrane phospholipids; this disturbance changes membrane fluidity and permits the structural changes of the release reaction to occur.

As the platelet release reaction proceeds, platelets change shape from disks to swollen spheres, extend spikelike pseudopods, and progress through a series of changes. The lentiform shape of the normal platelet is maintained by a **marginal band** of microfilaments and microtubules at the periphery. Under stimuli, microtubules depolymerize and reassemble and are important in forming pseudopods and releasing granules. During the release reaction, the marginal band contracts, forcing organelles to the cell center. Contents of dense bodies and α-granules are extruded from the platelet; the released substances promote aggregation of other platelets (Fig. 8.3).

Fibrinogen is a cofactor in platelet aggregation

Activated platelets develop new receptors (see Fig. 8.6) for fibrinogen on their surfaces. Contact of activated platelets with fibrinogen thus enhances platelet aggregation. This phenomenon was first noted when stimuli that aggregated platelets from normal animals failed to do so in plasma from patients with hereditary afibrinogenemia. Experimentally, washed platelets suspended in defibrinated plasma fail to aggregate in response to stimuli such as ADP or epinephrine, but addition of fibrin supports aggregation. Both stimuli are required; neither a single external stimulus nor fibrinogen alone can cause platelet aggregation.

Other peptides are involved in strengthening platelet-fibrin binding. **Thrombospondin**, the large glycoprotein secreted by platelets upon activation, binds to receptors on the platelet surface (fibrinogen may be a platelet-bound receptor for thrombospondin) and enhances the rate and firmness of fibrin binding.

Von Willebrand factor is required for platelets to adhere firmly to subendothelial collagen at sites of vascular injury. Circulating in blood and also present in α-granules, von Willebrand factor binds both to collagen exposed at the site of blood vessel injury and to receptors on the platelet surface (referred to as glycoprotein Ib, or GpIb). In addition (a second function), von Willebrand factor binds to and stabilizes coagulation factor VIII flowing in the bloodstream and, by doing so, provides another link between platelets and the coagulation system in the clotting process. Endothelial cells in different vascular beds vary in their production of von Willebrand factor. Von Willebrand factor acts as an acute phase protein; its concentration in plasma rises several-fold in response to tissue injury.

Platelets internalize debris and microorganisms

Platelet aggregation can also occur without defects in endothelium. When circulating platelets contact bacteria, bacterial mucopeptides, or cell debris, they are capable of internalizing this material into the canalicular system of the platelet. As bacteria-bearing vacuoles form, platelets degranulate, aggregate, and are phagocytized by macrophages. Although these platelets are not truly phagocytic, some researchers believe that platelets are deputized in inflammatory reactions, especially when neutrophils are missing or defective. This commonly occurs in the terminal stages of severe systemic infectious diseases.

Hyperlipidemia enhances platelet aggregation

Elevations in plasma concentration of lipids and cholesterol are associated with thrombosis in various diseases. Hypercholesterolemia alters the lipid content of platelet surface membranes and endothelial cells (which is the more important is not clear), and platelets become hyperresponsive to substances that stimulate the platelet release reaction.

Thrombocytopenia

Thrombocytopenia is a drop below 100,000 platelets/ml circulating blood. In most species, a drop below 10,000/μl is accompanied by abnormal bleeding tendencies. The point to which platelets must drop for bleeding to occur is highly variable. Vascular perfusion experiments clearly demonstrate the perpetual function of these cells in maintaining a closed vascular system. When an organ is perfused with platelet-poor plasma, it develops hemorrhages; organs perfused with platelet-rich plasma do not.

The diagnosis of platelet deficiency is based chiefly on three criteria: a history of bleeding, low platelet counts, and increased bleeding time. The history should include a tendency for bleeding, because it is impossible for platelet deficiency to exist for even brief periods without affecting hemostasis. The platelet count should be low, but platelet deficiency can also exist when platelets themselves are abnormal (the count may be normal and even elevated, but the platelets do not function normally). To confirm the diagnosis of platelet deficiency, the establishment of an abnormal bleeding time is essential.

Mechanisms of thrombocytopenia include (1) deficient formation of platelets in bone marrow (e.g., estrogen toxicosis); (2) excessive utilization of platelets, which occurs in any disease with widespread endothelial damage; and (3) premature destruction of platelets, either by intravascular lysis or by removal by the monocyte-macrophage system. **Acquired thrombocytopenia** may occur in systemic infectious diseases, in acute radiation injury, during drug treatment, and as part of some immunologic diseases involving antiplatelet antibodies. When known mechanisms of thrombocytopenia are not identified as causes of bleeding, the condition is referred to as **idiopathic thrombocytopenic purpura**.

Viruses cause thrombocytopenia

The widespread hemorrhagic diatheses that characterize several peracute viral diseases are due to diffuse **virus-induced endothelial damage** (e.g., infectious canine hepatitis, hog cholera, African swine fever, simian hemorrhagic fever, and epidemic hemorrhagic disease of deer). Thrombocytopenia is severe because platelets attach to sites of endothelial injury throughout the body (Fig. 8.4). When platelets are depleted and sites of endothelial injury cannot be covered, hemorrhage occurs.

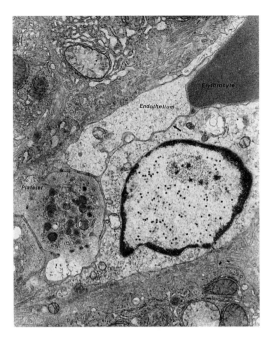

FIGURE 8.4. Platelet trapping, liver sinusoid, infectious canine hepatitis (canine adenovirus 1). Marked swelling of sinusoidal endothelial cells with obliteration of lumen *(arrow)*. Platelet apposed to endothelial cell surfaces is in early phase of release reaction: α-granules have pale areas, and smaller dense granules are at periphery.

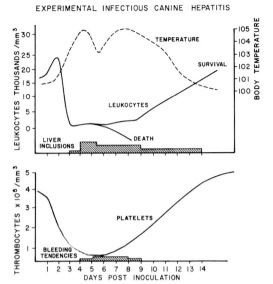

FIGURE 8.5. Relation of platelet deficiency to bleeding, pathogenesis of infectious canine hepatitis.

In most viral hemorrhagic diseases, thrombocytopenia results from the combined effects of direct viral injury to platelets and endothelium (e.g., the petechial and ecchymotic hemorrhages in the skin and below the serosal surface in acute hog cholera). Thrombocytopenia from endothelial damage is the major event in hemorrhages of African swine fever.

Bleeding into submucosal and subserosal areas is characteristic of terminal phases of **infectious canine hepatitis**. The occurrence of erythrocyte extravasation correlates with the lowest points in the thrombocyte count curve (Fig. 8.5). Although the liver is injured and decreased prothrombin and fibrinogen concentrations in plasma have been detected, these factors are less significant in promoting bleeding. They merely exaggerate the tendency to hemorrhage. Examination of liver lesions in early disease reveals the nature of the thrombocytopenia; platelets are trapped in hepatic sinusoids by damaged endothelium to such a great extent that they disappear from circulation.

Thrombocytopathy

Thrombocytopathy is defective platelet function. Acquired thrombocytopathy is common (usually subclinical) as a side effect of therapy with aspirin and phenylbutazone. Aspirin causes a primary release defect that irreversibly acetylates and inactivates the enzyme cyclooxygenase, thus inhibiting secretion mediated by prostaglandins and thromboxane. Aspirin prolongs bleeding time only slightly in normal animals but drastically in animals with other disorders of platelet function.

Hereditary thrombocytopathy is more severe than the acquired forms (Table 8.2). Rare specific congenital platelet defects are termed **thrombasthenia** (weak platelets) or **thrombopathy**. These have been seen in otter hounds, basset hounds, Simmental cattle, domestic cats, Aleutian mink, and fawn-hooded rats. In blood smears, severe structural distortions of platelets are present, and most affected animals have defective platelet granules. Platelets of some thrombasthenia patients lack platelet surface glycoprotein receptors and do not bind fibrinogen; they do not aggregate normally.

Several genetic diseases with major problems in other tissue systems also have defective platelets as an accompanying abnormality. Platelets of mice, cattle, and mink with Chédiak-Higashi disease are deficient in dense granules, serotonin, and ADP; affected animals have prolonged bleeding times.

BLOOD COAGULATION

Clotting (blood coagulation) results when blood vessel walls are injured, especially when endothelium is destroyed. The clot is formed by an enzymat-

TABLE 8.2. Platelet defect diseases

Defect	Association
Thrombocytopenia	
Platelet production	Neoplasms
	Estrogen therapy
	Hypothermia
	Drug toxicity
Platelet destruction	Antiplatelet antibodies
	Viral disease
	Uremia
	Drug toxicity
Thrombocytopathy	
Adhesion	Von Willebrand's disease
	Thrombopathy (Bernard-Soulier syndrome)
Aggregation	Afibrinogenemia
	Thrombasthenia (Glanzmann's disease)
	Hereditary predisposition[a]
Granule factors	Chédiak-Higashi syndrome
Secretion	Aspirin and other nonsteroid drugs

[a]In Aleutian mink, basset hounds, and Simmental cattle.

ic cascade, a series of zymogen activations in which an activated form of one coagulation factor catalyzes the activation of the next. Only small amounts of early factors are needed, because of the catalytic nature of the process. **Coagulation** (the formation of fibrin) is initiated when activated factor X (Xa) cleaves the circulating protein **prothrombin** into two large fragments. One fragment is no longer functional and is released into blood; the other is **thrombin**, a proteolytic enzyme that converts plasma **fibrinogen** to **fibrin**. This is the common final pathway of coagulation. The Xa-catalyzed generation of thrombin is the central focus of blood coagulation. Xa is produced by proteolysis of factor X, which occurs at the terminus of both intrinsic and extrinsic coagulation pathways.

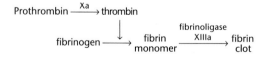

Coagulation pathways

Two enzyme pathways, extrinsic and intrinsic, cause activation of factor X. These two pathways are integrated at several points. The end products of both pathways are proteolytic enzymes that initiate the final common pathway of fibrin formation shown above. In vivo, clotting typically involves a mixture of intrinsic and extrinsic mechanisms.

Extrinsic coagulation pathway

The extrinsic coagulation pathway occurs outside the blood vessel wall when shed blood contacts tissue debris. Clotting is triggered by substances not normally present in flowing blood. **Thromboplastin** (tissue factor, or factor III) is a glycoprotein embedded in plasma membranes of most cells and plays the major role in extrinsic coagulation. It is released by trauma to endothelium and by the potent cytokines TNF and IL-1. Thromboplastin modifies the enzyme proconvertin (factor VII), which in turn activates factor X to initiate the final common pathway of fibrin formation. Experimentally, the extrinsic pathway can be demonstrated by adding a few drops of a dilute suspension of brain tissue extract to normal plasma; clotting is rapidly induced. The prothrombin time test is used to evaluate this pathway (see Table 8.3).

Tissue factor III + Ca^{2+}
↓ factor VII
X ⟶ Xa
↓ factor V
platelet factor III
prothrombin ⟶ thrombin

Intrinsic coagulation pathway

Intrinsic coagulation is triggered by the effects of abnormal surfaces on components normally present in blood. All the factors of the intrinsic system are present in normal plasma. The intrinsic pathway involves a cascade of complex enzymatic reactions, each of which activates the next until factor X is activated. Activated partial thromboplastin time testing is done to evaluate the intrinsic pathway (see Table 8.3).

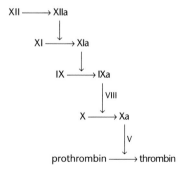

Factor XII activation on platelet surfaces

Commonly, factor XII is activated by contact with negative charges on the surfaces of aggregating

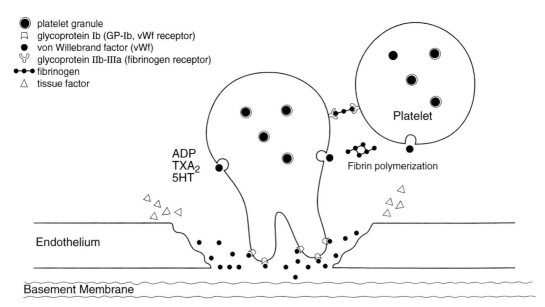

● platelet granule
⌂ glycoprotein Ib (GP-Ib, vWf receptor)
● von Willebrand factor (vWf)
Ψ glycoprotein IIb-IIIa (fibrinogen receptor)
●●● fibrinogen
△ tissue factor

Platelet

ADP
TXA₂
5HT

Fibrin polymerization

Endothelium

Basement Membrane

FIGURE 8.6. Platelet attachment at a site of endothelial injury. Von Willebrand factor, released by damaged endothelial cells, binds to GP-Ib receptors on platelet surfaces. Circulating fibrinogen binds to $\alpha_{IIb}\beta_3$ (GP-IIb-IIIa) receptors to link platelets together.

platelets. When the blood vessel wall is disrupted, subendothelial collagen, basement membrane material, and other connective tissue elements are exposed to plasma. Free carboxyl groups of the exposed collagen activate factor XII, which then initiates the rapid, complex sequence of clotting that terminates in cleavage of prothrombin and ultimately in fibrin polymerization.

In addition to activation on platelet membranes (or solid phase activation), factor XII is also cleaved in fluid phase by proteolysis to yield fragments active in fibrinolysis and kinin release. Thus, plasma deficient in factor XII not only clots abnormally but also shows reduced ability to generate fibrinolysis.

Common pathway

Activated factor X (Xa) is produced by proteolysis of factor X, which occurs at the terminus of both intrinsic and extrinsic coagulation pathways. Xa is a prothrombinase complex that converts prothrombin to thrombin. Factor X may also be activated by a calcium ion (Ca^{2+})–dependent mechanism on platelet surfaces. Prostaglandins released by damaged endothelium are intimately associated with coagulation; that is, tissue injury → endothelial PGI_2 release → factor X activation → coagulation. Factor Xa is a potent inhibitor of thromboxane A_2 synthesis in platelets and prostacyclin (PCI_2) synthesis in endothelial cells. PGI_2 inhibits platelet aggregation but does not significantly affect coagulation.

Prothrombin is a zymogen for thrombin

Prothrombin is synthesized in hepatocytes and released into the bloodstream by the liver. At one end of the prothrombin molecule is a string of carboxylated glutamates. These peculiar amino acids, arising by the carboxylation of terminal glutamates by a vitamin K–containing series of enzymes, are strong chelators of Ca^{2+}. By binding Ca^{2+}, prothrombin is anchored to phospholipid membranes derived from platelets, bringing it in proximity to factors Xa and V, which accelerate prothrombin cleavage. During activation of prothrombin, the terminal Ca^{2+}-binding fragment is cleaved away, leaving active thrombin free on the membrane surface to activate fibrinogen.

Thrombin cleaves peptides from fibrinogen

Fibrinogen is a soluble plasma protein with a molecular weight of nearly 340,000. The molecule is nodose and consists of three beads held together by a thin strand of protein (Fig. 8.6). Running throughout the molecule are three different chains (α, β, and γ), interconnected by disulfide bonds. There is an excess negative charge on the molecule, with a disproportionate amount of charge on the central region.

The triggering event for transformation of fibrinogen to fibrin monomer is the thrombin-catalyzed removal of small polar peptides (called fibrinopeptides A and B) from the central regions of the α and β chains. Cleavage of fibrinopeptides reduces the negative charge on the central region, so the fibrin monomer assumes an overall positive charge. Because the terminal regions retain a negative charge, the fibrin monomers spontaneously polymerize in overlapping, staggered patterns that give the typical periodicity to fibrinogen in electron micrographs.

Fibrin is stabilized by factor XIII

Establishment of covalent bonds between fibrin monomers by the enzyme factor XIII (fibrinoligase, or fibrin stabilizing factor) strengthens fibrin strands and stabilizes the fibrin gel. Factor XIII is activated by thrombin from a precursor in plasma and in platelets. The enzyme stitches neighboring fibrin monomers together by forming peptide bonds between side chains to create cross-links (it catalyzes formation of amide bonds between glutamine and lysine).

Factor XIII cross-links not only fibrin to fibrin but also fibrin to collagen, fibrin to fibronectin, and fibronectin to collagen. By these cross-links, the clot is firmly anchored into place in the tissue.

Coagulation disorders

Absence or defectiveness of any of the clotting factors may result in inadequate blood coagulation. Alternatively, coagulation may be impaired by inhibitors or by the proteolytic action of plasmin. The clinical signs of these diseases involve hemorrhage. In general, large hematomas suggest a coagulation disorder, whereas chronic bleeding from a mucosal surface indicates a platelet deficiency. An accurate differential diagnosis is largely a laboratory exercise. It is usually necessary that the coagulation time, bleeding time, partial thromboplastin time, prothrombin time, and platelet count be determined (Table 8.3).

Hereditary deficiencies in coagulation factors

Disorders arising from hereditary deficiencies in coagulation factors are discovered after excessive bruising, hematoma formation, and continued bleeding after minor trauma or surgery. In severe cases there may be melena, lameness due to periarticular hemorrhage, or prolonged estral bleeding.

Hemophilia is the bleeding diathesis resulting from a lack of procoagulant proteins in plasma. Affected animals develop localized hemorrhages in various tissues, particularly in joints. The defects are temporarily corrected by transfusions of normal plasma. Laboratory findings include prolonged clotting time and activated partial thromboplastin time (aPTT); platelets and prothrombin times are usually normal.

TABLE 8.3. Coagulation tests in dogs

Test	Normal value	Definition
Coagulation time	1–5 minutes	Time for blood to coagulate in vitro after withdrawal from vein
Bleeding time	<6 minutes	Time for bleeding to stop after puncture wound with periodic removal of blood with filter paper
Prothrombin time (PT)	<15 seconds	Time required for clotting of oxalated plasma by addition of calcium (in presence of excess thromboplastin)
Activated partial thromboplastin time (aPTT)	<25 seconds	Measurement of intrinsic and common coagulation systems

Hemophilia A is a factor VIII deficiency

Hemophilia A is the most common severe hereditary coagulation defect of animals and has been reported in most breeds of dogs and cats, Hereford cattle (in Australia), and in standardbred and thoroughbred horses. It is caused by decreased synthesis, secretion, or abnormal forms of factor VIII. Hemophilia is a recessive, sex-linked disease; that is, it is carried by the female and manifested by the male. In dogs, hemophilia A may be mild, moderate, or severe.

Factor VIII is produced in the liver. After activation by trace amounts of thrombin, it accelerates the rate of factor X activation by factor IX. In circulating blood, factor VIII is carried by a large adhesive glycoprotein called von Willebrand factor (vWF). This **factor VIII complex** thus has two components: VIII (antihemophilic factor) and vWF. It plays roles in both clot formation and platelet adhesion, and two of the most common bleeding disorders of animals are a result of a deficiency in the activity of one or the other of these components.

Von Willebrand's disease may be a factor VIII component deficiency

In plasma, **von Willebrand factor** is part of a huge multimer of several molecules. It is an adhesive glycoprotein synthesized by endothelial cells and megakaryocytes and serves as a carrier for factor VIII (Fig. 8.7). By binding to both platelet surfaces and to subendothelial collagen, von Willebrand factor promotes platelet adhesion to blood vessel walls.

In von Willebrand disease (vWD), this endothelial and platelet component is deficient. This is a

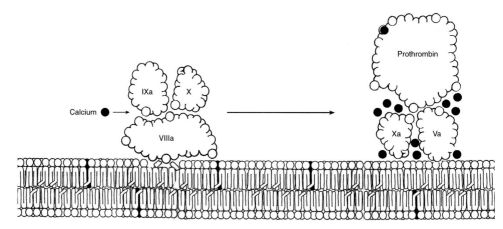

FIGURE 8.7. The role of coagulation factor VIII in converting coagulation factor X to Xa on platelet surfaces. Activated factor VIII (VIIIa) is shown attached to the phospholipid bilayer that forms the plasma membrane. Coagulation factor X is the substrate for the active enzyme (coagulation factor IXa) and the reaction accelerator (coagulation factor VIIIa). By incorporating calcium (black-filled circles), factors IXa and Xa bind to platelet surfaces. After binding the accelerator Va, factor Xa converts prothrombin (II) to thrombin (IIa).

common mild hereditary bleeding disorder of animals. It is an autosomal trait with two forms of genetic expression: an autosomal **recessive disease**, in which individuals are homozygous for the vWD gene and have two asymptomatic heterozygous parents, and an autosomal **incompletely dominant disease** with variable expression, in which both homozygotes and heterozygotes can have bleeding disease (homozygosity is usually lethal).

The incompletely dominant disease is common and occurs in more than 28 breeds of dogs. Scottish terriers have a high prevalence of gene frequency. The recessive disease has been reported in Poland China swine, Scottish terriers, and Chesapeake Bay retrievers.

vWD presents as a bleeding diathesis involving mucosal surfaces and is often associated with physical stresses or other diseases. Signs include gastrointestinal hemorrhage, recurrent hematuria, epistaxis, and bleeding from gingiva, vagina, penis, and nose. Affected dogs may bleed to death after surgery. They have long bleeding times and variable factor VIII-C levels. In dogs, bleeding diathesis becomes less severe with age and during pregnancy. The disease may be subclinical, despite prolonged bleeding times and reduced platelet adhesiveness.

TABLE 8.4. Blood coagulation factors

Factor	Common name	Deficiency
I	Fibrinogen (I_a = fibrin)	Congenital afibrinogenemia in goats, humans, and dogs
II	Prothrombin (II_a = thrombin)	Acquired deficiencies common; congenital deficiencies in English cocker spaniels
III	Thromboplastin	Tissue product; concentrated in brain and lung
IV	Calcium	If plasma Ca^{2+} is bound by oxalates or citrates, clotting is stopped
V	Proaccelerin	Deficiency not recognized in animals
VII	Proconvertin	Hereditary deficiency in beagles
VIII	Antihemophilic factor A	Classic hemophilia in cats, cattle, swine, horses, dogs (in males, sex-linked)
IX	Antihemophilic factor B	Hereditary deficiency, rare, in cats and dogs; depressed by coumarin-type drugs
X	Stuart factor	Deficiency hereditary or acquired; depressed by coumarin-type drugs
XI	Plasma thromboplastin antecedent*	Hereditary deficiency in Holstein cattle and English springer and Great Pyrenees dogs
XII	Hageman factor*	Hereditary deficiency in cats, standard poodles, German shorthaired pointer
XIII	Fibrin stabilizing factor	None reported

*Activity not established in lower vertebrates.

Hemophilia B is a factor IX deficiency

Also a sex-linked recessive disease, **hemophilia B** is rarer than factor VIII deficiency. Most cases have less than 1% of the normal amount of factor IX. It has been reported in several breeds of dogs: coonhound, Saint Bernard, cocker spaniel, bulldog, Alaskan malamute, Shetland sheepdog, and cairn, Airedale, and Scottish terriers. It also occurs in cats (Table 8.4). Blood test results are similar to those in factor VIII deficiency, but the activated partial thromboplastin time defect is corrected by addition of normal serum (because serum contains factor IX activity but not factor VIII coagulant activity).

Acquired deficiencies of coagulation

Acquired deficiencies of coagulation accompany many severe diseases, often with serious consequences. There may be transitory depression of factor synthesis, excessive utilization of factors for hemostasis, or consumption of factors during pathologic intravascular clotting. Factor deficiency may cause prolonged coagulation and prothrombin times even though the thrombocyte count is normal.

Acquired disorders may be general or specific. Severe **trauma** or deep **burns** produce consumption of most coagulation factors. In contrast, some snake venoms and plant toxins precisely affect only one coagulation factor.

Liver failure is associated with low coagulation factor levels

The liver is the important site of synthesis of many coagulation factors, and vitamin K plays an important role in this process. Acute destruction of hepatocytes or chronic liver disease can result in bleeding tendencies. For example, **hypoprothrombinemia** secondary to liver failure can be responsible for a clotting disorder.

Hemorrhage is severe in vitamin K deficiency

Vitamin K is required for synthesis of coagulation factors II, VII, IX, and X. Vitamin K deficiency,

---

FOCUS

Dicumarol and Sweet Clover Poisoning

IN THE EARLY 1900s, sweet clover became a popular crop among early settlers in the northern Midwest and the upper plains area of Canada. Simultaneously, outbreaks of a new hemorrhagic bovine disease began to appear. Cattle were prone to bleed to death after castration or dehorning. Pregnant cows aborted, and newborn calves bled during the first few days of life.

Frank Schofield, the veterinary pathologist at the Ontario Veterinary College at Guelph, first recognized that this disease occurred only in cows that had eaten moldy sweet clover silage. He showed that feeding the spoiled sweet clover to rabbits caused them to bleed and that, at the time of bleeding, the clotting time of the blood was prolonged. He also noted that transfusions of clotted, defibrinated blood briefly stopped the hemorrhage and shortened the clotting time. Lee Roderick of Fargo, North Dakota, confirmed this work in 1929 and added that the plasma prothrombin level was depressed in cattle with sweet clover poisoning.

The disease persisted wherever sweet clover was harvested and allowed to turn moldy in silos. In 1938 a second crucial link was put into place. A farmer strode down the corridors of the University of Wisconsin, sloshing unclotted blood from a pail onto the floor. He wanted action because his castrated and dehorned cattle were bleeding to death. Biochemists shortly thereafter identified the toxic substance: two coumarin molecules linked by formaldehyde.

▶

▶

Called dicumarol, this compound was quickly developed as an anticoagulant for humans. Soon after, it appeared as a rodenticide called warfarin. Poisoned rats bleed from body orifices, especially into tissue around the eyes. Death results from massive bleeding into the abdominal cavity.

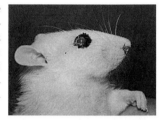

Warfarin markedly decreases the prothrombin concentration in circulating blood. Serum from poisoned rats has a pronounced depressant effect on prothrombin convertibility. Dicumarol acts primarily by inhibiting the conversion factor and only secondarily by depressing prothrombin.

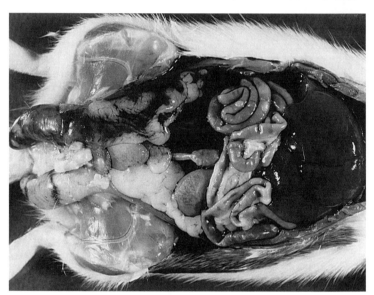

Marked hemorrhage in warfarin toxicity in a rat.

either dietary or due to malabsorption, is accompanied by defects in clotting. Vitamin K acts at the translational level of protein synthesis in the hepatocyte to regulate biosynthesis of prothrombin and other factors.

Abnormal prothrombin is synthesized in the absence of vitamin K or in the presence of vitamin K antagonists such as dicumarol. Although its amino acid sequence is normal, the carboxyglutamate amino terminus that binds Ca^{2+} is defective because vitamin K is an integral part of the enzymes that carboxylate the glutamate residues. Cattle fed dicumarol (which occurs naturally in lush sweet clover) produce this abnormal prothrombin that cannot bind Ca^{2+}.

Anticoagulating rodenticides are usually deriva-

tives of 4-hydroxycoumarin (warfarin, dicumarol) or of indan-1,3-dione (diphacinone, pindone). These drugs inhibit coagulation by suppressing hepatic synthesis of coagulation factors II, VII, IX, and X. There is no effect on circulating coagulation factors, so that a latent period of 24 hours occurs between consumption and clinical signs; in this period, circulating coagulation factors are depleted.

The rat poison **warfarin**, a coumarin derivative, inhibits the hepatic enzyme system responsible for synthesis of coagulation factors. Poisoned dogs have pallor of mucous membranes, petechiae or ecchymoses, epistaxis, and hemoptysis. In severe cases, hemorrhages in pulmonary and enteric tracts occur. Poisoning is characterized by progressive lowering of plasma concentrations of factors II, VII,

IX, and X, leading to a hemostatic defect with prolonged coagulation times. Treatment with vitamin K corrects the deficiency, reversing hypoprothrombinemia. Coumarin derivatives produced by toxigenic fungi growing on clover cause similar bleeding diseases in animals eating contaminated hay.

Viruses cause hemorrhage by depressing coagulation factors

Several of the viruses that attach to endothelium produce clinical signs of hemorrhage that are a result, in part, of excessive consumption of coagulation factors. For example, hog cholera virus replicates in endothelium, platelets, and leukocytes and induces degeneration and cellular death. One of the consequences of the widespread endothelial damage is the exhaustion of coagulation factors in an attempt to repair the vascular endothelium. The hemorrhages that typify the terminal stages of hog cholera, therefore, are due not only to the direct virus-induced damage to capillaries and platelets but also to the superimposition of coagulation factor deficiency and exhaustion thrombocytopenia. The same process is true for infectious canine hepatitis and several other systemic viral infections.

THROMBOSIS

Thrombosis is the formation within a vascular lumen of a **thrombus**, an aggregate of coagulated blood containing platelets, fibrin, and entrapped cells. Thrombi differ from simple clots, which involve only the activation of the coagulation cascade and can develop in vitro or in tissue postmortem. Thrombosis is a pathologic process that represents a blood clot within the uninterrupted blood vascular system.

Platelet-endothelial interaction is tightly coupled to coagulation. That is, activation of the coagulation system is inseparable from the interaction of the platelets with injured endothelium. A summary of the steps, although artificial, helps in understanding some of the mechanisms involved in thrombosis:

- Endothelial injury releases vWF and exposes collagen to platelets
- Activation of platelets leads to the platelet release reaction
- Platelet release reaction stimulates coagulation and aggregation
- Platelets adhere to endothelium or subendothelial collagen
- Added vWF from platelets and serum enhances adhesion and aggregation

- Aggregation—clumping of the platelet plug and interaction with fibrin—occurs
- The clot is consolidated by formation of firm platelet-fibrin binding

When the fibrin around a platelet thrombus becomes fully polymerized, circulating platelets no longer adhere to it readily. However, the chemotactic factors produced by plasmin-fibrin interaction and the release of platelet factors that interact with complement combine to attract additional platelets and to cause neutrophils to stick to the fibrin-platelet mass (Fig. 8.8). The invading neutrophils are important in dissolution of the thrombus and in repair of the endothelial surface.

Arterial and venous thrombi differ

Thrombi are heterogeneous structures, and their heterogeneity is a reflection of both the site where they are formed and their age. Thrombi that develop in slow zones of blood flow such as veins are composed of fibrin strands with entrapped erythrocytes, because the dominant mechanism of formation is coagulation. In contrast, arterial thrombi are generally due to endothelial injury, and the initial thrombus is composed of aggregated platelets.

Arterial thrombi

Arterial thrombosis is enhanced by three factors: endothelial damage, blood flow alterations (stasis, turbulence), and increased coagulability of the blood. Early arterial thrombi are soft, friable, and dark red with bands of yellow-buff that are due to platelets and fibrin. The latter elements stabilize the structure. If arterial thrombi grow, the flow patterns adjacent to the thrombi cause fibrin to be deposited, and the platelet mass that persists is transformed into a fibrin mass. Fibrin strands polymerize between the separating and degenerating platelets.

Venous thrombi

Venous thrombi are typically red because of the high numbers of erythrocytes. They resemble postmortem clots except that they are firmer, have a point of attachment, and on section have subtle fibrin laminae. Venous thrombi are caused by the same factors as arterial thrombi. Small thrombi do not generally induce clinical signs of disease. Occlusive thrombosis of the veins of the limbs causes lameness and edema, and thrombi may be released into the major veins as emboli.

Portal venous thrombi are large thrombi that may occur just as the portal vein enters the liver. In dogs, they are associated with pancreatic necrosis,

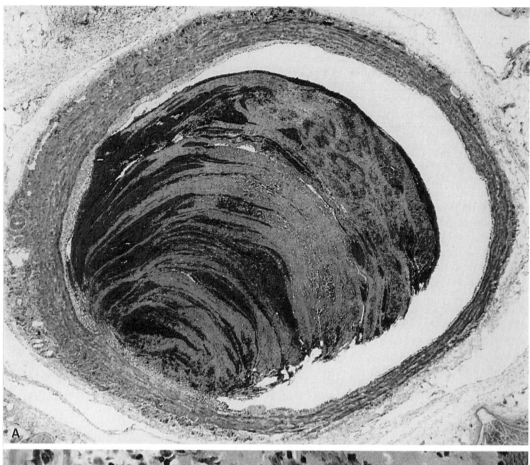

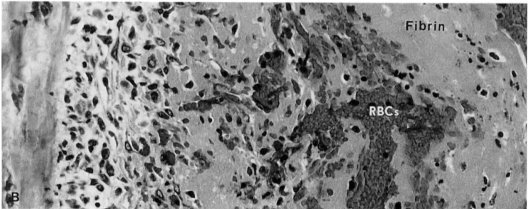

FIGURE 8.8. Venous thrombosis, dog with histoplasmosis. A. Thrombus attached to the wall of a vein draining the hepatic lymph node. B. Enlargement of *A:* thrombus contains fibrin and entrapped leukocytes and erythrocytes (RBCs). Fibroblasts are at the site of attachment to endothelium *(left).*

peritonitis, neoplasms, and steroid therapy. Dogs with portal venous thrombi will often have thrombi in pulmonary arteries. If thrombi extend into mesenteric veins, infarction of the jejunum may occur. If veins are blocked for several days, secondary **portosystemic shunts** develop to bypass the thrombus.

Occlusive thrombi are those that totally occlude the blood vessels; they are most often found in small muscular veins and venous plexuses. **Mu-**

ral thrombi form plaquelike masses attached to walls and are seen in the heart and aneurysms of larger arteries.

Postmortem clots, formed after death, are rubbery and homogeneous. Depending on whether the red blood cells have settled out after death, they are either solid red-blue (currant jelly clots) or clear yellow (chicken fat clots). Commonly, the upper part of the postmortem clot is clear yellow, and the lower part, into which erythrocytes have settled, is red.

Predisposition to thrombosis

Several clinical situations are prone to involve thrombosis. Some of the major predispositions to thrombosis include the following:

- Endothelial injury
- Stasis of blood flow
- Hypercoagulation

Stasis promotes thrombosis

During immobilization (as in surgery), procoagulant materials circulate and become trapped in areas of stasis. If stasis is prolonged, coagulation reactions may proceed to completion and form small intravascular clots. In normal animals these small thrombi fail to enlarge (to form significant venous thrombi), probably because of clotting suppression by inhibitors in plasma such as antithrombin III. Microthrombi are removed by the liver as they circulate.

Consequences of thrombosis

The consequences of thrombosis are obstruction of blood vessels (with infarction) and embolization. Thrombi can be fatal if they occur in blood vessels of visceral organs, particularly lung, heart, and intestine. The progression of events is tissue thrombosis → embolism → infarction. One of the most important sources of thromboemboli that lead to infarction is valvular endocarditis. Small thrombi that form vegetative attachments to endocardium of the heart valves break away, circulate in the bloodstream, and lodge in the microcirculation of the kidney and other organs (Fig. 8.9).

Partial obstruction of large arteries is one of the more common types of thrombosis, particularly in horses, in which thrombosis of the major arteries is associated with strongyle infestation (Fig. 8.10). When thrombosis occurs in the splanchnic arteries, the intestine is at risk of gangrene, and colic is an early sign. When the aorta is markedly involved, signs include exercise-induced hindlimb lameness, which disappears on rest (even if aortic lesions are severe). The affected limb is cool, fails to sweat during exercise, and has diminished arterial pulse and

decreased filling of saphenous veins. Studies of thrombosis of the terminal aorta and iliac arteries of horses suggest that organization of strongyle-related thromboemboli is the cause of lameness.

Suppression of natural vascular thromboresistance

As platelets adhere to an injured vessel wall, a plug forms and enlarges by aggregation of other circulating platelets. The two systems of thromboresistance are overwhelmed by the great facility with which platelets synthesize the opposing prostaglandins that initiate aggregation (thromboxane A_2 and PGI_2). As the fusing platelets discharge granule factors and thromboplastin into the plug area, fibrin polymerization is initiated. Platelet stimulation by ADP, epinephrine, and thrombin exposes binding sites specific for fibrinogen on the platelet surface, where the large, intact, symmetric fibrinogen molecules immediately bind the platelets together in a stable thrombus. Formation of alternating bands of fibrin and platelets may impart a laminated appearance to the thrombus. With time, the platelets disintegrate, and the thrombus appears as a friable, heterogeneous mass of fibrin. Anticoagulant drugs such as heparin have little effect on the platelet component but can effectively depress the deposition of fibrin.

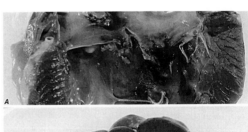
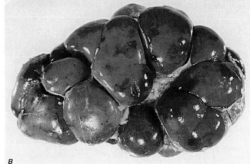

FIGURE 8.9. Thrombosis: association of thrombosis, embolism, and infarction, cow with purulent metritis. A. Vegetative valvular endocarditis with thrombosis of heart valves. B. Acute pale infarcts in the lobulated kidney of the cow. These arise from thrombi that sloughed from the heart valve, circulated, and lodged in the renal arcuate arteries.

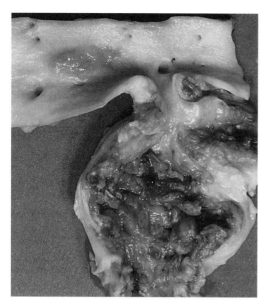

FIGURE 8.10. Pseudoaneurysm of anterior mesenteric artery as it originates from the aorta *(top)*, horse. Rugose endothelial surface and thrombosis are due to invasion by the parasite *Strongylus vulgaris*.

Fate of thrombi

The fate of thrombi (and the clinical consequences that arise from it) depends on several factors, including the extent of vascular injury, the size of the injured vessel, the rate of blood flow, and the effectiveness of intravascular clotting. Once an arterial thrombus is formed, it may progress through one of the following pathways:

- **Dissolution** (lysis) associated with thrombolytic activity
- **Progression** to further thrombosis (extension of the primary thrombus)
- **Embolization** to distant sites (with serious consequences of infarction)
- **Organization** (healing) by invasion of connective tissue
- **Canalization** by new blood vessels that extend through the thrombus

Contraction occurs as thrombi age

As condensed bands of fibrin and platelets attach to the vascular wall and become overgrown by endothelium, the clot becomes infiltrated with invading fibroblasts and new blood vessel sprouts, a process called **organization**. During organization of the clot, platelets contract, causing the thrombus to retract against the vascular wall. In this way, the vascular lumen is expanded to increase blood flow.

The contractile property of platelets resides in a peripheral band of cytoplasmic microfilaments and in microtubules. These cytoskeletal structures, which contain a contractile protein called **thrombosthenin**, not only direct platelet shape during the platelet release reaction but also are the force that causes contraction of the clot as it organizes.

Recanalization of thrombi permits blood flow

If significant occlusion of the blood vessel has taken place, **recanalization** permits blood to flow again through the vessel. This occurs by invasion of the thrombus mass by newly formed capillaries, which then anastomose (Fig. 8.11).

Causes of thrombosis

Any agent that extensively damages endothelial surfaces of blood vessels will cause thrombosis. Infectious agents are important causes. They include viruses that replicate in and destroy endothelial cells, and bacteria and fungi that cause tissue lesions that erode through blood vessel walls.

Morphologically, thrombi must be differentiated from clots that form extravascularly and from clots that form in vessels after death (postmortem clotting). If clots are found at multiple sites in the body, the pathologist must search for other evidence of the very serious systemic process called disseminated intravascular coagulation.

Disseminated intravascular coagulation

Coagulation within the intact vascular system accompanies some severe systemic diseases in which clotting mechanisms are activated. During this widespread coagulation disorder, the blood is depleted of platelets and coagulation factors; the syndrome is sometimes called **consumption coagulopathy**. Fibrinogen polymerizes within the capillary bed, and although the fibrinolytic system is activated, it cannot effectively deal with the large deposits of fibrin.

Animals with **disseminated intravascular coagulation** (DIC) have bleeding tendencies. The findings of the clinical pathologist are thrombocytopenia, hypofibrinogenemia, deficiency of prothrombin complexes, and depletion of factors V and VIII; there are also excess split products of fibrin in the blood (because of fibrinolysis). The first three deficiencies are required for the diagnosis.

The clinical consequences of disseminated intravascular coagulation are generalized hemorrhages and dysfunction of critical organs such as kidney and lung because of circulatory interference by fibrin thrombi. Fibrin-filled neutrophils are trapped in the capillary bed of the lungs, causing fatal inter-ference with respiration.

The development of disseminated intravascular coagulation indicates a severe disease process of rapid progression. Deposition of fibrin occurs at such a high rate that the fibrinolytic system cannot degrade it. Experimentally, when small amounts of thrombin are injected intravenously, aggregates of fibrin form in the blood and are removed by circulating neutrophils. These fibrin-filled cells lodge in the liver, spleen, and lung. The fibrin is degraded, and no signs of disease occur.

Intravenous thrombin

Thrombin, in addition to being the enzyme that polymerizes fibrinogen, is one of the most important activators of platelets—it can induce the platelet release reaction directly. When large amounts of **thrombin** (or thromboplastin) are quickly injected intravenously, the circulating blood clots rapidly and the animal dies. The explosive induction of thrombin sets off intravascular clotting and fatal interference with circulation. When the same quantity of thromboplastin is injected slowly, however, the animal survives. The slower and more incomplete formation of fibrin is removed rapidly enough by the monocyte-macrophage system that survival is possible. The animal is depleted of fibrinogen in the process, and its blood is incoagulable. There is often activation of the intravascular plasminogen. The plasma proteolytic enzyme plasmin degrades fibrin, and fibrin split products are removed by the kidney.

Tissue necrosis

Embolization of necrotic tissue during **septic disease** may induce coagulation. Disorders associated with **parturition** are common examples. Sepsis during abortion, intrauterine retention of dead fetuses, and the embolism of amniotic fluid and epithelial cells may be associated with a hypofibrinogenemia secondary to intravascular clotting.

Heparin treatment suppresses DIC and, experimentally at least, has a striking preventative effect in diseases involving tissue necrosis (which release massive amounts of thromboplastin). For example, heparin decreases mortality in carbon tetrachloride toxicity by inhibiting the following sequence: necrosis → thromboplastin release → intravascular coagulation → tissue hypoxia.

Tissue necrosis plus abnormal coagulation

Diseases characterized by large amounts of tissue destruction plus suppression of coagulation are prone to lead to DIC. Thus DIC commonly occurs

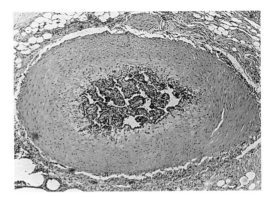

FIGURE 8.11. Recanalization of the pulmonary artery, dirofilariasis, cat. New vascular channels have formed in the artery previously blocked by an organized thrombus.

in severe burns, widespread metastatic tumors, systemic viral disease, heatstroke, and shock. In dogs, it may also accompany severe pneumonia, congestive heart failure, and heartworm disease. Dogs so affected bleed from the nose and gingiva because of thrombocytopenia and depletion of factors V, VIII, and X and fibrinogen.

Burns

Severe local lesions induce consumption of coagulation factors without evidence of DIC. Intense but local thermal injury is accompanied by marked, prolonged consumption within the burn wound of platelets, fibrinogen, and plasminogen. Later, hyperfibrinogenemia, thrombocytosis, and elevated split products occur in circulating blood and are evidence of local intravascular coagulation in the burn wound rather than of DIC.

Neoplasia

Neoplastic cells are the source of procoagulant factors in some types of vascular tumors and in leukemia. Metastasis of solid tumors may be accompanied by intravascular coagulation, but the direct cause is not known.

Snake venoms

Snake venoms are mixtures of as many as 30 different peptides, most of which are toxic. All poisonous venoms contain phospholipase A_2 (which has direct lytic action on plasma membranes of platelets and erythrocytes) and hyaluronidase (which cleaves glycosidic bonds of glycosaminoglycans and facilitates toxin spread). Venom of the tiger snake behaves as an activated factor X, whereas venom of the copperhead clots fibrinogen directly. The end result in both cases is defibrination with intravascular clotting. DIC is enhanced by the direct platelet damage caused by phospholipases.

Not all defibrinating syndromes lead to DIC. Crotalase, an enzyme fraction of rattlesnake venom, converts fibrinogen to an abnormal fibrin that is ineffective in clotting; the result is hemorrhage rather than DIC. Some venom toxins specifically block removal of fibrinopeptides from fibrinogen by thrombin. Reptilase (a toxin of *Bothrops atrox* venom) blocks removal of fibrinopeptide A. Enzymes in *Agkistrodon contortrix* venom block fibrinopeptide B removal. Other venom peptides have antithromboplastin activity.

Viruses that damage endothelium

Most cases of DIC in viral disease are due to liberation of procoagulant factors from tissue necrosis. Viral-induced endothelial loss exposes subendothelial matrix to attract platelets, and the degenerating endothelial cells are a source of tissue thromboplastin and other procoagulant factors. Hemostatic defects of acute **infectious canine hepatitis** include thrombocytopenia, abnormal platelet function, prolonged prothrombin times, depressed factor VIII activity, normal thrombin times, and increased circulating fibrin degradation products. These defects suggest that the mechanism is DIC.

The reduced number of platelets reflects both increased consumption (to repair virus-induced endothelial injury) and direct damage to platelets by viruses. Depressed factor VIII levels are probably due to consumption caused by vascular lesions.

Immunologic reactions may contribute to DIC in systemic viral disease. Cats with **feline infectious peritonitis** (FIP) can develop widespread vasculitis and thrombosis accompanied by thrombocytopenia, hyperfibrinogenemia, and increased fibrin degradation products in plasma. When FIP virus is experimentally inoculated, kittens with antibody develop more rapid and more severe disease than do kittens infected for the first time. Viral antigens and immunoglobulins are present in fibrinonecrotic lesions, which suggests an immunologic process.

Protozoal disease

Endothelial damage occurs in parasitemic phases of malaria and other protozoal diseases. In massive infection, DIC may lead to death. In cattle, the intraerythrocytic parasite *Babesia* sp. causes alterations in fibrinogen catabolism and in coagulation and kinin systems. There is no evidence of fibrin deposition or fibrinolysis and little evidence that the disease progresses to DIC. **Trypanosomiasis** in

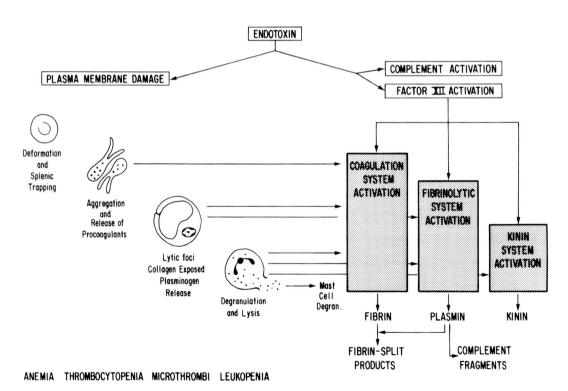

ANEMIA   THROMBOCYTOPENIA   MICROTHROMBI   LEUKOPENIA

FIGURE 8.12. Hemostatic alterations in endotoxic shock.

calves caused by *Trypanosoma congolense* leads to marked thrombocytopenia and hypofibrinogenemia. There is ineffective thrombopoiesis and increased megakaryocyte mass, which indicates that in chronic disease there is a partially compensated DIC.

Septicemia

Widespread vascular damage occurring when pathogenic bacteria circulate is the most common cause of DIC. Intact bacteria initially activate Hageman factor, and bacterial endotoxins produce endothelial damage that both increases vascular permeability and sustains the intravascular coagulation defect. **Septicemic salmonellosis** in swine is frequently accompanied by vascular necrosis in renal interlobular arteries and afferent glomerular arterioles, with widespread thrombosis in glomeruli. Similar lesions occur in epidermal capillaries. **Leptospirosis** is characterized by thrombocytopenia, increased fibrinolytic split products in blood, and endothelial injury. Damaged endothelium releases plasminogen activators, which stimulate the fibrinolytic system.

Bacterial endotoxins activate both extrinsic and intrinsic systems of coagulation. Hageman factor (XII) is activated, and monocytes are induced to release factors that activate factor VII. Furthermore, endotoxin has a direct action on platelets that leads to aggregation and platelet release reactions (Fig. 8.12). Factor VII plays a key role in the development of endotoxin-induced DIC. Infusion of endotoxin into factor VII–deficient dogs results in greater fibrin deposition and focal tissue necrosis than in normal dogs. Corticosteroids make blood vessels very sensitive to endotoxin by inhibiting catechol methyltransferase and thereby promoting α-adrenergic stimulation.

Platelets disappear rapidly after intravenous endotoxin and are trapped in capillary beds of lung and liver. In experiments using ^{51}Cr-labeled platelets in dogs, thrombocytopenia has been shown to be biphasic; that is, a rapid drop in circulating platelets is followed by partial recovery and then a second drop. The initial rapid drop requires participation of **complement**, especially in dogs and cats whose platelets contain immune adherence receptors.

Endotoxin DIC can be suppressed by deleting circulating platelets or neutrophils or by injecting heparin to prevent coagulation. DIC is induced with one endotoxin injection if lysed neutrophil granules are given simultaneously. Neutropenic animals are fully susceptible to endotoxin but do not develop some of the lung damage that normal animals do.

Although deposition of fibrin thrombi is most prominent in the kidney and lung during endotoxin-induced DIC, progressive microthrombosis also occurs in the splenic red pulp and hepatic sinusoids. Impairment of phagocytic function in these organs adds to the severity of endotoxic injury.

ADDITIONAL READING

Baker DC, Green RA. 1987. Coagulation defects of aflatoxin intoxicated rabbits. *Vet Pathol* 24:62.

Bertram TA. 1985. Quantitative morphology of peracute pulmonary lesions in swine induced by *Haemophilus pleuropneumonia. Vet Pathol* 22:598.

Casey HW, Splitter GA. 1975. Membranous glomerulonephritis in dogs infected with *Dirofilaria immitis. Vet Pathol* 12:111.

Collen D. 1998. Staphylokinase: a potent, uniquely fibrin-selective thrombolytic agent. *Nature Med* 4:279.

Cramer EM, et al. 1986. Absence of tubular structures and immunolabeling for von Willebrand factor in the platelet α-granules from porcine von Willebrand disease. *Blood* 68:774.

Doolittle RF. 1981. Fibrinogen and fibrin. *Sci Am* 245:127.

Edwards JF, et al. 1985. Megakaryocyte infection and thrombocytopenia in African swine fever. *Vet Pathol* 22:171.

Esmon CT. 1987. The regulation of natural anticoagulant pathways. *Science* 235:1348.

Fay WP, et al. 1996. High concentrations of active plasminogen activator inhibitor–1 in porcine coronary artery thrombi. *Atherosclero Thromb Vasc Biol* 16:1277.

Feldman BF, et al. 1981. Disseminated intravascular coagulation: antithrombin, plasminogen, and coagulation abnormalities in 41 dogs. *J Am Vet Med Assoc* 179:151.

Feldman BF, et al. 1983. Hemorrhage in a cat caused by inhibition of factor XI (plasma thromboplastin antecedent). *J Am Vet Med Assoc* 182:589.

Green RA, et al. 1985. Hypoalbuminemia-related platelet hypersensitivity in two dogs with nephrotic syndrome. *J Am Vet Med Assoc* 186:485.

Healy AM, et al. 1998. Intravascular coagulation activation in a murine model of thrombomodulin deficiency. *Blood* 92:4188.

Lenting PJ, et al. 1998. The life cycle of coagulation factor VIII in view of its structure and function. *Blood* 92:3983.

Maxie MG, Physick-Sheard PW. 1985. Aortic-iliac thrombosis in horses. *Vet Pathol* 22:238.

Meyers KM. 1985. Pathobiology of animal platelets. *Adv Vet Sci Comp Med* 30:131.

Meyers KM. 1992. Canine von Willebrand's disease: pathobiology, diagnosis, and short-term treatment. *Clin Hematol* 14:13.

Momotani E, et al. 1985. Histopathological evaluation of disseminated intravascular coagulation in *Haemophilus somnus* infection in cattle. *J Comp Pathol* 95:15.

Morley PS, Allen AL, Woolums AR. 1996. Aortic and iliac artery thrombosis in calves: nine cases (1974–1993). *J Am Vet Med Assoc* 209:130.

Morris DD, Beech J. 1983. Disseminated intravascular coagulation in six horses. *J Am Vet Med Assoc* 183:1067.

Nash R, et al. 1995. GM-CSF–associated thrombocytopenia in dogs: increased destruction of circulating platelets. *Blood* 86:1765.

Schulman A, et al. 1986. Diphacinone-induced coagulopathy in the dog. *J Am Vet Med Assoc* 188:402.

Shattil SJ, et al. 1998. Integrin signaling: the platelet paradigm. *Blood* 91:2645.

Slauson DO, Gribble DH. 1971. Thrombosis complicating renal amyloidosis in dogs. *Vet Pathol* 8:352.

Topol EJ, et al. 1999. Platelet GPIIb-IIIa blockers. *Lancet* 353:227.

Turk JR. 1998. Physiologic and pathophysiologic effects of endothelin. *J Am Vet Med Assoc* 212:265.

Williams DA, Maggio-Price L. 1984. Canine idiopathic thrombocytopenia. *J Am Vet Med Assoc* 185:660.

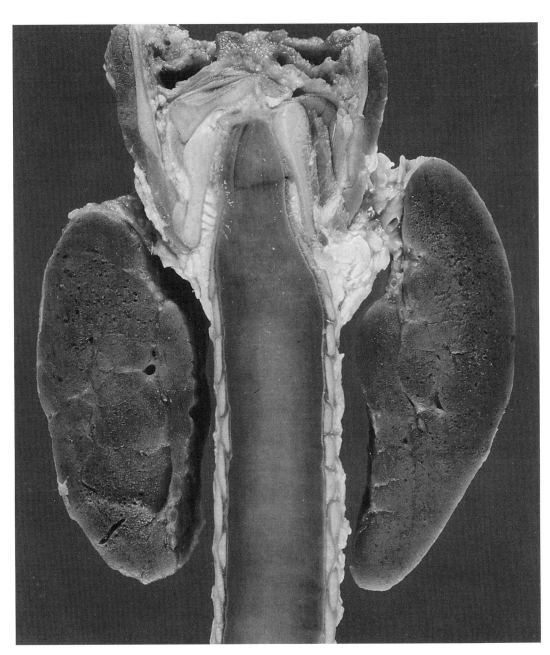

Thyroid hyperplasia.

PART 4

Disorders of Growth

AN UNDERSTANDING OF CELL GROWTH centers on the mechanisms whereby cells divide and differentiate. All cells in the body possess the capacity to undergo mitosis, because all have the same genome as the zygote. Some cells divide with extraordinary speed, such as hematologic stem cells in bone marrow, progenitor cells in crypts of the small intestine, and basal epidermal cells in active hair follicles. Other cells such as neurons and cardiac myocytes do not effectively undergo mitosis.

The controlling factors, which make only some cells divide, reside in the genome in the cell nucleus. These factors turn genes on or repress them so that the cycle of mitosis is closely regulated. **Growth factors**, soluble peptides secreted by cells, initiate differentiation, control migration, and can even regulate the speed and activity of mitosis. Cell growth is initiated by binding of a growth factor to specific receptors at the cell surface. Binding of receptor and growth factor at the cell surface transmits a signal to subsurface proteins that activate a protein phosphorylation cascade that causes the resting cell (called phase G_0) to enter G_1 and to proceed through the growth cycle.

The cell cycle extends from one mitosis to the next. The normal cell cycle is compartmentalized into four discrete periods, called G_1, S (synthesis), G_2, and M (mitosis). DNA is duplicated in the S phase, and G_1 and G_2 are gaps between S and M during which important preparatory events occur.

The standard cell cycle is long, lasting more than 12 hours for fast-growing mammalian tissues. The greatest variation occurs in G_1, during which cells can pause in the cycle to enter a specialized resting state, G_0. Cells can remain in G_0 for weeks or years before resuming proliferation. The shortest eukaryotic cycles are early embryonic cycles that occur immediately after fertilization. No growth occurs, the G_1 and G_2 phases are markedly shortened, and the time from one division to the next may take only 8 minutes, half spent in the S phase and half in the M phase.

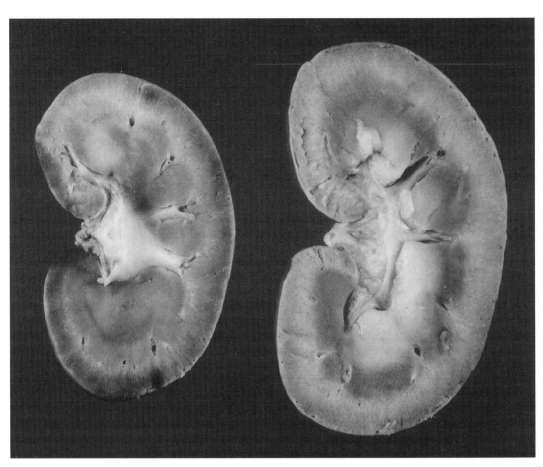

FIGURE 9.1. Renal hypertrophy. Kidney removed by unilateral nephrectomy in dog *(left)*; hypertrophic kidney *(right)* removed from the same dog 14 days later.

▦ CHAPTER 9

Disturbances of Cell Growth and Replication

HYPERTROPHY

Hypertrophy is an increase in size of a tissue or organ without an increase in number of cells (Fig. 9.1). Although it may occur in any tissue, it is seen in pure form only in tissues composed of cells that do not reproduce readily. The most common examples of hypertrophy arise from increased workload or from endocrine stimulation. In hypertrophic cells, increased metabolic activity is reflected in increased size of nucleus and cytoplasm and in increased numbers of organelles.

Muscle hypertrophies during increased work

The size of muscle cells increases progressively with work (e.g., the large muscle masses and large heart of the racing greyhound). In hypertrophic skeletal and cardiac muscle cells, the contractile myofilaments are increased in length and number. The phenotype of hypertrophying muscle is altered. There is a switch of contractile proteins to fetal or neonatal forms—for example, the activation of β-myosin heavy chains and repression of α-myosin heavy chains result in hypertrophied fibers that have slower velocity of contraction. The stimulus for increased production of new myofilaments is a growth factor that, when extracted from hypertrophic muscle, induces normal muscle to hypertrophy.

Kidneys have cycles of hypertrophy

Renal hypertrophy and regression occur during normal diurnal and nocturnal cycles of urine secretion. Substances that stimulate renal metabolism (antidiuretic hormone, catecholamines, and adrenocorticosteroids) produce this subtle, transient hypertrophy.

Surgical removal of a single kidney because of neoplastic disease or congenital defects results in marked and rapid hypertrophy of the remaining kidney. When one kidney is surgically removed from a dog, hypertrophy can be detected within a few days (see Fig. 9.1). All parts of the renal tubule enlarge, including the glomeruli. As in myocardium, the stimulus for renal hypertrophy involves some circulating factor.

Hormones stimulate hypertrophy

Hormones cause hypertrophy by increasing metabolism in cells bearing appropriate hormone receptors on their surfaces. **Thyroid hormones** have a general anabolic effect, manifested as increased oxygen consumption and activation of protein synthesis. Hyperthyroidism in most species is accompanied by cardiac hypertrophy, caused in part by general workload demands of the excessively active hyperthyroid animal but mostly by direct stimulation of protein synthesis in the myocyte.

The same hormone may produce different effects in different tissues. While the hyperthyroid animal has cardiac hypertrophy, it also develops atrophy of skeletal muscle and liver. This atrophy is caused in part by generalized protein drain of gluconeogenesis, which drains amino acids more easily from skeletal muscle and liver, and by different effects that thyroid hormone has on muscle and liver through its stimulation of tissue-specific lysosomal hydrolases.

Adrenal corticosteroids stimulate cells by inducing production of enzymes crucial for mitochondrial exudation, glycogen formation, and lipogenesis. In liver, small doses of cortisol induce hepatocyte hypertrophy. Large doses, as used in treatment of shock, produce massive glycogen deposits. Glycogen accumulation results from stimu-

235

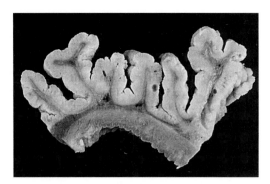

FIGURE 9.2. Gastric hyperplasia, dog. The gastric mucosa is markedly thickened.

lation both of enzymes of glycogen synthesis and of enzymes that cause amino acid degradation and gluconeogenesis.

Androgens stimulate muscle growth

Part of the body weight difference of males and females is attributed to testosterone-dependent muscle mass. **Androgenic steroids** are used as growth stimulants by weight lifters and other athletes to build muscle mass. Skeletal muscle cells contain specific receptors for androgens and show a selective response to these hormones.

Estrogens initiate genital hypertrophy

Some of the most striking examples of hypertrophy occur in glands when they are stimulated by the appropriate hormones. In females, for example, the acinar cells of the **mammary gland** undergo marked hypertrophy in late gestation under the influence of the steroid hormones of pregnancy and the pituitary peptide hormone prolactin.

Protein production in mammary epithelial cells is initiated when estrogens diffuse into the cells and combine with specific cytoplasmic estrogen receptor molecules. The **estrogen-receptor complex** migrates to the nucleus, where it activates the gene with codes to produce specific proteins (prolactin stimulates genes for milk proteins). The activated gene produces mRNA, which migrates through nuclear pores to the cytoplasm, where it joins ribosomes to initiate production of the appropriate protein.

Cycles of **uterine endometrial hypertrophy and regression** typify the mammalian estrous cycle. In the bitch, endometrial cells markedly enlarge under the influence of both estrogen and progesterone. At the end of anestrus, as serum estrogen rises, endometrial cells grow in the crypts and differentiate from glandular epithelial cells to well-developed, mucus-secreting cells. As estrogens decline and progesterones rise in metestrus, cells become hyperplastic and develop characteristics of absorptive and secretory cells. The uterine effects of progesterone are dependent on prior exposure to estrogen; that is, estrogen "priming" increases the concentration of progesterone receptors in the cytoplasm of endometrial epithelial cells.

Estrogens have an anabolic effect on liver

Estrogens have a pronounced general anabolic effect on liver. They increase protein synthesis and induce hypertrophy. Potent **anabolic steroids** with estrogenic activities are used as subcutaneous implants to increase growth rates of ruminant farm animals. They increase nitrogen retention in liver and promote protein synthesis. In sheep and cattle, the hepatocyte partitions amino acids between protein synthesis and deamination to yield substrates for energy production. In the latter case, amino groups are incorporated into urea by liver enzymes. Anabolic steroids reduce the urea entry rate in cattle and sheep, leading to more amino acids available for protein synthesis.

Injection of exogenous estrogen stimulates different hepatic proteins in different species. In avian liver, the egg yolk protein vitellogenin is stimulated. In mammals, plasma proteins and coagulation factors increase; the latter are particularly important in liver disease during human use of estrogenic contraceptive agents.

HYPERPLASIA

Hyperplasia is an increase in the number of cells in a tissue. As in hypertrophy, the hyperplastic cells and its organelles are not qualitatively abnormal. They are simply present in greater numbers.

One of the most common causes of hyperplasia in epithelial surfaces is **chronic irritation**. Mechanical or toxic injury induces epithelial cells to proliferate and accumulate, and the thickened epithelium forms a protective barrier against the inciting causal agent. Parasite infestation of the skin, gut, respiratory tract, or urogenital system usually causes epithelial hyperplasia. A callus in the skin is due to hyperplasia of keratinocytes within the epidermis.

A syndrome of gastric hyperplasia develops in aged dogs with severe systemic disease. The gastric mucosa is thrown into thickened folds (Fig. 9.2), and there is an increase in HCl-producing parietal cells and in chief cells. Mucous hyperplasia of the fovea or neck regions of the gastric glands occurs, and dilatation deep in the gland creates a cystic appearance in the mucosa. The lesions seem to arise from the influence of hormones (chiefly gastrin) and by action of some of the epithelial growth factors.

Hyperplasia of endocrine origin

Tissues that are target organs of the sex hormones show cyclical growth and regression according to hormone levels in the bloodstream. The mammary gland undergoes hyperplasia during lactation. Rarely, excess production of mammary gland tissue occurs during nonlactating periods. A unique condition occurs as a rapid, benign growth of one or more mammary glands of young estrus-cycling or pregnant cats. It is called **fibroepithelial hyperplasia** because of its proliferation of stroma and mammary ductal epithelium.

In the bitch, **cystic endometrial hyperplasia** arises from an arrest in the estrogen-progesterone–induced cycle of endometrial hypertrophy and regression. Prolonged hormonal stimulation causes the uterus to expand, with marked increases in secreting cells and accumulation of secretions in the lumen. The uterus becomes infected, usually with *Escherichia coli,* and is filled with pus. Inflammatory exudates block the ducts of hyperplastic glands to cause cysts in the endometrium. Lesions of endometrial hyperplasia can be induced experimentally by treating dogs with large amounts of progesterone or estrogen-progesterone combinations.

Thyroid hyperplasia

Thyroid hyperplasia of young, iodine-deficient animals illustrates the progression from hypertrophy to hyperplasia. Initially, deficiency of iodine leads to the diminished output of thyroid hormones and the compensatory increase in pituitary production of thyroid-stimulating hormone (TSH). Increased circulating TSH causes hypertrophy of thyroid epithelium. If iodine deficiency is sustained and excess TSH is not fully compensatory, hypertrophy progresses to thyroid epithelial hyperplasia. Hyperplastic thyroid glands are enlarged and highly vascular. Follicular lumens are small because of encroachment of epithelium. In older animals the uniformly hyperplastic thyroid gland gives way to a cystic and papillomatous growth pattern of "colloid goiter," an involutionary variant of thyroid hyperplasia.

Prostate hyperplasia

In several species, **prostate hyperplasia** develops in intact males of advancing age. Epithelial cells increase in size and number, and fibromuscular tissue markedly expands the interstitium. Prostatic epithelial cells are filled with secretory granules, and there is reduplication of organelles involved in protein synthesis.

Chronic prostatic hyperplasia, which is common in aged dogs, develops in the presence of a functioning testis and is produced by testosterone and its metabolites. Hyperplasia of prostate tissue regresses after castration but can be restored by administration of androgens (Fig. 9.3). The pathogenesis of canine prostate hyperplasia involves unbalanced testosterone metabolism and complex synergism with hormones. Circulating in blood, testosterone diffuses into prostate cells, where it can act directly or be converted to other steroids that are more androgenic, estrogenic, or inactive on the reproductive tract.

Testosterone binds to receptors in the cytoplasm

After testosterone binds to androgen receptors, the testosterone-receptor complex is conveyed to the nucleus, where it binds to chromatin and causes gene transcription. The new mRNA that is produced exits through nuclear pores into the cytoplasm, where it initiates (in ribosomes) synthesis of new peptides for growth of the prostate epithelial cell.

The pathway that forms 5α-dihydrotestosterone (5α-DHT) is more important in males: testosterone —(5α-reductase)→ 5α-DHT → 5α-androstanediol. 5α-DHT amplifies the androgenic action of testosterone. Androstanediols are also androgenic, but their activities depend on back conversion to 5α-DHT. Both testosterone and 5α-DHT bind to the same androgen receptors, although 5α-DHT–receptor complexes are more efficient in action on the chromosome and hence more androgenic. In adult male dogs, production of 5α-DHT from testosterone occurs rapidly in the prostate, and when measured biochemically, prostate hyperplastic tissue from adult dogs contains five times more 5α-DHT than does prostate tissue of young dogs.

Estradiol is synergistic with androgens in prostate

Estradiol arises via the enzyme aromatase and acts, after combining with specific **estrogen receptors**, either in the tissue where it is produced or at distant sites. In adults, the actions of testosterone on muscle and brain are mediated through its conversion to estradiol. In prostate, estradiol increases the number of androgen receptor complexes in the nucleus and causes progesterone receptors to appear in the cytoplasm.

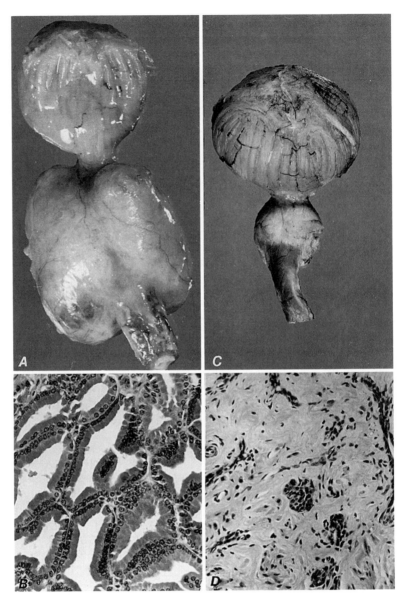

FIGURE 9.3. Hypertrophy *(left)* and atrophy *(right)*, canine prostates. A. Hypertrophic gland, aged intact dog. B. Tall columnar epithelial cells, little stroma. C. Atrophy of prostate gland, aged castrated male dog. D. Small epithelial cells surrounded by masses of collagen and fibrocytes.

5β-Androgen stimulates liver metabolism

5β-Androgen is a metabolite of testosterone that arises by action of the enzyme 5β-reductase. It has no growth-promoting effects on the male reproductive tract and thus is not a true androgen. It stimulates metabolism in liver and bone marrow and acts after combining in the cytoplasm with specific β-steroid receptors.

Steroid receptors and hyperplasia

Both androgen and estrogen receptors occur in canine prostate epithelium. With age, **androgen receptors** diminish and become unequally distributed. Hyperplastic prostates have proliferation of both androgen receptor–bearing and receptor–free cell populations. When androgenic receptors are measured in cytoplasmic extracts of canine hyperplastic prostate tissue, total content is not diminished. In contrast, nuclear extracts show marked increases in androgen receptor complexes, possibly arising from estrogenic stimulation. Hyperplasia of fibromuscular components is an estrogen-dependent phenomenon.

There are also hypothalamic-pituitary alterations in prostate hyperplasia. Affected dogs have increased serum growth hormone and diminished prolactin. Hyperplastic prostate tissue has markedly increased numbers of cells bearing receptors for prolactin (which may explain the low amounts in serum), and prolactin is known to facilitate uptake of testosterone in prostate.

Virus-induced hyperplasia

Hyperplasia is induced specifically by some viruses. Pox viruses, herpesviruses, and other DNA viruses produce a curious preliminary hyperplastic response that precedes the degenerative changes typical of cytolytic infection. Papillomaviruses, however, induce massive hyperplastic responses with little cytolytic effect. Hyperplasia of the stratum germinativum of epidermis results in massive keratin formation (hyperkeratosis), with a very small number of virus-producing cells discretely placed at the superficial junction where keratinocytes are cornified. Papillomaviruses elicit two different processes. First, they stimulate increased cell activity, mitosis, and proliferation (i.e., papilloma formation). Later, selected cells are usurped to produce virus. Hyperplasia is initiated by contact of virus with cell nucleoproteins, which either directly stimulate mitosis or induce production of peptides that act as epidermal growth factors to enhance proliferation and differentiation of keratinocytes.

FOCUS

Anabolic Steroids and Hyperplasia

THE RACEHORSE STEROID EQUIPOISE (bodenone), widely prescribed in equine medicine, has been used illegally in racehorses, and prescriptions have been diverted to human use. The abuse of this and other androgenic steroids has a long history in athletic conditioning, in misdirected attempts to create superathletes.

Ben Johnson, a Canadian track star, won a gold medal at the 1988 Olympic games in Seoul. In the 100-meter race, he ran past other runners to take the victory in 9.79 seconds. But 72 hours later, Olympic officials announced that his performance was drug driven and his medal was rescinded. There were traces of the anabolic steroid stanozolol (Winstrol, Winthrop Pharmaceuticals) in a urine sample taken after the race. Testosterone was only 15% of normal, a sign of long-term steroid use.

Anabolic steroids are synthetic variants of testosterone. The Nazi government under Hitler developed and used anabolic steroids to promote the anabolic effects of testosterone without its androgenic masculinizing qualities. Although androgenic effects were reduced, they were not eliminated, and this remained a serious problem. Beginning in the 1940s, anabolic steroids were used clinically to treat human female breast cancer and to combat anemia. The Soviets began using steroids as power boosters in weight lifters for Olympic competition in the 1950s. American use began in the 1960s, often in doses 100 times larger than recommended.

Anabolic steroids cause masculinization. High doses suppress natural testosterone and cause the testes to shrink and, in long-term use, are associated with damage to the liver and kidneys, heart disease, hepatocellular carcinoma, and carcinoma of the prostate.

Reference
Marshall E. 1988. *Science* 242:183.

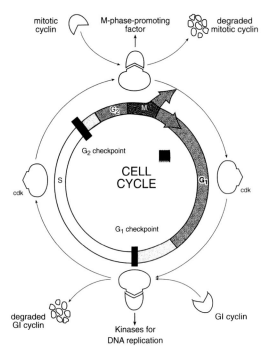

FIGURE 9.4. Phases of the cell mitotic cycle.

Control of mitosis

The **cell cycle** is the period extending from one mitosis to the next (Fig. 9.4). The normal cell cycle is compartmentalized into four discrete periods, called G_1, S (synthesis), G_2, and M (mitosis). G_1 and G_2 are gaps between S and M during which important preparatory events occur.

G_1 is the resting phase; RNA and protein synthesis are necessary for cells to progress through it. DNA is duplicated in the S phase, which is initiated by a new set of regulators. Subsequent progress through the cycle is governed by a temporal sequence of genetic transcriptions held in sequence by the dependency of one on the next.

Cell activities are geared to the nuclear cycle of chromosome replication and segregation that define the four periods. Control, regulation, and inhibition of cell replication are achieved by interruption of the nuclear cycle. The three major chromosomal events in cell division (reproduction, movement, and cleavage) all occur with strict continuity in the cycle. If one is blocked, the others do not occur (Table 9.1).

Timing of the cell cycle is controlled by **cyclins**. Cyclins increase in amount during one phase of the cycle and then decline in another, all in a period manner. There are many cyclins, which are grouped in categories noted by letters. The B cyclins accumulate in G_2 and are degraded in M. The E and D cyclins act in G_1, whereas the A cyclins function during the S phase. Cyclins regulate **protein kinases**, which are referred to as Cdks (cyclin-dependent kinases).

Combinations of cyclin E with Cdk2, and cyclin D with Cdk4, lead to phosphorylation of several critical proteins and allow the S phase of the cell cycle to begin. Before a cell enters the S phase, it is important that its DNA be intact and not damaged. Duplication of defective DNA leads to an enhanced frequency of mutations.

The S phase is recognized cytochemically by supplying cells with labeled thymidine, a compound that cells use exclusively for DNA synthesis. The label can be radioactive H^3 or a chemical probe, usually the artificial thymidine analog bromodeoxyuridine. From the fraction of cells that are labeled (the labeling index), one can estimate the duration of S phase as a fraction of the whole cycle. From the fraction of cells in mitosis (the mitotic index), one can estimate the duration of M phase as a fraction of the whole cycle. Fluorescence-activated cell sorters facilitate the measurement of DNA content, which doubles during S phase.

There are two major checkpoints in the cell's cycle: the G_1-S checkpoint, just before entry into S phase (this checkpoint prevents the cell from replicating damaged DNA); and the G_2-M checkpoint, at

TABLE 9.1. Indexes of mitotic activity

Term	Definition	Comment
Mitotic index	Percentage of cells in a population in mitosis at a given time	Low mitotic index may indicate a few cells dividing rapidly or all cells dividing slowly
Mitotic time	Time from prophase to telophase	
Generation time	Prophase to prophase (mitotic time + interphase time)	
Turnover time	Time required for the production of a number of cells equal to number already present	Does not equal cell cycle time unless all cells are dividing
Labeling index	Number of cells taking up thymidine-H^3 over total number of cells	Analogous to mitotic index but greater, because DNA synthesis duration is greater than mitotic time

the entry into mitosis (this checkpoint prevents chromosome segregation if the chromosome is not intact). In eukaryotic cells, signals that arrest the cycle usually act at the G_1 control point. Little is known about the G_2-M checkpoint in mammalian cells.

The cell cycle control system is based on two key families of proteins: (1) **cyclin-dependent protein kinase** (Cdk) family, which induces downstream processes by phosphorylating serine and threonine molecules of selected proteins; and (2) **cyclins**, which bind to Cdk molecules and control their ability to phosphorylate targets. There are two main classes of cyclins: **mitotic cyclins**, which bind to Cdk molecules during G_2 and are required for entry into mitosis, and the G_1 **cyclins**, which bind to Cdk molecules during G_1 and are required for entry into S phase. Cdks associate successively with different cyclins to trigger successive phases of the cycle.

Mitotic cyclin accumulates gradually during G_2 and binds to Cdk to form **M-phase promoting factor** (MPF), a complex that triggers mitosis. The ultimate activation of MPF is explosive—the MPF concentration builds to a critical flash point, whereupon a flood of active MPF triggers events that propel the cell to mitosis.

Progression from one stage to the next in the cell cycle requires that cyclins from the previous stage be destroyed while those cyclins needed for the next stage are activated. The proteolytic destruction of mitotic cyclins occurs by ubiquitinization. Cyclins are covalently conjugated to multiple molecules of the polypeptide **ubiquitin**, which marks them for rapid hydrolysis by directing them to the **proteasome**, a 26S (2000-kd) complex that inactivates and degrades the active cyclin. These events are important because mutations that alter proteasome degradation may lead to neoplasia; for example, papilloma viruses induce tumors by stimulating ubiquitin-mediated degradation of the tumor suppressor p53.

Primordial cells normally undergo mitosis to provide populations of differentiated cells. Epithelial cells of the epidermal stratum germinativum, crypt cells of the intestine, and stem cells in bone marrow undergo mitosis via influence from humoral substances. Feedback control circuits exist between functions of the differentiated cells and proliferation of the primordial cells.

Growth factors and chalones

Decreased functional need (as in atrophy) leads to diminished amounts of mitotic stimulants. In hibernation, the kinetics and metabolism of cells in animals are markedly suppressed. Proliferating cells are blocked in the G_1 phase, and they cannot synthesize DNA. Transcription and translation are suppressed, and permeability of plasma membranes is diminished. Shrunken mitochondria with only a few short cristae reflect the low metabolic activity of the cell.

Growth factors stimulate mitosis. Mitosis is maintained by tissue-specific peptide factors that promote or suppress the cell cycle (Table 9.2). Blood and tissue fluids contain a number of peptide growth factors that induce mitosis. Similar peptides are present not only in blood but also in urine, tears, saliva, and colostrum. They are given names according to the system used in their study and detection (e.g., **epidermal growth factor**, or EGF, and **platelet-derived growth factor**, or PDGF). **Insulin** is also a growth factor. To function, growth factors bind to specific plasma membrane receptors, enter the cell, and assert their effect on the mitotic cycle. Their control is tightly regulated by gene action during their profound effects in the developing fetus. In contrast, their role in wound healing, hyperplasia, and neoplastic disease is determined by acquired characters; that is, their production can be turned on according to body needs.

Chalones are mitosis-inhibiting factors. Chalones permeate tissue and inhibit the cell at various points in the G phase of the cell cycle. In theory, chalones in the keratinocyte suppress mitosis and permit the cell to become cornified. In epithelial injury, chalones are missing, inhibition of the G_1 phase is weakened, and cells enter the S phase. Chalones are studied only in crude extracts of tissue and have not been adequately purified, so their activities have not been clearly identified in the living animal.

TABLE 9.2. Families of growth factors

Growth factor (GF)	Source	Molecular weight	Other members
Platelet-derived GF (PDGF)	Platelet α-granule	30,000	Osteosarcoma-derived GF Fibroblast-derived GF Transforming protein of several viruses
Epidermal GF (EGF)	Urine (human) Saliva (mouse)	6,000	Transforming GF
Insulin	Pancreatic β cells	5,700	Somatomedin C

METAPLASIA

Metaplasia is the substitution of one type of fully differentiated adult cell in a tissue for another adult cell type normally found there. It represents replacement of vulnerable cells by cells more resistant to an inciting stress. Like hyperplasia, it is a form of controlled, abnormal cell growth that is reversible. The change is orderly, and there is faithful reproduction of the new cell type.

A common form of metaplasia is the development of squamous from columnar epithelium. **Squamous metaplasia** of the trachea, bronchioles, gallbladder, and glandular excretory ducts often occurs when these tissues are chronically irritated or inflamed. Stones in these ductal systems typically induce squamous differentiation. In human smok-

---

FOCUS

Hepatectomy and Hepatic Hyperplasia

THE CLASSIC MODEL of hepatic regeneration, developed in rats by Higgins in the 1930s, involved surgical removal of about 70% (all but two lobes) of the liver. Liver regeneration was striking and rapid—the liver doubled in size by 48 hours and growth ceased in about 10 days, when the liver mass reached the original size. This model was confirmed in dogs and underlies our understanding of events that follow massive surgical resection of the liver.

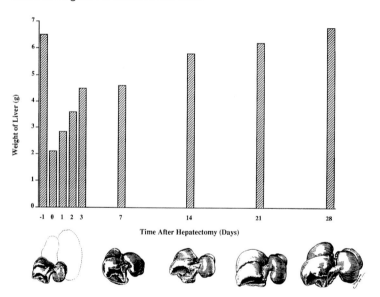

Hepatocyte DNA synthesis begins at about 12 hours after partial hepatectomy and reaches a peak at 24 hours. After massive removal of the liver, the remaining hepatocytes undergo a partially synchronous wave of DNA synthesis and cell division. Proliferation begins in periportal areas, and new hepatocytes move outward to form sinusoids. Mitotic activity peaks at 48 hours. Sinusoidal cells and Kupffer cells undergo marked regenerative responses but lag behind hepatocyte DNA synthesis by 1 to 3 days.

▶

ers, squamous metaplasia of bronchioles is a protective response to chronic injury.

Metaplasia develops from a genetic reprogramming of undifferentiated stem cells. Growth factors and other regulators of cell growth and differentiation bring about the metaplastic change. Vitamin A exerts a controlling influence on epithelial differentiation, and its deficiency leads to widespread squamous metaplasia throughout the body.

Metaplasia often occurs in organs undergoing atrophy. Long-term treatment of male animals with estrogens causes atrophy of the prostate with squamous metaplasia of prostatic glandular epithelium. Secretory cells shrink and disappear, and basal reserve cells proliferate and undergo squamous metaplasia.

ATROPHY

Atrophy is the decrease in size of cells that have gained full development. The muscle wasted in disuse, the mammary gland shrunken in old age, and the diminished size of genitalia after castration are all examples of atrophy. Atrophy represents adaption to a changed cellular environment. Cells shrink when their level of work is diminished or when their source of nutrition or stimulation is removed. Obviously, when large numbers of parenchymal cells shrink, the organ involved decreases in size commensurably.

Some examples in which cells decrease in size after once functioning in full capacity follow. The prefaces used indicate the various causes associated with the process but do not reflect the complex interplay that often exists among them.

- **Disuse atrophy** may result from inactivity or a limitation in movement. It is particularly important in muscle when limbs are restrained by casts or other mechanisms.
- **Neurogenic atrophy** is loss of innervation due to peripheral nerve injury or loss of central control due to brain or spinal cord injury.
- **Endocrine atrophy** results from lack of pituitary trophic hormones and decreased metabolism.
- **Vascular atrophy** is a consequence of loss of blood supply. **Pressure atrophy** comes from direct pressure on the cell; most instances involve pressure on the blood supply or blockade of a duct.

The term **senile atrophy** is sometimes applied to changes that involve the slowly progressive loss of parenchymal cells with advancing age. The repro-

---

In the newly formed hepatocytes, there is marked increase in organelles that facilitate cell growth—nucleolus, nuclear sites of transcription, nuclear pores, and the cytoplasmic machinery of protein synthesis. During rapid growth, intercellular junctions are disassembled and re-form as new cell-to-cell relationships are stabilized.

Biochemical changes in serum and liver reveal the striking metabolic changes that drive hepatic hyperplasia. Serum of partially hepatectomized rats contains several powerful growth factors. Plasma level of hepatocyte growth factor (HGF) rises sharply by 1 hour after surgery (probably as a result of decreased clearance by the liver); the rise in HGF is a major stimulus for transfer of hepatocytes from G_0 to G_1 of the cell cycle. The initiation of early gene expression then begins a remarkable spectrum of growth factor action that drives hyperplasia.

Upon examination of slices of regenerating liver tissue, one finds a large increase in many factors that stimulate growth—for example, transforming growth factors (TGFs). Growth factors that originate outside the liver also influence growth of regenerating hepatocytes during circulation in the bloodstream—for example, epidermal growth factor (EGF). The hormones insulin, glucagon, vasopressin, norepinephrine, and thyroid and parathyroid hormones are important adjuvants in liver regeneration.

ductive organs atrophy first, followed by muscles, bone, and later the nervous system. The term **physiologic atrophy** is applied by some to the programmed disappearance of embryonic tissues that degenerate as part of their normal life cycle, a process here referred to as **programmed cell death**.

Atrophic cells are smaller than normal. Organelles of atrophic cells are small and sparse. Appropriate stimuli for cell metabolism are lacking. **Mitochondria are small** in atrophic cells. The reduction in transcription, translation, and conjugation of secretory proteins results in **loss of**

rIbosomes and endoplasmic reticulum, with disappearance of secretory granules. **Autophagy** (autophagocytosis), the process in which degenerating organelles are taken into lysosomes, is exaggerated, so that atrophic cells are often filled with large secondary lysosomes called residual bodies. Programmed cell death contributes to atrophy, especially with endocrine organs.

When prostatic epithelial cells are deprived of androgens by castration, they cannot produce secretory granules (see Fig. 9.3). The rough endoplasmic reticulum is strikingly diminished in vol-

---

FOCUS

Vitamin A Deficiency and Metaplasia

VITAMIN A ALCOHOL (retinol) or its precursors, the carotenes, occurs in most normal diets. Both are present in plants containing yellow pigments and in animal fats and liver (e.g., cod liver oil). Beta carotene, the most important, is cleaved in the gut mucosa into two molecules of retinal (vitamin A aldehyde). After absorption, large amounts are stored in stellate, interstitial cells of the liver (liver disease impairs storage).

Squamous metaplasia of epithelial surfaces is the dominant lesion in vitamin A deficiency. Throughout the body there are widespread changes of simple types of epithelium to stratified squamous epithelium. This is most easily detected at body orifices but also occurs in viscera such as the pancreas, the bladder, and other organs. It is especially important in ductal structures and has been established as a cause of urolithiasis in cats, although this has not been confirmed.

Studies on vitamin A deficiency in calves during the 1960s concluded that metaplasia of the parotid duct was pathognomonic. In calves, clinically significant changes occur in arachnoid villi of the meninges; outflow of cerebrospinal fluid is inhibited, causing increased intracranial pressure.

Vitamin A exerts a controlling influence on development of epithelial cells. It has a steroidlike effect on nuclear transcription that causes dedifferentiation of cells followed by redifferentiation along a different pathway. In **respiratory epithelium,** goblet cells are eliminated and replaced with keratin-synthesizing squamous cells. Foci of hyperplastic basal cells develop and expand, causing cells to desquamate. As basal cells enlarge, they gradually convert to keratin production.

Teeth are often abnormal in young animals with vitamin A deficiency. Ameloblasts show abnormal differentiation, which in turn adversely affects odontoblast development. Lesions induce hypoplasia of enamel, deficient mineralization of teeth, and retarded eruption.

Vitamin A deficiency in pregnant animals has been associated with stillbirth and abortions, particularly in swine.

ume. Loss of prostatic epithelial cells involves a shift in protein synthesis to protein degradation and is often accompanied by an increase in stromal connective tissue.

Endocrine atrophy

In the natural cycling of sexual activities, the ovary and testis alternately become hypertrophic and atrophic. Changes are most striking in animals with seasonal breeding and sexual cycles. During involution, parenchymal cells shrink, interstitial spaces expand, and activated monocytes invade and differentiate to macrophages as they scavenge cell debris.

In the testicles of carnivores, blood vessels expand during the breeding season and regress during the long months of sexual inactivity (Fig. 9.5). Testicular atrophy in these species is governed by light-dark cycles. Exposure to darkness stimulates the pineal gland to release antigonadotropic substances that inhibit release or synthesis of hypothalamic-releasing hormones, luteinizing hormone (LH), and follicle-stimulating hormone (FSH).

Atrophy of cachexia

Wasting syndromes that occur in senility, nutritional deficiencies, and prolonged chronic infections often result in diffuse atrophy of skeletal muscle. In cachectic atrophy, muscles are small and pale. Myofibers vary considerably in size, and shrunken atrophic fibers are intermingled with normal fibers.

Muscle wasting in various catabolic states is due to activation of the ubiquitin-proteasome pathway. In this system, muscle protein is selectively identified and degraded by a process called **ubiquitinization**. Signals released by the pathologic process induce formation of the potent cytokines interleukin-1 (IL1) and tumor necrosis factor α (TNF-α), which in turn induce the muscle cell to produce all the components of the system—ubiquitin, a carrier molecule, and the proteasome components. At the molecular level, the protein to be degraded is identified, carried to the proteasome, and inserted into its inner chamber, a reactive site where only unfolded proteins can be admitted and degraded.

$$Stimulus \rightarrow TNF\text{-}\alpha \rightarrow ubiquitin \rightarrow$$
$$protein\ degradation \rightarrow muscle\ wasting$$

This pathway is common to many conditions, such as fasting, uremia (renal failure), cancer, severe burns, sepsis, and other severe infections.

As the atrophying myofiber diminishes in size, it becomes pyknotic, with clumps of undegraded myoglobin through the length of the fiber. Destruction of myoglobin incites the lysosomal-endosomal pathway, a second major proteolytic system that is activated to degrade other proteins in the cell and to expel them from the atrophic cell.

Fat atrophy

When lipid mobilization is excessive and extended over long periods, lipolysis induces characteristic changes in adipose tissue. These lesions are commonly present in starving hypoproteic animals, particularly in the very young and very old. Fat around the coronary band of the heart is prominently affected. The watery and translucent appearance of atrophic fat is responsible for the term **serous atrophy of fat**.

Microscopically, lipid globules of the adipose cell break up and decrease in size when fat undergoes atrophy. There is an increase in glycosaminoglycans, which is best seen as thickened basement membranes around adipocytes. In the interstitium, large mesenchymal cells appear that actively synthesize and release large amounts of collagen and basement membrane material. Glycosaminoglycan granules increase, and the tissue stains intensely with alcian blue for mucopolysaccharides.

Atrophy of inflammation

Many of the cytokines that mediate inflammation cause atrophy of parenchymal organs, and it is not uncommon to see atrophy in chronic inflammatory lesions caused by bacteria and viruses. In the nasal cavity, an effect on growing cartilage causes **turbinate atrophy**, and in some species, particularly the dog and pig, loss of turbinates is associated with specific bacterial toxins. In the intestine, replication of some enteric viruses in the intestinal crypts, the site of progenitor cells for maintaining villous epithelium, causes **villous atrophy** (Fig. 9.6).

HYPOPLASIA

Hypoplasia is the failure of organs or tissues to obtain full size. Hypoplastic organs are typically discovered in young animals. They are caused by events that occur in late stages of the developing fetus and neonate. Often the etiologic agent cannot be determined. Known causes of hypoplasia include (1) deletion of critical cell populations by viruses and toxins that produce degeneration and necrosis and (2) genetic mutations that alter the proper differentiation and migration of cells in the embryo.

Virus-induced hypoplasia

Congenital cerebellar hypoplasia occurs in young animals and is manifest clinically as ataxia. Although no evidence of cause may be present at

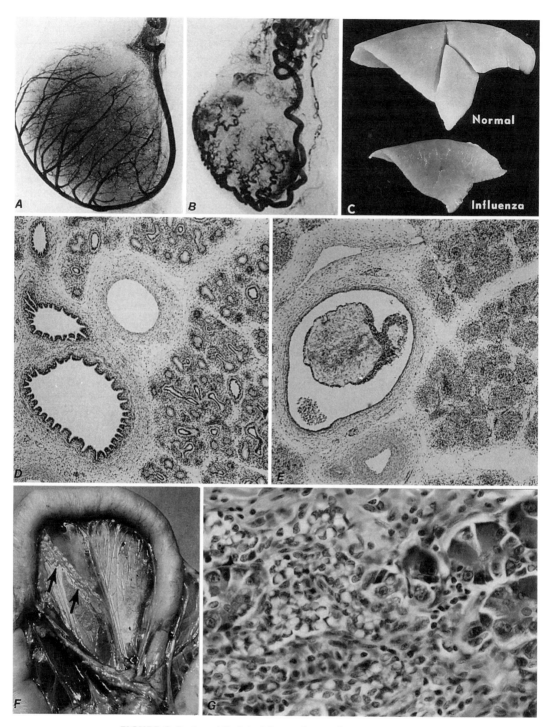

FIGURE 9.5. A and B. Arterial tree, fox testis. A. During breeding season. B. During sexual inactivity. C–E. Lungs of fetal pigs. C. Normal and influenza virus–infected lungs. D. Normal lung. E. Degeneration and necrosis of developing bronchiolar epithelium and primordial alveoli in influenza-infected lung. F and G. Pancreatic hypoplasia, dog. F. Only remnants of pancreatic tissue remain in the mesoduodenum. G. Hypoplastic and degenerate pancreatic acinar cells. (Photographs A and B: M. Joffre, *Anat Rec* 183:599, 1975; photographs C–E: Talmadge Brown, *Vet Pathol* 17:455, 1980)

necropsy, viral infections during pregnancy clearly can cause cerebellar hypoplasia (e.g., feline panleukopenia virus, bluetongue virus in lambs and calves, and bovine viral diarrhea virus in calves). The actively mitotic cells of the external germinal layer are specifically destroyed and fail to migrate to form the definitive internal granular layer of the cerebellum. Cerebellar folia are stunted and fail to function properly.

Hereditary hypoplasia

Hypoplasia of pituitary, thyroid, pancreas, and kidney occurs spontaneously. Causes are not known but presumably involve a hereditary tendency. Pancreatic hypoplasia in the German shepherd leads to a complex of intestinal malabsorption, with wasting, polyphagia, and abnormal feces. Pancreatic tissue is rudimentary (see Fig. 9.5), and although the dog may survive early life, it will succumb in early adulthood. During rapid growth of the young dog, the few remaining normal acinar cells progressively degranulate, leaving dark hypoplastic cells around an intact ductal system. Islet cell destruction and diabetes mellitus often accompany exocrine pancreatic failure.

Familial renal hypoplasia follows the same pattern. Pups may survive for a time with partial kidney function but succumb during the first crisis involving increased demands on renal excretion.

APLASIA

Aplasia is the complete failure of an organ to develop. The organ may be totally absent (**agenesis**) or may be represented by a rudimentary structure composed of connective tissue. Thymic aplasia and gonadal aplasia are two clinically important examples.

Aplasia is most common and best understood in the reproductive organs, particularly in the male genital system. Chromosomal sex, established at the time of conception, directs development of the indifferent gonad to testis or ovary. The Y chromosome initiates testicular development; in its absence, ovaries form.

When testes are produced by action of the Y chromosome, two secretions are essential for the male reproductive organs: (1) **müllerian inhibiting substance** (from primordial spermatogenic tubules), which causes regression of the müllerian ducts; and (2) **testosterone** (produced slightly later by the interstitial cells), which stimulates the wolffian duct system. If these hormones are not produced, the fetal gonad secretes estradiol and promotes the female system (the castrated embryo develops as a female).

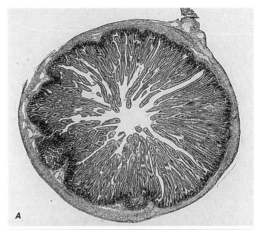

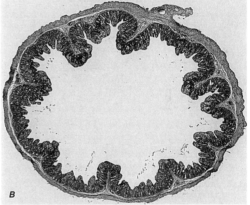

FIGURE 9.6. Jejunum, pig. A. Normal villi. B. Severe villous atrophy. (Micrographs: Harley Moon).

Aplasia may arise from defects in the primitive gonad: (1) defective synthesis of müllerian inhibiting substance by spermatogenic tubules and (2) defective testosterone production by interstitial (Leydig) cells (Table 9.3). Several syndromes of testosterone deficiency occur in humans, each with a defect involving an enzyme required for conversion of cholesterol to testosterone.

Single-gene mutations and testosterone synthesis

If testosterone synthesis is missing or suppressed in the developing fetus, the wolffian duct system will not develop, and there may be aplasia of the male genital tract. The epididymis, vas deferens, and seminal vesicles may be missing or rudimentary (see Table 9.3).

Defects may occur not in the gonad but in **testosterone metabolism** in the genital target tissue. Inside cells, testosterone can act directly or be converted by the enzyme 5α-reductase to dihydro-

TABLE 9.3. Mechanisms of aplasia in fetal reproductive tracts

Defect	Phenotype	Müllerian duct (oviduct, uterus)	Wolffian duct (epididymis, vas deferens, seminal vesicles)	Urogenital sinus (vagina, clitoris; penis, scrotum)
Genetic male				
Müllerian-inhibiting substance synthesis in spermatogenic tubules (persistent müllerian duct syndrome)	♂	+	+	Penis
Testosterone synthesis in Leydig cells (various syndromes of incomplete virilization in humans)[a]				
Severe form	♀	−	−	Vagina
Slight form	♂	−	±	Penis (hypospadias)
5α-Reductase synthesis in genital tissue (absence of 5α-DHT)	♀	−	+	Vagina
Androgen receptor synthesis in genital tissue (testicular feminization [Tfm] mutation in humans, rats, mice)	♂ and ♀	−	+	Vagina
Genetic female[a,b]				
Androgen exposure during fetal development (female virilization)	♀	+	±	Vagina, hypoplastic
Female born co-twin with male, fused placental circulation (bovine freemartin)	♀	−	±	Vagina, hypoplastic
Congenital adrenal hyperplasia, defect in 21-hydroxylation and cortisol synthesis with compensatory androgen production (humans)	♀	±	±	Vagina, hypoplastic
Maternal androgenic tumors or androgen therapy	♀	±	±	Vagina

Note: +, present; −, absent; ±, may be present.

[a]Several single-gene mutations causing defective testosterone synthesis are known; no mutations have been identified that cause deficient estrogen synthesis or tissue resistance to estrogen action.

[b]Female embryos have same androgen receptor system in genital tissues as male; sexes differ only in gonadal production of hormones.

testosterone. Although these two androgens are both bound to cytoplasmic androgen receptors, they do not uniformly affect the male genital primordia; that is, their effects are organ specific. Testosterone receptor complexes cause virilization of the wolffian ducts. Dihydrotestosterone receptor complexes induce virilization of the urogenital sinus and external genitalia.

Persistent müllerian duct syndrome

Male pseudohermaphroditism, the most common form of intersexuality in dogs, occurs in male miniature schnauzers with the persistent müllerian duct syndrome. Müllerian duct derivatives persist, and there is unilateral or bilateral cryptorchidism. Affected dogs have normal male chromosome patterns (i.e., 38 pairs of autosomes, a large X chromosome, and a small Y chromosome). Biosynthesis of testosterone proceeds normally because affected

males are masculinized and the wolffian system is present. A genetic basis for this syndrome is likely, given that it is seen in siblings, but the mode of inheritance is not known.

DYSPLASIA

Dysplasia, meaning abnormal development, is a deliberately vague term used to describe tissues with cell populations that are affected by different processes and are improperly arranged. In most cases it is uncertain whether the condition is truly hypoplastic or has undergone a programmed degenerative change or atrophy induced by an abnormal genome. The term *dysplasia* is most commonly used in reference to developmental defects in the eye, skin, brain, and skeletal system. By definition, the term applies to tissues malformed during maturation. For example, spermatozoa are dysplastic when the head and tailpiece are struc-

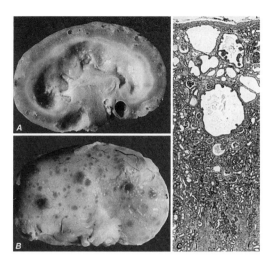

FIGURE 9.7. Renal cysts in an aged dog associated with hydronephrosis. A. Cut surface of the kidney, showing marked dilatation of the pelvis. B. Various sized cysts on the surface of the kidney. C. Histology. Cysts are present in renal tubules.

turally abnormal or improperly aligned.

Classically, although somewhat erroneously, *dysplasia* is also applied to disorganized tissues that have peculiar cells but are not clearly neoplastic. **Fibrous dysplasia** in bone indicates that fibrous connective tissue has replaced normal bone, but its growth will not progress in the manner of a tumor.

TERATOLOGY

Teratology is the study of congenital malformations. **Congenital** implies only that the disease was present at birth. **Malformations** involve a seemingly endless list of unrelated syndromes whose causes are found in the vague borderland between environment and genetics. Although some malformations are clearly associated with abnormal genes, many are acquired in utero when differentiating cells are destroyed by viruses or toxins.

Early in embryogenesis, cells become committed to specific developmental pathways. When genes are expressed sufficiently to alter cell structure or function, the cell has **differentiated**. Differentiation, which is usually irreversible, involves a change in genetic expression, not gene structure. Thus it seems that malformations can be acquired not only by deletion of critical primordial cells but also by drugs that influence genetic expression during early phases of fetal development.

Small defects in tissue architecture that block secretory ducts or excretory pathways may lead to large, life-threatening lesions (Figs. 9.7 and 9.8). For

example, renal malformation can be produced by the anatomic obstruction of the fetal urinary tract, a manipulation that disturbs the complex changes in morphogenesis by altering gene expression, cell turnover, and urine composition. Nephrogenesis is controlled by genes that enhance or inhibit growth, and shifts in the expression of these genes lead to abnormal cellular proliferation, differentiation, and morphogenesis. The following are some terms useful in describing malformations:

- **Atresia**—absence of an opening
- **Stenosis**—narrowing or stricture of a duct or canal
- **Ectasia**—dilatation, distension, or expansion of a space
- **Dilatation**—an orifice or tubule stretched beyond normal dimension

Viral infections cause fetal malformations

Viruses that produce systemic infection and that cross the placenta to infect the fetus are often teratogenic, especially in the brain. Multiple organ systems are commonly affected (Table 9.4). Anomalies are caused by intracellular viral replication and necrosis of a specific group of cells.

Cerebellar ataxia

In **feline panleukopenia**, the causal parvovirus destroys an entire layer of the cerebellum during development in utero. Viremia develops during infection of the pregnant cat, the fetal brain is infected, and virus replicates in developing cells of the cerebellum. When fetuses are examined, inclusion bodies, viral antigens, and other evidence of

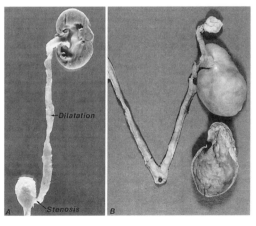

FIGURE 9.8. A. Stenosis of the vesiculo-ureteral orifice, resulting in dilatation of the ureter and renal pelvis. B. Cyst of the uterine wall, dog.

TABLE 9.4. Viral causes of malformation

Species	Virus	Malformation
Cat	Feline panleukopenia	Cerebellar atrophy
Pig	Influenza	Pulmonary hypoplasia[a]
Cow	Bovine viral diarrhea	Cerebellar hypoplasia, hypomyelinogenesis, arthrogryposis, porencephaly, retinal atrophy, hypotrichosis
	Akabane virus	Hydranencephaly, arthrogryposis
	Bluetongue	Hydranencephaly
Human	Rubella	Cataracts, deafness, cardiac anomalies
	Varicella	Growth retardation, limb atrophy, neurologic and ocular defects
	Cytomegalovirus	Hearing loss
	Mumps	Placentitis and abortion[a,b]
	Influenza	Placentitis and abortion[b]

[a]Experimental evidence only; no clear evidence of naturally occurring defect.
[b]Loss of embryo or fetus; no malformations.

infection can be found. However, these disappear by the time the animal is born; the only evidence remaining is a badly malformed brain. Cerebellar ataxia of newborn calves is a complication of herpesvirus infection of the fetus in **bovine infectious rhinotracheitis.**

Hydranencephaly

Congenital cavitary anomalies of the brain appeared in the later 1960s after vaccination of pregnant ewes with bluetongue vaccines. **Hydranencephaly**, in which cerebral hemispheres are reduced to membranous, fluid-filled sacs (the head is of normal size, in contrast to the size in hydrocephalus), was common. By injecting bluetongue vaccine virus directly into fetal lambs at different stages of gestation, it was shown that these lesions were due to virus-induced necrosis. Lambs infected at 50–58 days developed severed necrotizing en-

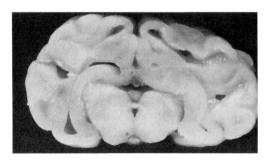

FIGURE 9.9. Porencephaly. Porous lesions involving subcortical white matter in the cerebrum of a 120-day fetal lamb inoculated with bluetongue virus vaccine at 77 days of gestation. (Photograph: Bennie Osburn, *Lab Invest* 25:197, 1971)

cephalopathy and by birth had severe hydranencephaly. Lambs infected at 75–78 days of gestation developed multifocal encephalitis, which presented at birth as porencephaly (discrete cystic defects). Lambs infected after 100 days of gestation developed only mild encephalitis and had no pathologic sequelae (Fig. 9.9).

Pulmonary hypoplasia

Influenza virus causes congenital malformations of fetuses whose mothers suffer infection during pregnancy. Although teratogenic effects have never been clearly confirmed, influenza virus given to pregnant swine causes striking hypoplasia of the lungs (see Fig. 9.5). Incriminating a particular virus after pregnancy is terminated is difficult, for the mother may not have exhibited clinical signs of viral infection. Hog cholera live-virus vaccines given to pregnant swine do not produce clinical disease, yet may cause multiple fetal malformations, including pulmonary hypoplasia, microencephaly, and liver nodules with ascites.

Plant toxins and fetal malformations

Cyclopia

Ingestion of the plant *Veratrum californicum* by pregnant sheep between the 10th and 15th day of gestation induces **cyclopia** in the fetus. Before and after this period, there is little effect of the plant toxin on the developing fetus. The teratogenic capacity of this toxin, unlike that of most plant toxins, is confined to a narrow period. Cyclopia (holoprosencephaly) is an absence of midline structures in embryonic development that results in a proboscis with fused nasal cavities that overlie a single eye. In the brain, the prosencephalic derivatives develop as a single, undivided vesicle consisting of fused remnants of dorsal telencephalic lobes, with an undivided eye tract and absence of ventral forebrain structures, including the optic stalk, optic chiasm, and pituitary.

Skeletal malformations

Calves born to cows that have ingested poison hemlock (*Conium maculatum*) during 40–70 days of gestation develop skeletal malformations. Coniine, the major toxic alkaloid in poison hemlock, is probably responsible for the defect, although other alkaloids are also teratogenic. Piglets develop cleft palate (palatoschisis) when pregnant sows are fed poison hemlock during gestation days 30–45.

Drugs are important causes of malformations

Drugs are only rarely associated with malformations in animals but are important human teratogens. The veterinary pathologist plays a significant role in prevention of human drug-induced malformations by testing and approving new pharmaceutical preparations. Widespread occurrence of **amelia** (absence of limbs) in human infants was traced to the drug thalidomide, given during pregnancy to prevent nausea. Thalidomide inhibits limb bud formation at a precise period of development.

Inhalation anesthetics were first incriminated as teratogens when operating room nurses were shown to have a high incidence of fetal malformations. Experimentally, exposure of pregnant rats to nitrous oxide causes fetal resorption and several types of malformations.

The teratogenic effects of drugs are not limited to pregnancy. Organs not fully developed at birth, such as brain, eye, and lung, are susceptible to damage in the neonatal period, especially to drugs that alkylate or interfere with DNA.

The etiologic factor in many congenital malformations remains unknown, especially for those diseases that permit survival. Because of the familial nature of these conditions, many are presumed to be of genetic origin. An environmentally caused disease, however, may masquerade as a Mendelian trait, and only careful analysis can establish a genetic origin.

AGING

Increased age is inevitably accompanied by degenerative disease. Many aging changes are secondary to diminished function of supportive structures. Bone joints and connective tissues become increasingly rigid. Interstitial spaces are expanded by deposition of collagen and ground substance. The cardiovascular system has a diminished capacity to

---

FOCUS

Cyclopia

CHANGES IN CYCLOPIA result from mutations that arise when teratogens block cholesterol biosynthesis, a complex mechanism that connects cholesterol metabolism to embryonic development in the brain. Teratogens that cause cyclopia specifically block a critical signaling pathway that originates in a gene locus known as **sonic hedgehog**. Proteins from the sonic hedgehog gene must be cleaved and bind to cholesterol to generate their signal. The teratogenic effect is not on the gene, but on the ability of the embryonic brain cell to respond to the sonic hedgehog signal. Disruption in cholesterol transport thus prevents embryonic cells from responding to the signal that directs cellular movement that is essential in the formation of the developing brain.

The major teratogens in *Veratrum californicum*, the corn lily, are the alkaloids cyclopamine and jervine, a distal inhibitor of cholesterol biosynthesis that can reproduce cyclopi-like defects in chick embryos. Exposure of a chick embryo (or of explants of chick embryo brain in vitro) to jervine at the intermediate to definitive streak stage induces cyclopia.

respond. Brain, muscle, and viscera suffer from the decreased perfusion by circulating blood. Neurons, myocytes, and other cells slowly accumulate metabolic products that remain in the cell. The progressing cycles of diminished function and structural change inevitably reach a point where tissue is more susceptible to injury. This in turn hastens the progression of tissue senescence.

In some specific diseases, the capacity of groups of cells to remain functional is related to factors of blood supply, innervation, endocrine stimulation, and combinations of these factors. If thyroid and adrenal hormones are diminished, so is the viability of the cells stimulated by these hormones.

Starvation is a common cause of death in aged animals. In some insects with short life spans, there is a genetically programmed loss of key enzymes in the digestive tract. In others, crucial mouthparts drop off during metamorphosis, and the insect dies after fat reserves are exhausted. These same mechanisms affect vertebrates, though less strikingly. Aged mammals, for example, may die from malnutrition brought about by loss of teeth. The complex interplay of age-related biological turnoffs and starvation is poorly understood.

Lymphoid tissue dysfunction is implicated in aging. Death may be hastened because of progressive loss of the capacity to rid the body of unwanted protein antigens. Disappearance of the thymus and its hormone **thymosin** allegedly leads to loss of immunologic surveillance. Aging is also associated with abnormal antigens on cell surfaces that predispose to autoallergic disease and malignancy.

Cell aging

Aging cells accumulate many abnormal gene products that can represent molecular mischief. Key enzymes (and mechanisms for their production) become increasingly sluggish. Repair mechanisms for the major macromolecules DNA, RNA, and protein become less efficient, and breaks that occur in these molecules are defectively repaired. In all of this the primary causes of aging are difficult to distinguish from secondary expressions of cell damage.

In addition to cellular damage, the relations within and between cells begin to break down, destroying the feedback mechanisms that orchestrate cell functions in the efficient multicellular organism. Although cellular aging ultimately leads to aging and death, the aging process is complicated by many factors, including the following:

- Diet
- Vascular disease
- Endocrine dysfunction
- Genetic factors

Error in DNA triggers cell senescence

Error theories, which involve errors in both DNA (somatic mutation) and protein synthesis, imply that cells accumulate nonlethal damage until reaching a threshold where biologic function ceases. The **somatic mutation theory** postulates a progressive accumulation, with age, of random errors in DNA of somatic cells, probably due to declining capacity for DNA repair. Evidence of defective protein synthesis can be readily detected in tissues of aged animals. Decreased quantities of crucial enzymes and of proteins that function as cell surface receptors are especially important in endothelium, macrophages, and leukocytes. Decreased activities of hydroxylases in fibroblasts cause production of collagen with abnormal ratios of α chains. The diminished sensitivity to insulin associated with aging affects liver, muscle, and adipose tissue.

Neuroendocrine clocks control aging

The central nervous system mediates aging through the hypothalamic-pituitary axis. This genetically controlled neuroendocrine clock slows with age, and the loss of its hormonal direction deprives supporting tissues of stimuli to repair and reconstruct. In some lower vertebrates, excess adrenal cortical activity is associated with senescence. Pacific salmon undergo an intriguingly rapid pattern of aging and death after their migration from the sea to freshwater rivers to spawn. After eggs are ejected and fertilized, the adults become increasingly sluggish and die within a few days. Adrenal cortical "toxicosis" has been reported to cause this rapid aging process. Changes that occur are associated with onset of sexual maturity; they include atrophy of the digestive tract, muscles, and viscera. Castration suppresses adrenal activity and allows an increased life span in these fish. The *clk-1* gene in the nematode *Caenorhabditis elegans* controls growth and development, and mutant forms of *clk-1* can markedly alter the life span of these worms.

Shortening of telomeres signals senescence

The accumulative effects of incomplete replications at the ends of chromosomes, called telomere shortening, appear to be one manifestation of cellular aging. The ends of each chromosome contain short repeated sequences of DNA referred to as telomeres. Telomeres protect the ends of the chromosome from abnormal fusion or loss during replication and assist in the termination of replication. The telomere sequence is formed by specific enzymes called telomerases whose function is to maintain and stabilize the proper length of the telomere. Loss of telomerase activity and shortened telomeres signal cell aging (conversely, unrestricted telomerase activity and elongated telomeres appear to have an association with cancer).

ADDITIONAL READING

Attar R, et al. 1998. Short-term urinary flow impairment deregulates PAX2 and PCNA expression and cell survival in fetal sheep kidneys. *Am J Pathol* 152:1225.

Bolande RP. 1979. Developmental pathology. *Am J Pathol* 94:627.

Bowden DM, Williams DD. 1984. Aging. *Adv Vet Sci Comp Med* 28:305.

Breider MA, et al. 1996. Cellular hyperplasia in rats following continuous intravenous infusion of recombinant human epidermal growth factor. *Vet Pathol* 33:184.

Edwards MJ. 1978. Congenital defects due to hyperthermia. *Adv Vet Sci Comp Med* 22:29.

Leipold HW, et al. 1983. Bovine congenital defects. *Adv Vet Sci Comp Med* 27:198.

Marshall LS, et al. 1982. Persistent müllerian duct syndrome in miniature schnauzers. *J Am Vet Med Assoc* 181:798.

Mitch WE, Goldberg AL. 1996. Mechanisms of muscle wasting. *New Engl J Med* 335:1897.

Molkentin JD, et al. 1998. A calcineurin-dependent transcriptional pathway for cardiac hypertrophy. *Cell* 93:215.

Panter KE, et al. 1985. Induction of cleft palate in newborn pigs by maternal ingestion of poison hemlock *(Conium maculatum)*. *Am J Vet Res* 46:1368.

Rewerts MJ, et al. 1997. Atraumatic rupture of the gastrocnemius muscle after corticosteroid administration in a dog. *J Am Vet Med Assoc* 210:655.

Rowland JM, Hendricks AG. 1983. Corticosteroid teratogenicity. *Adv Vet Sci Comp Med* 27:99.

Schwartz K, et al. 1992. Switches in cardiac muscle gene expression as a result of pressure and volume overload. *Am J Physiol* 252:R364.

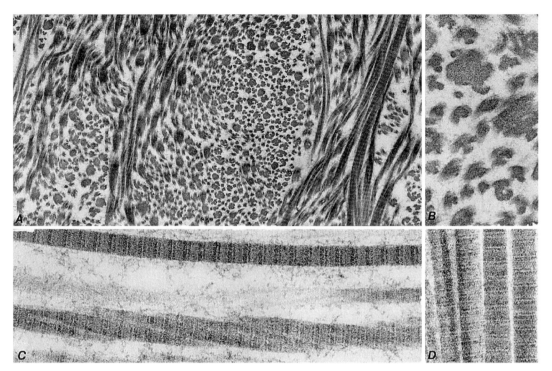

FIGURE 10.1. Abnormal collagen fibrils, dermatosparaxis, cat. A. Collagen fibers with fibrils in various planes of section. B. Bizarre shapes in cross section. C. Longitudinal section shows loosely woven bundles of filaments that spiral around one another. D. Collagen fibrils, normal cat. (Micrographs: Karen A. Holbrook, *J Invest Dermatol* 74:100, 1980)

CHAPTER 10

Genetic Disease

Genetic disease develops from abnormalities in DNA, the cell's genetic material. The total genetic information, or genome, is partitioned into specific numbers of chromosomes, which are transmitted by gametes through generations according to the laws of Mendel. In this chapter, we are concerned with **germ-line defects**, hereditary disorders that, by definition, are transmitted in the gametes from one generation to another. They arise from mutations that are considered familial when passed through several generations. Stable alterations of genes within mitotically active **somatic cells** also occur. These changes are not transmitted to future generations and will not be discussed. Genetic diseases may be placed in three major categories:

- Single mutant genes of large effect
- Multifactorial inheritance
- Cytogenetic disease

Diseases related to **mutant genes of large effect**, the so-called Mendelian disorders, include the rare inborn errors of metabolism that result from mutation of a single gene (Fig. 10.1). The defects are so small that chromosomal analysis does not reveal abnormal structures.

Diseases of **multifactorial inheritance**, often called polygenic inheritance, involve traits that are solely due to two or more genetic loci—for example, neural tube defects, cleft palate, and some congenital heart defects. Multifactorial inheritance involves traits governed by the additive effect of many genes of small impact and usually involves nongenetic environmental factors that influence the phenotypic expression of disease. Diabetes mellitus and congenital hip dysplasia of dogs are diseases in which multifactorial inheritance, coupled with predisposing environmental influences, underlie development of disease.

Diseases due to **abnormalities of chromosomal structure or function** are detected by the analysis of cellular chromosomes, that is, cytogenetic analysis. Change in chromosomal structure implies breakage followed by rearrangement. Abnormal numbers of chromosomes are due to nondisjunction, either during meiotic division (which results in an aneuploid gamete) or during postzygotic mitotic division (anaphase lag). Many of these changes are incompatible with life and result in death of the fetus.

Inherited traits are passed from one generation to the next in a predictable manner. Visible or measurable properties—the appearance of the animal—are called the **phenotype**. Genetic factors (which are inferred) that create the phenotype are called the **genotype**. Some phenotypic traits are determined by simple genes, and others are determined by several genes that act in concert.

A **gene** is simply a specific sequence of base pairs in DNA. Genetic information for synthesis of peptides is not arranged in a continuous sequence of DNA codons. Genes are split, and patches of coding sequences are separated by noncoding DNA. When a gene is transcribed onto mRNA, the new transcript mRNA must be cleansed of the noncoded parts and the cleansed molecule spliced together so that the coding sequences are joined directly to form a coherent mRNA. The many different proteins produced in cells require more information than can be provided by an unaltered linear gene. This diversity is provided by shuffling various combinations of gene segments and by selective RNA transcription.

The DNA in different cells of an individual contains the same genetic information, but only a limited amount is expressed. The cell's genetic program can be switched on and off or can be **selectively expressed**. Thus the neuron and keratinocyte have the same genome, but very different expressions of it. Selective expression is illustrated by classic nuclear transplantation experiments done in the 1960s. Nuclei extracted from tadpole gut epithelium were transplanted into frog ova from which the nuclei had been removed. Some ova developed into normal adults, showing that intestinal epithelial nuclei contained all the genes required for development. These studies provided the foundation for experiments that control genetic expression by injecting ova with purified extracts of mRNA, which can instruct the cell to make specific proteins.

MUTANT GENES OF LARGE EFFECT (MENDELIAN DISORDERS)

Pedigree analysis based on mendelian laws is used to establish probable genetic cause, to predict the degree of risk of individuals, and to indicate possible abnormal genetic mechanisms even when biochemical mechanisms are unknown. Mendel's concepts of dominance and recessivity were derived from phenotypes and not from molecular mechanisms of inheritance.

Rediscovered in 1900, Mendel's laws of 1860 stated that (1) a unit of genetic information is transmitted unchanged from one generation to another and (2) alternate forms of this gene (later called an allele) must segregate during gamete formation and recombine independently in the offspring to provide a 1:2:1 ratio. Mendel's observations were made on the self-fertilizing pea plant, of which he had many true-breeding varieties. He crossed hybrids derived from true breeders and made quantitative calculations of disparate characters that appeared in succeeding generations. When plants containing wrinkled seeds were crossed with plants containing smooth seeds, he found that only smooth-coated seeds were present in the F_1, or first, hybrid generation. When he self-fertilized smooth-seeded F_1 plants, the result was one-fourth true-breeding smooth-seeded plants and two-fourths smooth-seeded, impure breeders, which, when self-fertilized, produced the same 1:2:1 ratio. The wrinkled coat, although phenotypically not present in the F_1 hybrid, was transmitted unchanged from parent seed to the F_2, or second-generation, hybrids. He thus proposed that the physical expression (**phenotype**) differed from the genetic constitution (**genotype**) and that the genotype must be determined by two transmissible characters or genes.

FOCUS

Belgian Blue Cattle

THE DOUBLE-MUSCLE MUTATION in Belgian Blue cattle was reported in 1807. In the 1950s, breeders in Belgium began to select for the double-muscle trait. In the face of high production costs and cheap meat, they wished to increase meat production. The breed that emerged has a striking degree of muscle hyperplasia, with many more myocytes than normal. This is in contrast to some heavily muscular individuals in other breeds in which muscle hypertrophy results from very large skeletal muscle cells but no increase in cell numbers, a condition in which the meat is tough. The neonatal Belgian Blue calf is so large that cesarean section is routinely done. In Belgian Blue cattle, the gene for **myostatin**, a protein that shuts down myocyte replication at the appropriate time (limiting skeletal muscle growth), is mutated. The myostatin gene has been mapped to a region of bovine chromosome 2. The defect is an inactivating mutation—an 11–base pair deletion—that results in complete truncation of the active region of the protein (*Science* 277:1922, 1997). Piedmontese cattle also have a mutated myostatin gene, but the lesser amount of muscle in Piedmontese cattle is due to other genes that compensate for loss of myostatin.

TABLE 10.1. Rules for inheritance

Autosomal dominant disease
1. Every animal with the phenotype has a parent that exhibits the phenotype (unless it is a mutation).
2. The trait usually exhibits no preference for one sex.
3. Approximately one-half of the descendants of an affected animal will have the trait.
4. If a descendant of an affected animal is free of the trait, all of its descendants will be free.

Autosomal recessive disease
1. Recessive traits may show in pedigrees in two different ways.[a]
2. Both sexes are affected about equally.
3. Autosomal recessive strains appear far more frequently as a result of related breeding.

Sex-linked dominant disease
1. An affected male gives the disease to all female offspring but to none of the male offspring.
2. An affected female gives the trait to one-half of her offspring, male and female.
3. More females are affected than males (the key to determination is the pattern of disease in offspring of affected males).

Sex-linked recessive disease
1. The disease will be in males (carried on the X chromosome).
2. All female offspring of affected males will be carriers and will give the recessive gene to one-half of their offspring.

[a]If the disease is rare (the usual case), then the animal having the trait may be the only one in the pedigree that has the trait (thus it is usually not possible to establish that an autosomal recessive disease is hereditary by family history). If the disease is common, there may be cases of the disease on both sides of the pedigree. There will still be a frequent skipped generation.

Dominance and recessivity

By examining pedigrees and plotting incidence of animal disease in a related population, the pattern of inheritance can be determined as one of the four models of simple mendelian inheritance: autosomal dominant, autosomal recessive, sex-linked dominant, and sex-linked recessive (Table 10.1). **Autosomal dominant** diseases are those in which heterozygotes express the mutant allele. Both males and females are affected, and both transmit the disease. When an affected animal is mated to an unaffected animal, one-half of the offspring will be affected. Some dominant conditions do not invariably manifest themselves in the heterozygote, a phenomenon called incomplete penetrance.

Pedigree analysis has shown that hereditary multiple exostoses in horses occur as an autosomal dominant condition. Three observations compatible with this analysis are that males and females are affected equally, that mating of affected and unrelated normals gives rise to a large number of affected offspring, and that mating of two affected horses can yield normal females. The last finding is incompatible with X-linked inheritance.

Only homozygotes express autosomal recessive traits

In transmission of **autosomal recessive** traits, disease typically occurs in offspring of unaffected parent animals (with a 1:4 risk). The great majority of inborn errors of metabolism are autosomal recessive, and the heterozygotes in many of these cases show a partial deficiency of the enzyme that is lacking in the homozygote.

Chondrodysplasia of Alaskan malamute dwarfs is transmitted as a simple autosomal recessive trait with complete penetrance and variable phenotypic expression. It is a generalized symmetrical defect in endochondral ossification of cuboidal bones (which have wide, flat, irregular physes). Hypertrophic and degenerative zones in affected bones are irregular and widened proximally to microfractures in the primary spongiosa. Histologically, dwarf proliferative chondrocytes occur in clumps separated by wide areas of extracellular matrix. Ultrastructurally, the proliferating chondrocytes are vesiculated and surrounded by a matrix that is deficient in matrix granules. Proteoglycans extracted from growth plate cartilage have abnormal glycosaminoglycan ratios; that is, there is increased chondroitin-6-sulfate and galactosamine, an indication of immature cartilage matrix.

Transmission of sex-linked diseases

Sex-linked (or X-linked) diseases are transmitted by heterozygous carrier females only to sons who are hemizygous for the X chromosome. Very rarely, a female is affected if the male transmits a mutant dominant gene or if both parents transmit mutant recessive genes. No Y-linked diseases are known.

The relationship between sex determination and the presence of abnormal genetic traits was founded in the early 1900s on the **hemophilia** model based on the lineage of Queen Victoria of England, in which females were unaffected carriers of classic hemophilia A. In 1950, Brinkhous showed that hemophilia of dogs was also sex-linked and that,

FOCUS

Albino Animals

ALBINISM RESULTS FROM a structural gene mutation at the locus that codes for tyrosinase; that is, albino animals have a genetically determined failure of tyrosine synthesis. Animals that inherit an albino gene from both parents (are homozygous for albino) are unable to make melanin because the albino gene fails to direct synthesis of the enzyme tyrosinase. Albino cats are homozygous for a c-locus tyrosinase-negative allele. Heterozygotes have normal pigments but abnormal vision and can be identified with a tyrosinase enzyme assay. Albinism in humans is an example of genetic heterogeneity—the same defect in pigmentation can be caused by different genes.

Some albino animals have no tyrosinase, and others form tyrosine but no melanosomes (there are least seven variants of human albinism). In **partial albinism**, there is a general reduction in skin pigmentation but no pigments are present in the eye. Epidermal melanocytes show retarded melanogenesis; their granules are immature fibrillar premelanosomes. It has been suggested that defective receptors for melanin-stimulating hormone are responsible for partial albinism.

The gene Himalayan, a variant of albino (and at the same locus on the chromosome), codes for an enzyme that can synthesize melanin at relatively low temperature only, so that affected mice, Himalayan rabbits, and Siamese cats (which have this gene) have pale or white bodies with darkened extremities.

Siamese cats, white tigers, albino rats, and pearl mink all have genetic mutations characterized by reduced pigmentation and abnormal vision involving central visual pathways (some optic nerve fibers go to the wrong side of the brain). In all Siamese cats, the **lateral geniculate nucleus** (LGN), the main cerebral group that relays messages from the retina to the cerebral cortex, is abnormal. These cats often have crossed eyes, since it is in the LGN that inputs from the two eyes are matched and passed to the cortex (in mammals, correct alignment of the eyes requires a normal LGN).

TABLE 10.2. Sex-linked traits and disease in animals

Gene product or disease	Animal species affected[a]
Glucose-6-phosphate dehydrogenase deficiency	Primate (human, gorilla, chimpanzee), horse, donkey, sheep, cattle, pig, hare, mouse, hamster, kangaroo
α-Galactosidase deficiency	Sheep, cow, pig, rabbit, hamster, mouse
Coagulation factor VIII deficiency	Dog
Coagulation factor IX deficiency	Dog
Phosphoglycerate kinase deficiency	Horse, hamster, mouse, kangaroo, chimpanzee
Hypoxanthine-guanine phosphoribosyltransferase deficiency	Horse, hamster, mouse, chimpanzee
Anhidrotic ectodermal dysplasia	Cow
Copper transport deficiency	Mouse (Menkes' kinky-hair syndrome)
Testicular feminization syndrome	Cow, dog, rat, mouse
Vitamin D–resistant rickets	Mouse
Ornithine transcarbamoylase deficiency	Mouse
Muscular dystrophy (Duchenne's)	Mouse

[a]All syndromes have been identified in humans.

TABLE 10.3. Defective proteins as mutant gene products

Defect	Example
Missing enzymes fail to catalyze metabolic pathways	
Accumulation of precursors due to enzyme block	Lipid storage disease
Deficiency of end products	Albinism
Accumulation of toxic by-products	Phenylketonuria[a]
Abnormal enzymes fail to catalyze membrane transport	
Sodium not absorbed in erythrocytes	Hereditary spherocytosis
Phosphate not absorbed in kidney	Hypophosphatemic rickets
Glucose not absorbed in kidney	Renal glycosuria
Cystine not absorbed in kidney	Cystinuria/renal lithiasis
Missing components of coagulation	
Factor VIII and IX deficiency	Hemophilia
Fibrinogen deficiency	Congenital afibrinogenemia
Failure to maintain structural proteins	
Collagen enzymes missing	Dermatosparaxis

[a]Reported only in humans.

through crossbreeding, hemophilic but viable homozygous females could be produced (negating the assertion that females bearing two hemophilic genes on their X chromosomes were probably inviable).

Sex-linked traits are known for many animal species. Glucose-6-phosphate dehydrogenase production is sex-linked in primates (human, gorilla, chimpanzee), horse, donkey, kangaroo, and several rodent species. The X-linked disease **glucose-6-phosphate dehydrogenase deficiency** is found in these animals. In general, a gene found to be X-linked in one mammal can be expected to be X chromosome–linked in other mammals. Many other X-linked traits of animals are known (Table 10.2).

Proteins as mutant gene products

Mutation of genes controlling protein synthesis, particularly of enzymes, can have widespread pathologic effects. The consequences of amino acid substitution vary from trivial to lethal. Some variants in protein do not produce functional impairment. For example, many normal, functioning variants have been reported for hemoglobin. The defects that arise from abnormal protein synthesis may be expressed in several different ways (Table 10.3).

The first molecular genetic disease to be described was human **sickle cell anemia**, in which an abnormal gene causes valine to be substituted for glutamic acid. This amino acid substitution results in the abnormal hemoglobin S. When deoxygenated, hemoglobin S polymerizes into aligned fibers, which form a gel and distort the erythrocyte into abnormal sickle shapes. Sickled erythrocytes have a short life span, and their lysis is manifested as hemolytic anemia.

Disorders of **amino acid metabolism** are among the most common (but less serious) of the inborn errors of human metabolism; very few have been reported in animals (Table 10.4). They are caused by a single enzyme deficiency based on a single genetic mutation. Most aminoacidopathies are subclinical disorders discovered during amino acid analyses of urine.

Myophosphorylase deficiency

Glycogen phosphorylase is a glycogenolytic enzyme required for the release of glucosyl units from glycogen stored in muscle, liver, and brain. Isoforms of glycogen phosphorylase in these tissues are the products of different genes. Hereditary deficiency of skeletal muscle phosphorylase (myophosphorylase) occurs in Charolais cattle and humans (McArdle's disease). Affected cattle show marked exercise intolerance, fatigue, and inability to walk for long distances. The diagnosis of glycogen phosphorylase deficiency is made by a total lack of enzymes as detected biochemically or in histochemical staining of muscle biopsy tissue.

Mutations in collagen IV genes

The component polypeptides of collagen IV, called α chains, contain long stretches of triple helical trimers that aggregate on three-dimensional lattices to form basement membranes. Six collagen IV α chains are present in mammals, and there is a clear genetic switch at birth from the "embryonic" to "adult" collagens. In the glomerular basement membranes of the kidney, α1 and α2(IV), present in the embryo, are replaced by α3–5(VI) chains as

TABLE 10.4. Aminoacidopathies

Amino acid detected	Primary disorder	Secondarily increased in . . .
Alanine	—	Lactic aciduria, hyperammonemia
Arginine	Arginase deficiency	Ornithinemia
Carnosine	Carnosine deficiency	—
Cystine	Cystinosis (transport defect)	Renal disease
Glycine	Hyperglycinemia (nonketotic)	Ketosis
Ornithine	Ornithine-oxoacid aminotransferase deficiency	—
Phenylalanine	Phenylalanine hydroxylase deficiency (phenylketonuria)	High-protein diet in newborn
	Dihydropteridine reductase deficiency (hyperphenylalaninemia)	—
Phosphoethanolamine	Hypophosphatasia (alkaline phosphatase deficiency)	Bone disease
Proline	Hyperprolinemia	—

development proceeds. Mutation of collagen 3, 4, and 5(IV) chain genes in mice and humans (and presumably dogs) results in a delayed onset renal disease called **Alport's syndrome**. This syndrome is characterized by retention of α1 and α2(IV) collagen, which causes marked thickening of the glomerular basement membrane, with a characteristic "basket weaving" appearance when examined ultrastructurally.

Dermatosparaxis is an inherited disease characterized by lose fragile skin easily torn with minor trauma. It results from a deficiency of procollagen peptidase, the enzyme that cleaves the amino-terminal nonhelical extension from the precursor procollagen molecules. Although procollagen has both carboxy- and amino-terminal extensions cleaved to yield collagen, procollagen with the amino terminus is the only precursor that accumulates in dermatosparaxis.

The degree of enzyme deficiency is a major species difference in this disease. Sheep have almost no collagen chains in skin and generally die at birth or within a few weeks. The defect is less severe in cats and calves, which have significant amounts of normal collagen chains. Newborn calves with dermatosparaxis have extremely fragile skin with large numbers of flat, twisted, unbanded collagen fibrils in disordered patterns. The striking deficiency of mature collagen fibers is demonstrable by their lack of birefringence under polarized light and by abnormal X-ray diffraction patterns.

Instead of the normal weaving of fibers, dermal collagen has a tangled organization of fibrils within the fiber and an abnormal weaving pattern (Fig. 10.1). The aberrant collagen molecules alter the structure of individual fibrils, the assembly of fibrils into fiber bundles, and the woven network in the reticular dermis of skin. In calves, the abnormal fibrils are embedded in excess ground substance, which may be responsible for the jellylike feel of the skin.

Lysosomal storage diseases

Genetic defectiveness in any part of the lysosome leads to serious disease that either kills the developing fetus or is manifested in neonatal or early life. The most serious diseases are those that involve defects in lysosomal enzymes that specifically metabolize cellular components. Major genetic storage diseases that involve accumulation of lysosomes include the following:

- Lipid storage disease
- Mucopolysaccharidoses
- Mucolipidoses
- Glycoproteinoses
- Lysosomal transport disorders
- Glycogen storage diseases
- Amino acid transport disease

Cellular changes that develop when substrates accumulate in lysosomal storage diseases lead to massively enlarged cells with foamy cytoplasm. Ultrastructural examination of these cells reveals giant, complex lysosomes filled with remnants of membranes and lipids (Fig. 10.2).

Lipid storage disease

Lipid storage diseases are the most common of the lysosomal storage diseases. The disease is manifested when the substrate for the missing enzyme accumulates in cells of the brain, liver, or other organs. The most important lipid storage diseases involve defective or missing enzymes that degrade components of membranes.

Because of the importance of myelin biosynthesis, lipid storage diseases typically involve the central nervous system. Deficits of enzymes that degrade **cerebrosides**, which are present in myelin, involve macrophages of the central nervous system. **Gangliosides** occur in neurons, and degradation defectiveness is reflected in those cells.

GM$_1$ gangliosidosis, caused by deficient activity of β-galactosidase, is one of the most common

Leukocyte Adhesion Deficiency in Cattle

LEUKOCYTE ADHESION DEFICIENCIES (LADs) are rare autosomal recessive disorders that result from mutations and greatly reduced expression of β_2 integrin adhesion molecules on leukocytes. The capacity of neutrophils to bind to a pass through endothelium in response to inflammatory stimuli requires β_2 integrin-endothelial cell interaction. Without β_2 integrins, neutrophils are unable to enter tissues from the bloodstream and cannot destroy invading pathogenic microorganisms. LAD patients suffer recurrent bacterial infections.

LAD in Holstein calves involves recurrent pneumonia, ulcerative stomatitis, enteritis, periodontitis, and delayed wound healing. Histologic examination of all of these lesions reveals large numbers of neutrophils within the capillary and venous blood vessels but none within the tissue spaces. Pedigree analysis of these animals revealed that all were offspring of a common sire.

The bovine LAD defect is specifically in the β subunit β_2 integrins, which include MAC-1, LFA-1 and p150.95. Two point mutations have been identified within the gene encoding bovine CD18 in a Holstein calf afflicted with LAD. One mutation causes an aspartic acid to glycine substitution at amino acid 128 (D128G) in the highly conserved extracellular region of this adhesion glycoprotein, a region where several mutations have been found to cause human LAD. The other mutation is silent. The carrier frequency for the D128G allele among Holstein cattle in the United States is approximately 15% among bulls and 6% among cows. This disorder is among the most common genetic diseases known in veterinary science.

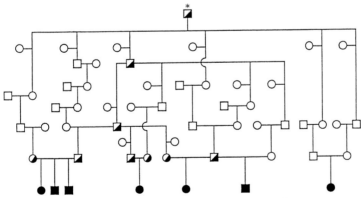

Pedigrees of LAD calves (filled symbols) showing their relationship to a common carrier sire, Osborndale Ivanhoe, listed as the "Father of the Holstein Breed," with thousands of registered offspring (*). All LAD calves are homozygous for the D128G mutation. Open symbols represent animals that were not tested for the D128G mutation, and half-filled symbols denote carriers.

References

Kehrli ME, et al. 1992. Bovine leukocyte adhesion deficiency. *Am J Pathol* 140:1489.

Shuster DE, et al. 1992. Identification and prevalence of a genetic defect that causes leukocyte adhesion deficiency in Holstein cattle. *Proc Natl Acad Sci* 89:9225.

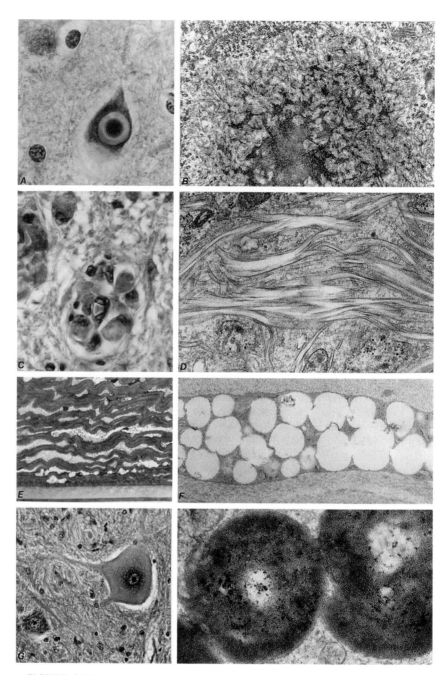

FIGURE 10.2. Lysosomal storage disease. A. Glycoprotein cytoplasmic inclusion, neuron, Lafora's disease, dog. B. Core and margin of neuronal inclusion, and surrounding ribosomes of Purkinje cell, Lafora's disease, dog. C. Perivascular macrophages filled with cerebrosides, globoid cell leukodystrophy, dog. D. Arched, twisted, and interdigitated membrane-bound, ribbonlike structures, globoid cell leukodystrophy, dog. E. Enlarged keratocytes filled with aggregates of inclusions, feline mucopolysaccharidosis VI. Descemet's membrane *(bottom)* is normal. F. Electron-lucent vacuoles filling keratocyte cytoplasm. G. Massively enlarged neuron *(right)* and normal neuron *(left)*, gangliosidosis, cat. H. Sulfatide-containing inclusions consisting of myelin figures, metachromatic leukodystrophy, brain, human infant. (Micrographs A and B: J. M. Holland, *Am J Pathol* 58:509, 1970; micrograph D: Eduardo J. Yunis, *Am J Pathol* 85:99, 1976; micrograph F: M. E. Haskins, *Am J Pathol* 101:567, 1980; micrograph H: A. Gregoire, *J Pathol Exp Neurol* 25:626, 1966)

lysosomal storage diseases. Reported in dogs, cats, cows, and sheep, it is manifested as a massive increase in lysosomes with accumulation of substrate, in the form of whorls and laminar arrangements of membranes within cells of the CNS and viscera.

Mucopolysaccharidoses

The mucopolysaccharidoses are a group of genetic diseases characterized by storage of incompletely degraded glycosaminoglycans (GAGs) in cells that normally degrade these substances. Storage results from diminished activity of specific hydrolases (in lysosomes) required for degradation. Massive accumulations of giant lysosomes bearing GAG polymers cause marked distortion of affected cells. Different lysosomal hydrolases can be demonstrated to be deficient or absent in fibroblasts cultured from the skin of affected animals.

Mucopolysaccharidosis type I, which results from an absence of α-L-iduronidase, occurs in Siamese cats and Plott hounds. Affected cats have facial and bony deformities and clouded corneas. Circulating leukocytes have abnormally large granules, and activity of the lysosomal enzyme α-L-iduronidase is less than 1% normal. The diagnosis is confirmed at weaning by detection of excess GAGs (dermatan sulfate, heparan sulfate) in urine.

Mucolipidoses

Cells from patients with mucolipidosis form large granulofibrillar vacuoles that represent accumulated glycolipids and glycosaminoglycans. The mucolipidoses include a genetic deficiency of ganglioside sialidase, the enzyme that cleaves sialic acid from gangliosides during glycosphingolipid catabolism.

Glycogen storage diseases

Glycogenoses are inherited syndromes caused by missing or defective enzymes of carbohydrate metabolism. Deposits of glycogen (or abnormally branched glucose polymers) accumulate to produce massive amounts of foamy cytoplasm. Most glycogenoses involve glycogen deposits in the cytosol and are not lysosomal storage diseases. In **glycogenosis type II**, which occurs in dogs, cat, cattle, and sheep, glycogen accumulates in lysosomes because the lysosomal enzyme glucosidase is missing. Hepatocytes and skeletal muscles cells are affected, and both have a foamy, swollen appearance.

Triplet-repeat diseases

Most genetic diseases result from a mutation that impairs a gene product. The triplet-repeat diseases are a small group of chronic disorders of skeletal muscle and brain that are associated with expansion of a repeated sequence of three nucleotides. With progressing replications, these nucleotide repetitions lengthen, eventually reaching a size that influences cellular function. In situ hybridization techniques on affected cells reveal aggregates of the trinucleotide repeat in nuclei. Disease appears to result from a "gain of function" effect—a new function arises from the genetic defect. The best known of these diseases are Huntington's disease and myotonic dystrophy.

In some of the brain disorders, grouped as polyglutamine diseases, the defect results from the expansion of the triplet CAG, which encodes the amino acid glutamine and creates a new protein with a polyglutamine component. Transcripts of the expanded gene accumulate as large, cytoplasmic polyglutamine inclusions in neurons.

MULTIFACTORIAL (POLYGENIC) INHERITANCE DISORDERS

Many genetic diseases are **polygenic, or multifactorial, disorders**. That is, the trait is determined by more than one gene and results from the blending of several genes. In Mendel's experiments the color trait was manifested in the following way. When purple-petaled and white-petaled plants were crossed, an intermediate mauve color resulted in the hybrid. When this F_1 hybrid was self-fertilized, a range in color was determined by more than one gene.

Many of the hereditary malformations have this kind of inconsistent mode of inheritance. **Polydactyly** (excess digits) of Simmental cattle develops as a polygenic disorder. **Porcine encephalocele** follows a similar pattern (Fig. 10.3). Cleft palate, spina bifida, and pyloric stenosis occur in human populations with frequencies suggesting a multifactorial genetic disease.

Multiple defects transmitted together

Several independent abnormal traits may be transmitted together, presumably because of their close relationship on the chromosome. In the gray collie syndrome, a condition called cyclic hematopoiesis is transmitted as an autosomal recessive disease. Blood cells, chiefly neutrophils, disappear from the bloodstream in 11-day cycles, and the affected animal eventually succumbs to bacterial infection. Affected dogs also have traits for abnormal gray silver coat color and microphthalmia, which are transmitted together with the blood disorder.

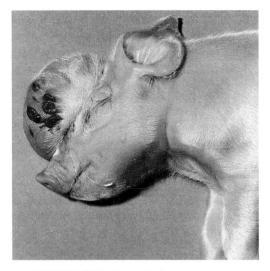

FIGURE 10.3. Growth disturbance: enceph-alocele in newborn pig. A bony defect in the cranium allows the protrusion of the meninges and nervous tissue into a skin-covered sac. Dark areas in the skin are vascular malformations with stasis of blood.

Polygenic inheritance complicates genetic analysis

Ocular dermoids are solid, skinlike masses in or on the eye. Typically, they occur as unilateral hairy growths adhered to the anterior surface of the globe, astride the ventrolateral limbus. They are especially common in some cattle breeds; it has been shown that in Hereford cattle, they are transmitted according to autosomal recessive and polygenic inheritance.

Genetic transmission is indicated by the following: (1) a high incidence in one geographic location without increased incidence in other breeds, (2) bilateral expression of the defect, (3) common ancestry of affected cattle, (4) occurrence in more males than females, (5) independence of season, and (6) inability to demonstrate teratogenic environmental patterns.

CHROMOSOMAL DISORDERS
Abnormal chromosomal numbers

By structural examination of chromosomes, subtle aberrations involving discrete changes within single genes (**point mutations**) cannot be detected. However, when large numbers of genes are rearranged, abnormalities can be seen on cytogenetic analysis. These gross chromosomal abnormalities may have several consequences. Fetal death with spontaneous abortion is common because most of

TABLE 10.5. Classification of chromosomal abnormalities

Abnormality	Description
Polyploidy	Abnormality in multiples of the haploid number
Triploidy	Three of each instead of normal pair
Tetraploidy	Four of each: occurs normally in some animal tissues
Aneuploidy	Increase or decrease in normal (euploid) number of chromosomes but not involving haploid sets; may involve autosomes or sex chromosomes
Monosomy	Only one chromosome in particular pair
Trisomy	One chromosome present 3 times instead of 2; congenital malformations associated with specific trisomies (Down's syndrome in humans involves number 21); trisomy in calves with brachygnathia; number 11 trisomy in fetal runted cats
Mosaicism	Presence of more than one karyotype variety of cell in same individual derived from single zygote; arises from postzygotic mitotic nondisjunction
Chimerism	Two genotypes present in one individual as a result of maternal-fetal cross circulation or postnatal transfusion (bovine freemartin)
Abnormal structure	
Translocation	Separated chromosomal fragments attached to another chromosome
Deletion	Absence of piece of chromosome
Isochromosome	Chromosome separated in wrong plane at centromere: short arms attached to short arms and long to long
Inversion	Segments within a chromosomal arm not arranged in proper order

these conditions are lethal. Only in rare instances is the animal born alive. In humans, in which several specific changes are known, congenital malformation syndromes often involve mental retardation (Table 10.5).

Cytogenetic analysis

Cytogenetic evaluation is done by examining the chromosomes of circulating lymphocytes. Blood samples collected by venipuncture are centrifuged to separate the cells. Lymphocytes are then incubated in culture medium to which a mitotic stimulant (mitogen) has been added. After 3 days, colchicine is added to stop all dividing cells in metaphase. The cells are fixed, dried, and flattened to spread out the chromosomes, which are then stained to emphasize the shape and banding patterns. The number of chromosomes of about 20 well-spread cells is counted, and the presence of the sex chromosomes noted. Chromosomes in metaphase appear in various structural patterns, according to the position of the centromere (kinetochore), which determines the length of the chromosomal arms. **Acrocentric** chromosomes have centromeres at one end and thus have two long arms. In **telocentric** chromosomes, centromeres are near the end. **Metacentric** chromosomes have centromeres approximately in the middle, and **submetacentric** chromosomes have two short and two long arms.

Special stains are used in banding techniques that help differentiate specialized portions of the chromosome for proper identification. **Q banding** utilizes quinacrine fluorochromes that bind specifically to adenine-thymine bases in DNA. Differences in base compositions of DNA segments provide variations in shades of brightness on ultraviolet fluorescence microscopy. **Giemsa (G) banding** gives patterns similar to those of Q banding. Other banding techniques are used to augment these common procedures (Fig. 10.4).

Sex chromatin detection

A useful technique for screening the number of X and Y chromosomes is the staining and evaluation of buccal smears. The female sex chromatin (Barr or X body) is a condensed chromatin mass about 1 μm in diameter along the nuclear membrane in nuclei of female cells. The X body is seen in about 20% of female nuclei; its presence indicates two X chromosomes, one of which is inactivated and condensed. The male Y chromosome in buccal smears can be detected only with special fluorescence microscopy. Only one X chromosome of the female is active during interphase; the second is inactive and pushed aside in the nucleus. This explains the equality of gene products in male and female. In

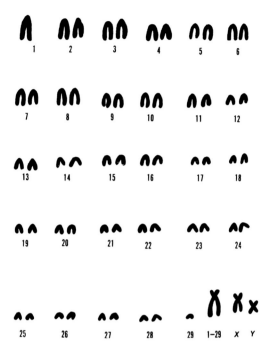

FIGURE 10.4. Chromosome spread of leukocytes from cow with Robertsonian chromosomal translocation. Chromosomes 1 and 29 have fused.

theory, if both female X chromosomes were active, females would have twice the amount of gene product as do males.

Karyotype: a code for chromosome numbers

The karyotype is designated by writing the total chromosome number and the sex chromosomes; for example, the normal male cat is 38,XY. In defining structural abnormalities, the short arm of a chromosome is designated *p* and the long arm *q*. Thus 38,XY,5p– indicates a male with 38 chromosomes and a deletion of the short arm of number 5. A female cat with trisomy of chromosome 18 would be designated 38,XX,+18. Chromosomal **mosaics** (the presence of more than one karyotype in one individual) are identified by separating the cell types with a slash: 38,XX/39,XXY is a mosaic with cells of normal female chromosomes and cells with an extra chromosome.

Species differences in chromosome types

Cattle have 60 chromosomes per cell (2*n*=60). All autosomes are telocentric (although sex chromosomes are metacentric), making it difficult to identify individual chromosomes.

Avian chromosomes fall into two distinct classes: macrochromosomes and microchromosomes. The microchromosomes are very small and easily lost in metaphase chromosomal spreads. In birds, the growing pinfeather has a very high mitotic index and provides material for the "feather pulp technique." Avian embryos at 16–72 hours of development can also be used for chromosome preparations.

Natural polyploidy in lower vertebrates

Triploidy is a rare but naturally occurring phenomenon in fish, amphibians, and reptiles. This development of diploid-triploid mosaic individuals has benefits that enhance reproductive output. Triploid populations are unisexual (all females) and reproduce by **pathogenesis** (reproduction by development of an unfertilized gamete) or **gynogenesis** (in which the embryo contains only maternal chromosomes because of activation of the egg by a sperm that degenerates without fusing with the egg nucleus.

Abnormal spermiogenesis in mules and hybrid horses

Hybrids between horses and donkeys are called mules or hinnies, depending on the species of the dam. If a jack (male donkey) is mated to a mare, the resulting offspring is a mule. If a stallion is bred to a jenny (female donkey), the offspring is a hinny. Spermatogenesis is arrested in male mules and hinnies. At meiosis there are markedly abnormal pairings of chromosomes at the pachytene stage of meiotic prophase because of the dissimilarity of the parental karyotypes; that is, the horse (*Equus caballus*, 2*n*=64), has 26 metacentric and 36 acrocentric autosomal chromosomes, whereas the donkey (*E. asinus*, 2*n*=62) has 38 metacentric and 22 acrocentric.

The Przewalski horse of Siberia has 66 chromosomes. F_1 hybrids between *E. caballus* and *E. przewalskii* (2*n*=66) are fertile and have a diploid chromosome number of 2*n*=65. A single Robertsonian translocation occurs, transforming 4 acrocentric chromosomes of *E. przewalskii* into 2 metacentric chromosomes in *E. caballus*. A trivalent chromosome is formed at meiosis by pairing of the three elements involved in centric fusion rearrangement.

Diseases related to chromosomal defects

Few diseases of animals are associated with identifiable abnormalities in karyotype. This may be largely due to the lethality of such large genetic errors and loss of the embryo without detection. Most embryos with abnormal karyotypes are lost at the time of implantation. In some breeds this may be a major cause of embryonic death. Chickens have up to 9% abnormal karyotypes (variation among breeds is from 0.5 to 9%), and pigs may have up to 12% abnormal karyotypes with coincident loss of embryos.

Chromosomal aberrations related to reproductive system

In **X monosomy**, one homologous X chromosome is missing, giving XO instead of XX. It has been seen most commonly in horses. Affected mares are infertile and have small reproductive organs: ovaries lack follicles, the uterus is small and flaccid, and there are irregular periods of estrus, often with no cyclic ovarian activity. Although the Arabian breed is chiefly affected, monosomy has been seen in Belgian mares and several other equine breeds. Known as Turner's syndrome in humans, XO monosomy has been reported in pigs, cats, sheep, monkeys, wallabies, and rodents.

In **trisomy** there is an additional (third) chromosome of one type in an otherwise diploid cell (2*n*+1). **Trisomy 17** in cattle is associated with brachygnathia (short jaw) and is called the lethal brachygnathia trisomy syndrome. Other trisomies have been suggested as being related to individual cases of cardiac anomaly, intersex, and arthrogryposis. In many instances, 100% of the cells are not trisomic, and most reports are too incomplete to provide a clinical understanding of these diseases.

X-inactivation

In 1961, Mary Lyon proposed the hypothesis of X-inactivation: only one of the X chromosomes is genetically active; inactivation of either maternal or paternal X occurs early in the blastocyst; and inactivation of the same X chromosome occurs in all cells derived from each precursor cell. From this hypothesis, we know that females are mosaic—two populations, one with an inactivated maternal X, the other with an inactivated paternal X chromosome. The inactive X chromosome can be seen as a dense eccentric Barr body in interphase cells of the female.

The molecular basis of X-inactivation is unclear, but we know that some genes escape X-inactivation. The X-inactive-specific transcript gene, or XIST (which does not code for protein—its mRNA never leaves the nucleus), prevents transcription of some genes on the X chromosome. Abnormal XIST genes that prevent normal X-inactivation explain the very rare female-to-female transmission of some X-linked traits.

X-inactivation and tortoiseshell and calico cats

In cats, the X-linked gene confers orange, brown, and black hair coats (white is an autosomal gene). The male cat with the recessive orange allele has orange fur. The female cat heterozygous for orange will be patched with orange and brown or black and is called tortoiseshell. The **calico cat** is white with patched orange and brown or black. The earlier the X-inactivation, the larger the color patches. The only way for a male to be calico is to inherit an extra X chromosome.

Male tortoiseshell cats are infertile because of hypoplastic testicular tubules and aspermatogenesis. Their chromosome anomaly is an additional X chromosome, 39,XXY. Karyotypes of these cats actually reveal several mosaic varieties, including 38,XX/38,XY and 38,XY/39,XXY. Male tortoiseshells may also be 38,XY/38,XY, presumed to be somatic chimerics, that is, to have arisen from early embryonic fusion of what should have been two separate individuals.

The term **tortoiseshell** signifies a mix of orange and black, usually blended together. Two sex-linked alleles determine color in the cat's hair coat, orange (O) and black (O+). These alleles are codominant, for each is expressed in the heterozygote, the tortoiseshell. The homozygous female may be black (O+O+) or orange (OO), but the hemizygous male must be orange (O) or black (O+). The normal heterozygous female (OO+) is tortoiseshell, but for the male to be tortoiseshell, there must be an additional sex chromosome and at least two sex chromosomes of differing color genes.

Modifying genes affect the pattern and intensity of black and orange, and the identification of the phenotypes must be done carefully. Calico (or tricolor, i.e., orange and black, plus white) cats are similar except for the white patches, which are inherited and do not influence orange-black color inheritance.

Male tortoiseshell cats are a model for Klinefelter's syndrome of human males, which includes testicular degeneration, infertility, enlarged breasts, and a karyotype of XXY. Similar syndromes of extra sex chromosomes and testicular abnormalities have been reported in mice, pigs, sheep, dogs, and cattle. The Y chromosome is male determining, promoting testicular development from the medullary part of the primitive gonad. With two X chromosomes, the cortex of the gonad develops into an ovary. The importance of the Y chromosome is seen in these XXY males, which are male despite the presence of two X chromosomes.

1/29 translocation of cattle

The 1/29 translocation of cattle was first found during studies of lymphocytes and bovine leukemia. This chromosomal abnormality has been reported in nearly 40 breeds. Its frequency is near 0 in major North American breeds but is 30% in some breeds and as high as 66% in some herds of British white cattle. The 1/29 translocation, which is transmitted for heterozygous parents in a standard mendelian pattern as a dominant, is associated with a subtle reduction of breeding ability. Affected females return to estrus early. The nondisjunction may occur during meiosis, and the resulting germ cells have a deficiency or duplication; zygotes resulting from such germ cells die early as embryos. No live monosomic or trisomic animals have been found in progeny of 1/29 parents.

In Sweden, screening all males to eliminate 1/29 heterozygotes and homozygotes from artificial insemination programs has reversed a trend to lowered fertility in Swedish red and white cattle. Approximately 25 other translocations in bovine chromosomes have been reported. None has been associated with defined clinical disease or altered reproductive function.

Chimerism and the bovine freemartin

Chimeras (or "allophanic animals") have cells of more than one genotype. The bovine freemartin is a genetic female with genital hypoplasia, born co-twin with a male. Anastomosing placental circulations allow exchange of blood-borne cells during fetal life. The newborn freemartin is normal except that chimerism results in an intersex phenotype. Tubular genitalia of the müllerian duct system fail to develop, because of the influence of androgens produced by the male twin, which arrived in the female as a result of fused placental circulation. The testicle develops earlier than the ovary, so that androgens of the male circulate to suppress development of female genitalia in the female twin. Ovaries are rudimentary and contain vestigial seminiferous tubules.

Evidence of mingling of blood supplies is found in circulating blood cells of freemartins. The hematopoietic chimerism can be shown by karyotyping bone marrow cells. If 100 cells are counted, more than half may contain XXY sex chromosomes, and the remainder will be normal female karyotypes with XX. The XX/XY karyotype is not found in solid tissues. The bull twin will also have XX leukocytes in its circulation; chimeric bulls are often sterile or produce only abnormal sperm. Freemartins also occur in swine, sheep, and goats.

Genetic testing

Heterozygote testing

Screening animal populations for heterozygosity is founded on the gene dosage phenomenon whereby the enzyme levels of heterozygous animals having one normal and one mutant gene are approximately midway between disease and normal levels. There is typically an overlap between heterozygous and normal values, so that equivocal diagnoses are expected. In most lysosomal hydrolase deficiencies, enzyme activity of these genotypes is also reflected in plasma levels. Testing is best done in age- and sex-matched peer groups from the same individual herds, flocks, or groups. Accuracy may be improved by using leukocytes rather than plasma.

Lysosomal disease control programs have been started using heterozygote detection for α-mannosidosis of Angus and Murray Grey cattle in New Zealand and Australia, for glycogen storage type II in shorthorn and Brahman cattle, and for β-mannosidosis in Salers cattle in many countries, and for fucosidosis in springer spaniel dogs in Australia and England.

DNA analysis and gene probes

DNA from semen, leukocytes, or hair roots can be used as samples for gene probes. The polymerase chain reaction, used in combination with methods for detection of genetic polymorphisms, provides definitive diagnoses of normal, heterozygote, or disease. Gene probes are especially important if there is a single mutation in the population being screened. It is currently used to control bovine α- and β-mannosidosis and bovine glycogen storage disease.

Genetic analyses require only a small amount of DNA because use of the polymerase chain reaction (PCR) allows for amplification of DNA up to a million times. In most genetic disease, all body cells contain the same DNA and every cell is affected. If the structures of the normal gene and its mutant counterpart are known, a **direct** method of DNA analysis can be used. However, in animal disease, one must resort to **indirect**, or "gene tracking," methods. Natural variations in DNA sequences are used to track individual chromosomes. DNA polymorphisms that are useful in these assays are **restriction fragment length polymorphism**, or RFLP (the variation in fragment length between individuals that results from DNA sequence polymorphisms), and **variable number of tandem repeats** (VNTRs). VNTRs are short sequences of DNA arranged in head-to-tail manner and repeated several times in tandem arrangements; the variation is so marked that individual animals can be identified.

In situ hybridization (ISH) involves binding (annealing) of complementary DNA and RNA sequences. ISH permits detection of specific nucleic acid sequences in morphologically preserved chromosomes, cells, and tissue sections. Gene activity at DNA, mRNA, or protein levels can be examined in combination with immunocytochemistry. Proteins labeled with biotin or digoxigenin are detected with fluorophores such as fluorescein or rhodamine. Uses of ISH include the following:

- Mapping of DNA sequences in specific chromosomes
- Detection of breakpoints (using probes for DNA sequences)
- Detection of numerical chromosome abnormalities in interphase/metaphase
- Direct detection of chromosomal rearrangements (repositioned sequences between chromosomes)

DEFINITIONS

Autosomal—transmitted with no relation to sex.

Diploid—having pairs of matching but not identical chromosomes. The cell's chromosome number is $2n$, the normal condition in somatic cells.

Dominant—expressed in both heterozygous and homozygous states.

Genotype—genetic makeup of an animal, consisting of a double set of information (except for that carried on the X chromosome in males).

Haploid—having a single set of unmatched chromosomes in a cell. The cell's chromosome number is $1n$, and each gene is unmatched, the normal condition in gametes.

Hemizygous—represented by only one gene (such as any X-linked trait in a genetic male with one chromosome).

Heterozygous—represented by a pair of different genes, one from each parent.

Homozygous—represented by a pair of the same genes, one from each parent.

Multifactorial inheritance—inheritance of a given characteristic determined by many genes.

Penetrance—the expression or nonexpression of a gene in the phenotype.

Phenotype—observable characters (i.e., expressed traits) of an animal. Recessive traits are not part of the phenotype unless they are homozygous and expressed.

Pleiotropy—the ability of one gene to have numerous effects on the organism.

Recessive—expressed only in a homozygous or hemizygous state.

Sex-linked—transmitted by a sex chromosome. All genes carried on the X chromosome are sex-linked.

Triploid—having three sets of chromosomes in a cell. The cell's chromosome number is 3n. The condition stems from an error in meiosis that results in a 2n gamete.

ADDITIONAL READING

Mutant genes of large effect

Benirschke K. 1970. Spontaneous chimerism in mammals. *Curr Top Pathol* 51:1.

Bergsjo T, et al. 1984. Congenital blindness with ocular developmental anomalies, including retinal dysplasia, in Doberman pinscher dogs. *J Am Vet Med Assoc* 184:1383.

Bilstrom JA, et al. 1998. Genetic test for myophosphorylase deficiency in Charolais cattle. *Am J Vet Res* 59:267.

Bingel SA, et al. 1985. Chondrodysplasia in the Alaskan malamute. *Lab Invest* 53:479.

Eaton KA, et al. 1997. Autosomal dominant polycystic kidney disease in Persian and Persian-cross cats. *Vet Pathol* 34:117.

Edwards JF, et al. 1994. Urethral atresia with uroperitoneum in a newborn bovine freemartin. *Vet Pathol* 31:117.

Elledge SJ. 1996. Cell cycle checkpoint: preventing an identity crisis. *Science* 274:1664.

Gitzelmann R, et al. 1994. Feline mucopolysaccharidosis VII due to β-glucuronidase deficiency. *Vet Pathol* 31:435.

Gopal T, et al. 1996. Congenital cardiac defects in calves. *Am J Vet Res* 47:1120.

Gundlach AL, et al. 1988. Deficit of spinal cord glycine/strychnine receptors in inherited myoclonus of polled Hereford calves. *Science* 241:1807.

Holmes NG, et al. 1998. DNA marker C04107 for copper toxicosis in a population of Bedlington terriers in the United Kingdom. *Vet Rec* 142:351.

Jolly RD, Walkley S. 1997. Lysosomal diseases of animals. *Vet Pathol* 34:527.

Kerlin RL, Van Winkle TJ. 1995. Renal dysplasia in golden retrievers. *Vet Pathol* 32:327.

Meyers-Wallen VN, et al. 1989. Testicular feminization in a cat. *J Am Vet Med Assoc* 195:631.

Minkus G, et al. 1994. Familial nephropathy in Bernese Mountain dogs. *Vet Pathol* 31:421.

Singer RH. 1998. Triplet-repeat transcripts: a role for RNA in disease. *Science* 280:696.

Vonderfecht SL, et al. 1983. Congenital intestinal aganglionosis and white foals. *Vet Pathol* 20:65.

Weber AF, et al. 1989. Low fertility related to 1/29 centric fusion anomaly in cattle. *J Am Vet Med Assoc* 195:643.

Yuzbasiyan-Gurkan V, et al. 1997. Linkage of a microsatellite marker to the canine copper toxicosis locus in Bedlington terriers. *Am J Vet Res* 58:23.

Multifactor inheritance disorders

Barkyoumb SD, Leipold HW. 1984. Nature and cause of bilateral ocular dermoids in Hereford cattle. *Vet Pathol* 21:316.

Gardner EJ, et al. 1975. Hereditary multiple exostosis. *J Heredity* 66:318.

Nicholas FW. 1987. *Veterinary genetics.* Clarendon Press, Oxford.

Chromosomal disorders

Buoen LC, et al. 1997. Arthrogryposis in the foal and its possible relation to autosomal trisomy. *Equine Vet J* 29:60–62.

Gelehrter TD, Collins FS, Ginsburg D. 1998. *Principles of medical genetics.* 2d ed., Williams and Wilkins, Baltimore.

Gustavsson I. 1980. Banding techniques in chromosome analysis of domestic animals. *Adv Vet Sci* 24:245.

Johnston SD, et al. 1983. X-chromosome monosomy (37,XO) in a Burmese cat with gonadal dysgenesis. *J Am Vet Med Assoc* 182:986.

Leipold HW, et al. 1983. Bovine congenital defects. *Adv Vet Sci Comp Med* 27:197.

McFeely RA. 1990. Domestic animal cytogenetics. *Adv Vet Sci* 34:1.

Pailhoux E, et al. 1994. Molecular analysis of 60,XX pseudohermaphrodite polled goats for the presence of SRY and ZFY genes. *J Reprod Fertil* 100:491.

Rousseaux CG. 1988. Developmental anomalies in farm animals. *Can Vet J* 29:23.

Smith FWK Jr, et al. 1989. X-chromosomal monosomy (77,XO) in a Doberman pinscher with gonadal dysgenesis. *J Vet Intern Med* 3:90.

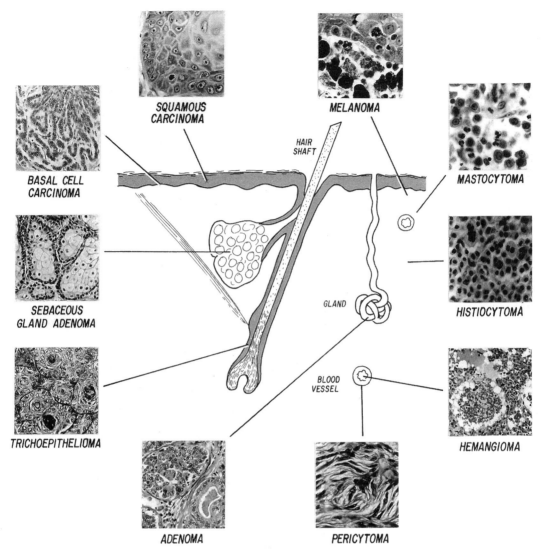

SQUAMOUS
CARCINOMA

MELANOMA

MASTOCYTOMA

BASAL CELL
CARCINOMA

HAIR
SHAFT

HISTIOCYTOMA

SEBACEOUS
GLAND ADENOMA

GLAND

TRICHOEPITHELIOMA

BLOOD
VESSEL

HEMANGIOMA

ADENOMA

PERICYTOMA

Histogenetic origin of different types of skin neoplasms.

PART 5

Neoplasia

A tumor is an abnormal mass of tissue, the growth of which exceeds and is uncoordinated with that of normal tissue and persists in the same excessive manner after cessation of the stimuli which evoked the change.
—Willis, 1942

A NEOPLASM, OR TUMOR, typically first appears as an unexplained, clinically silent mass in tissue. When the patient enters the clinic, there is an expectation that the veterinarian will make a thorough clinical examination and work through a logical progression of appropriate tests that will end in the correct diagnosis and an accurate prognosis. The first question you must answer is, Is the mass a neoplasm?

A tissue biopsy (or in some cases a cytologic aspirate) is required to determine if the mass is a neoplasm. If tissue is neoplastic, the client wishes to know if it is benign or malignant and, if malignant, the degree of malignancy. Each organ and tissue has its own spectrum of neoplasms. For example, skin tumors can arise from basal or squamous epithelial cells or any component of dermal connective tissue. Tumors arising from different cell types will behave differently as they grow in the animal.

Combining the clinical data with the pathologic diagnosis made from the tissue biopsy leads to an estimate on the likelihood of recurrence at the surgical sites and of metastasis to the regional lymph node or other organs. The client will probably ask what cancer is, what causes cancer, and how it develops. Where did the tumor come from? Is the mass a primary tumor formed from tissues at the site, or is it a secondary, metastatic tumor that migrated from a primary tumor elsewhere in the body?

Neoplasia involves an intrinsic genetic abnormality in somatic cells that gives rise to autonomous growth. Neoplastic cells do not behave as integrated, interdependent populations. The regulatory mechanisms that control mitosis, differentiation, and cell-to-cell interactions are defective. Cells grow in rapidly expanding masses that impinge upon adjacent tissues, and that may ultimately compromise host survival.

What is it that endows these cells with such aberrant behavior? First, and most important, is the capacity for uncontrolled mitosis. The expansive growth of a neoplasm is due directly to an increase in the rate of cellular replication. Other attributes that contribute to neoplastic growth are changes that give the cell an ability to dissociate from its neighbors and to grow and move in its new environment. As the neoplastic cell moves away from the expanding tumor mass, it must alter connective tissue ground substance and stimulate angiogenesis, the growth of new vascular tissue. If new capillaries do not develop for nourishment, the developing tumor will not thrive.

Neoplasms occur as a spectrum of entities that vary from dense solid masses to the diffusely mobile cells of the leukemias. Solid neoplasms may be small, well-demarcated discrete nodules or diffuse infiltrating lesions with ill-defined borders. In characterizing tumors, the term **benign** is applied to a neoplasm that remains localized, does not invade surrounding tissues, and does not spread to new sites. In contrast, **malignant** neoplasms disseminate, invade, and metastasize to new sites in the body. The word **tumor**, used classically to describe any mass or swelling, is now used synonymously with neoplasm.

Cancer (a term used for any malignant tumor) is a chronic disease and begins many months before clinical signs first appear. The clinical phases of the disease represent only a fraction of the pathogenic process. Some epithelial lesions, termed precancerous, smolder silently for months or even years before malignant foci of cells can be demonstrated. We now know that neoplastic cells arise from normal cells through a series of discrete mutations. That is, the progressive development of a tumor is characterized by the evolution of successive clones of cells, each coming one step closer to the overt cancer cell type that proliferates, stopping only with the death of the host.

What causes cancer? We know that biological, chemical, and physical agents can promote and even initiate tumor development. We are now learning that all of these causes have a common cellular basis. They induce genetic instability that leads to somatic mutation, and the disrupted gene product in turn influences organelles that function in growth, movement, and death of cells. The clinical behavior of naturally occurring neoplasms is now being explained by experimental neoplasms in animal models. The mutation of specific genes in rodents has led to tumors that parallel those found in a clinical setting.

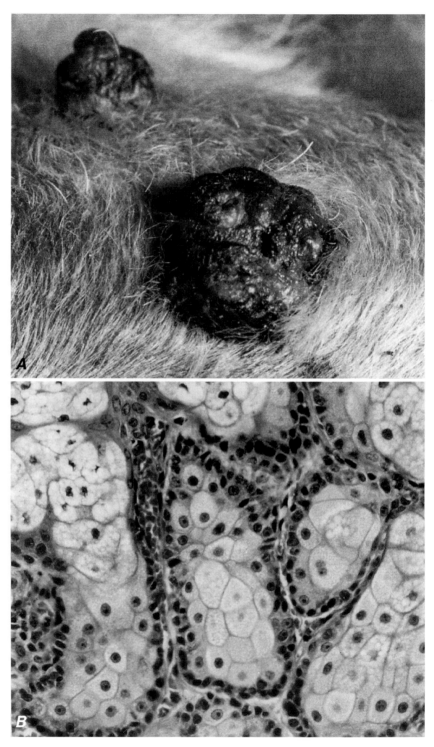

FIGURE 11.1. Sebaceous gland adenoma, dog. A. Nodular growths project above skin surface. B. Large, lipid-filled sebaceous cells surrounded by small, dark germinal cells, closely resembling tissue architecture of normal sebaceous glands.

▦ CHAPTER 11

Characterizing the Neoplasm

CLASSIFICATION OF NEOPLASMS

Neoplasms are classified so that the pathologist can communicate precisely with the clinician who must provide a prognosis for the patient. Histologic analysis is used to examine cellular structure and tissue architecture of tumors to answer two important questions: what is the cell of origin, and how will the neoplasm behave clinically in the patient? Studies are thus directed to **histogenesis** to determine the tissue of origin of the neoplasm and to **cellular characteristics** to determine if the tumor is benign or malignant. The tumor arises from a single tissue cell and will usually have enough characteristics of that cell type to be recognized morphologically. In skin, for example, tumors can arise either from cells that originate in epithelium or in connective tissue. The squamous cell carcinoma originating from epidermal cells will differ in growth from the fibrosarcoma, a stromal tumor. The cumulative knowledge from more than a century of study allows us to make reasonable predictions of tumor behavior on the basis of histologic appearance.

Benign neoplasms

Neoplasms that are well differentiated, grow slowly by expansion, and do not invade below basement membranes are called **benign** (L. *benignus,* kind or friendly). A neoplasm is benign when its cellular characteristics are considered innocent and closely resemble those of the parent tissue. The designation *benign* implies that the tumor will remain localized and will not recur after simple excision. Benign tumors typically develop a rim of compressed fibrous tissue that is derived from normal connective tissue stroma. Tumors surrounded by such a fibrous capsule are said to be **encapsulated**. However, the lack of capsule does not imply malignancy. Cutaneous histiocytomas and hemangiomas, both benign tumors, are not encapsulated, and neoplastic cells may appear to infiltrate along the edges of the tumor.

Benign tumors are classified according to their histologic appearance. They are designated by adding the suffix **-oma** to the cell type of origin. A benign tumor of epithelium is an **epithelioma**; of fibrocytes, a **fibroma**; and of chondrocytes in cartilage, a **chondroma**. In all of these, tumor cells closely resemble their normal counterparts.

Benign epithelial tumors that produce glandular patterns are called **adenomas**. For example, sebaceous gland adenomas are common tumors in dogs. They grow in polypoid or lobular forms that extend through the skin surface. Typically, these adenomas will continue to grow slowly by expansion but will not invade into the dermis or metastasize (Fig. 11.1).

Benign tumors can cause serious disease by exerting pressure on ducts, arteries, or the nervous system. Parathyroid adenomas are benign and may be tiny, yet they can cause lethal disease in the animal through secretion of hormones by the neoplastic cell.

Location is an important factor in the effect of a benign tumor. A tumor may have little clinical effect at one site, yet be life-threatening in another. Lipomas (benign tumors of adipose cells) are common tumors on the skin of a dog, where they can produce unsightly lumps but are of no consequence to the general health of the animal. In contrast, lipomas in the mesentery of the horse, equally benign in growth, can cause strangulation of the intestine.

Tumor classification is based on the clear separation of benign versus malignant, and epithelial ver-

TABLE 11.1. Classification of neoplasms

Organ of origin	Cell of origin	Benign tumor	Malignant tumor
Epidermis	Squamous cell	Epithelioma	Squamous cell carcinoma
	Basal cell		Basal cell carcinoma
Adnexa	Hair follicle	Trichoepithelioma	Adenocarcinoma
	Sweat gland	Adenoma	Adenocarcinoma
	Sebaceous gland	Adenoma	Adenocarcinoma
	Perianal gland	Adenoma	Adenocarcinoma
Other glands	Salivary gland	Adenoma	Adenocarcinoma
			Mixed tumor, malignant
	Mammary gland	Adenoma	Adenocarcinoma
		Mixed tumor	Mixed tumor, malignant
			Duct tumor
Neuroectoderm	Melanoblast	Melanoma	Malignant melanoma
Connective tissue	Fibrocyte	Fibroma	Fibrosarcoma
	Adipose cell	Lipoma	Liposarcoma
	Undifferentiated cell	Histiocytoma	Reticulum cell sarcoma
		Myxoma	Myxosarcoma
	Mast cell	Mastocytoma	Mast cell sarcoma
	Schwann cells	Neurilemmoma	Malignant neurilemmoma
	Nerve sheath cell	Neurofibroma	Neurofibrosarcoma
Vascular tissue	Endothelium	Hemangioma	Hemangiosarcoma
	Pericyte	Hemangiopericytoma	Malignant hemangiopericytoma
Muscle tissue	Skeletal muscle	Rhabdomyoma	Rhabdomyosarcoma
	Smooth muscle	Leiomyoma	Leiomyosarcoma
Skeletal tissue	Cartilage	Chondroma	Chondrosarcoma
	Bone	Osteoma	Osteosarcoma
Other	Synovium	Synovioma	Synovial sarcoma
	Mesothelium	Mesothelioma	Mesothelial sarcoma
	Meninges	Meningioma	Malignant meningioma

sus connective tissue origin (Table 11.1). To the beginning student of pathology, enormous lists of neoplasms can be overwhelming. Understanding the difference between benign and malignant seems simple enough, but this is complicated by the use of special terms for unique neoplasms. For example, the terms **mixed mammary gland tumor** and **transmissible venereal tumor** have been established by precedent for neoplasms that do not fit comfortably within a rigid classification scheme based on histologic appearance.

Certain clinical and histological characteristics separate malignant neoplasms from their benign counterparts (Table 11.2). These are not requisites of malignancy but are general characteristics of malignant neoplasms. Although most neoplasms can be definitively classified as benign or malignant, it is important to recognize that the borderland between the two is blurred in some cases. The common mammary tumors of dogs may appear generally benign yet contain small foci of atypical cells that make the pathologic interpretation difficult.

As a clinician, you must understand these danger zones and make clear to the owner of a tumor-bearing animal that the surgical site of removal and the regional lymph node must be closely monitored for a year or longer.

Malignant neoplasms

At the other extreme of tumor behavior are the **malignant** neoplasms, whose cells are anaplastic and which metastasize and invade. **Anaplasia** is defined as the loss of differentiation of cells and of their orientation to one another (syn: dedifferentiation). Anaplastic cells typically are **pleomorphic**—they vary in size and shape; in highly anaplastic tumors, some cells are very large and others very small. The aggressive neoplastic cells of malignant tumors reproduce rapidly, resulting in highly cellular masses that infiltrate (and in some cases destroy) normal tissues.

Malignancy is a clinical concept (cells in culture cannot be considered malignant), and its characteristics and behavior must relate to the growth

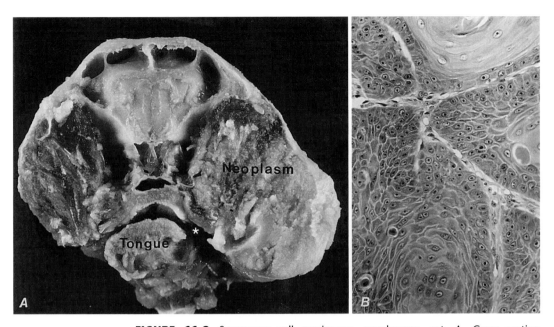

FIGURE 11.2. Squamous cell carcinoma, oropharynx, cat. A. Cross section through posterior sinuses and frontal brain. The primary tumor originated in the right dorsolateral surface of the palate *(white asterisk)* and spread through masseter muscles and salivary glands. B. Moderate differentiation of neoplastic keratinocytes with keratin whorls.

of the neoplasm within the animal.

A "cancer" is a malignant neoplasm. Those of epithelial derivation are called **carcinomas,** and those of mesodermal origin, **sarcomas.** In most malignant neoplasms, cells have some resemblance or similarity to the cell of origin. For example, the squamous cell carcinoma of the skin will have many structural characteristics of squamous epithelium, even when it invades deeply into other tissues (Fig. 11.2).

Adenocarcinoma is a term applied to carcinomas that derive from glandular epithelium and that typically form glandular patterns during growth. In some tumors, early divergence of the developing neoplastic cell gives rise to **mixed tumors.** A common example is the malignant mixed mammary

gland tumor of dogs, in which islands of epithelial cells that behave as a carcinoma are mixed with areas of myxomatous stroma, cartilage, and bone typical of a sarcoma.

Sarcomas resemble components of mesenchymal tissue from which they arise. The fibrosarcoma is composed of undifferentiated fibroblast-like cells that are spaced too closely together, are haphazard in arrangement, and lack orderly associations with other tissue structures. Malignant neoplasms of vascular tissue (hemangiosarcomas) originate from endothelial cells of small blood vessels and typically form distorted vascular channels. Hemangiosarcomas are common in dogs (Fig. 11.3) and may have spread to other tissues by the time they are noticed by the owner. Sarcomas are often highly malignant and can be difficult to classify.

Malignant neoplasms range from well differentiated to undifferentiated. The well-differentiated mammary gland adenocarcinoma forms acini in which cells are tightly connected by relatively normal intercellular junctions and have secretory granules that contain proteins similar to normal mammary secretions. In contrast, cells of the anaplastic mammary adenocarcinoma show great variation in size and shape, have pleomorphic nuclei and cytoplasmic organelles, and have much less tendency to form structures that resemble normal mammary

TABLE 11.2. Differences in benign and malignant tumors

Benign	Malignant
Slow growth	Rapid growth
Expansive but circumscribed	Invasive and infiltrative
Encapsulated	Nonencapsulated
No metastases	Metastasis
Well differentiated	Anaplastic
Few mitotic figures	Many mitotic figures

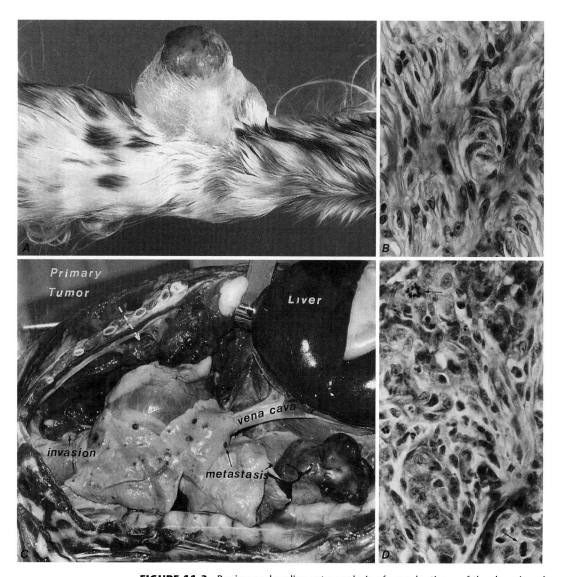

FIGURE 11.3. Benign and malignant neoplasia of vascular tissue of the dog. A and B. Hemangiopericytoma: benign vascular tumor originating from pericytes that surround capillaries, forelimb. Neoplastic cells resemble and produce collagen, as do normal pericytes. C and D. Hemangiosarcoma: malignant vascular tumor of endothelial cells. Primary tumor on the skin has invaded the chest wall, producing intrathoracic secondary tumors. Metastatic tumors from hematogenous dissemination occur as dark spots on the lungs. Malignant cells are highly pleomorphic, contain mitotic figures *(arrows)*, and lack any resemblance to normal cell types.

gland acini. Frequently, a cancer is composed of such primitive anaplastic cells that it must be designated **undifferentiated carcinoma, undifferentiated sarcoma**, or even **highly undifferentiated neoplasm**.

In their biological behavior, malignant cells have certain features in common that make them different from mature or differentiated normal cells.

These include (1) mitotic structures that are readily activated, (2) cell surfaces that are designed for movement and migration (at the expense of intercellular communication), (3) production of abnormal secretory granules and proteins that resemble embryonic products, and (4) simplified energy production via fermentation of glucose, with oxygen and the mitochondrial respiratory chain less effective. These are also characteristics of undifferentiated embryonic cells. Indeed, the common thread among cells of various malignant neoplasms is a failure of differentiation.

Differentiation refers to the extent to which cells resemble the cells of their tissue of origin (in embryology, *differentiation* is used to indicate a change from a lower to a higher state of specialization). **Anaplasia**, synonymous with **undifferentiation**, refers to the loss of specialization and organization, with anarchic changes in cellular organelles. Cell differentiation, the derivation of specialized cells from less specialized ones, is an expression of specific gene activity. As cells switch to differentiated forms, genes that control embryonic characters are switched off, and genes for the most differentiated characters are activated.

Mitosis is uncontrolled

The growth rate of a tumor depends on two major inherent determinants of growth: mitosis and cell death. Mitotic rates are associated with both the fraction of cells in a tumor undergoing mitosis and the length of the cell cycle (i.e., the interval between mitosis and completion of subsequent mitosis in daughter cells). The length of the tumor cell cycle is usually (but not always) shorter than that of its normal cellular counterpart.

The capacity to undergo mitosis is inherent in all cells. Throughout life, mitotic activity is repressed or controlled in some way. Neoplastic cells lack this repression and must be considered cells unresponsive to the controlling mechanism or in which the mechanism itself is imperfect. For neoplastic cells to gain immortality, they must grow unrestrained and uncontrolled by the host.

The developing neoplastic cell gains the attributes of malignancy by the progressive misprogramming of gene function at any step of differentiation or the selective reactivation of genes involved in early development. These genes need not be abnormal (in the sense of directing faulty protein synthesis). Instead, control of gene expression may be defective, leading to synthesis of gene products in excess or at the wrong time.

Cell surfaces are abnormal

One important distinguishing feature of malignant cells is the loss of cohesiveness with neighboring cells. Decreased adhesiveness, which results from a major defect of cell surface adhesion molecules, is manifested as the capacity of malignant cells to spread by invasion of tissue, by implantation on new surfaces, and by metastasis to new sites through lymphatic or blood vessels.

One of the major changes in tumor cell surfaces is the presence of abnormal glycoproteins that are embedded in the plasma membrane of the cell. These are abnormal receptors and other integral membrane proteins whose dysfunction leads to defects in intracellular signal pathways. A second major change at cell surfaces is the release of collagenase, elastase, and other enzymes that degrade structures that normally promote cell-to-cell adhesion. A third defect in tumor cell surfaces is a more negative surface charge associated with abnormal amounts of sialomucopeptides, which tend to repel cells from one another.

Because of these surface changes, cellular contact inhibition is abnormal in neoplasms. In normal tissues, there are control mechanisms that inhibit cell movement and growth when cells are in contact with one another. Contact in some way allows the exchange of signals and the establishment of gap junctions and desmosomes for maintaining contact. Even when normal cells grow in culture, there is inhibition of movement and mitosis when they contact each other. When tumor pieces are placed in culture, cells migrate away from the explant more quickly than do cells from normal tissue. They grow outward, not in organized radial strands but in random, haphazard patterns.

Cytoskeleton is dysfunctional

The cytoskeleton is abnormal in most neoplastic cells. Abnormal **microfilament** and **microtubule** functions are reflected in aberrant cell shape, movement, and chromosomal instability. The abnormal contours of malignant cells have been found to correlate with an abnormal polymerization of tubulin, the protein that makes up microtubules. Perhaps the most important result of a dysfunctional cytoskeleton is a failure of cell-to-cell adhesion, a function that the cytoskeleton plays in its connections to intercellular junctions.

Intercellular junctions are abnormal in most neoplasms. Alterations in **tight junctions** correspond with tumor differentiation but are not implicated in tumor growth promotion. They are a result, not a cause, of malignant changes. In epithelial tumors that produce basement membranes, hemidesmosomes may develop in an attempt to anchor the tumor cell temporarily.

Gap junctions are often broken in neoplastic cells; the absence of this direct communication between cells alters the behavior of the tissue as a homogeneous unit and removes the mechanism whereby cells can share metabolites and control molecules. When cancer cells have fewer gap junctions, they are unable to send and receive signal molecules from neighboring cells. This may promote uncontrolled growth. Even though cancer cells may have normal gap junctions, they may possess some internal defect in their ability to respond normally to transferred signal molecules. It has been hypothesized that vitamin A impedes the development of epithelial neoplasms because of its ability to maintain epithelial differentiation and to block preneoplastic dedifferentiation by causing a significant proliferation of gap junctions.

Metabolism is shifted

Regulation and flexibility of protein synthesis are lost in neoplastic cells. Reprogramming of gene expression and mRNA translation in the cytoplasm is directed to purine synthesis and utilization to supply the requirement for mitosis. Altered plasma membrane components are skewed to excessive or abnormal receptor molecules and abnormal surface glycoproteins. Altered mechanisms of energy production develop, and there is dominance of glycolysis in the cytoplasmic matrix over mitochondrial oxidative phosphorylation (Table 11.3).

Borderland between benign and malignant

Preneoplastic lesions

Preneoplastic, dysplastic lesions precede several types of epithelial neoplasms—for example, squamous cell carcinomas, transitional tumors of the bladder, and malignant melanomas of the skin. Preneoplastic lesions may appear at first to be hyperplastic cells but on close microscopic examination they are seen to contain dedifferentiated and anaplastic changes typical of malignancy. In cases where it is known that these changes will progress

to true carcinoma, they are referred to as **carcinoma in situ**.

The livers of aged dogs often contain multiple, discrete, well-differentiated hyperplastic nodules (the lesion is called nodular regeneration). These nodules are formed of hyperplastic hepatocytes that closely resemble normal hepatocytes. They are not neoplastic, and most nodules will not develop neoplastic change. However, these nodules are considered **preneoplastic**; in some nodules, hepatocytes will undergo mutations that lead to neoplasia. We do know that dogs with nodular livers have a much higher incidence of hepatocellular carcinoma than do dogs with normal livers.

Benign tumors with atypia

Pathologists are frequently faced with large neoplasms that appear benign in almost all aspects yet have one or two small foci of atypical cells. These tumors are probably benign but do have some subtle evidence of malignancy, placing the clinician and the pathologist in the dilemma of choosing excessive or inadequate treatment. A few nests of anaplastic cells in an otherwise benign neoplasm may drive the diagnosis to malignancy. As a clinician, you must understand this dilemma and caution the patient's owner accordingly—that is, surgery to remove a neoplasm with a low risk of recurrence may be declined, yet failure to remove the tumor leaves the animal susceptible to recurrence.

Neoplasia-like malformations

Special terms (which are rarely used but are entrenched in the literature) are sometimes applied to malformations and tumors derived from them. A

TABLE 11.3. Characteristics of anaplasia

Defect and manifestations	Detected by
Pleomorphism	
Loss of cell contact, cohesiveness	Histology
Adhesion molecule defects	Histochemistry
Cytoskeletal defects	Electron microscopy, histochemistry
Mitotic index increase	
Mitotic figures present	Histology
Abnormal amounts of DNA	DNA ploidy analysis, image analysis
Excess of proliferation markers	Immunostaining (Ki67, PCNA)
Presence of oncogenes	In situ hybridization
Gross chromosome defects	Karyotype analysis
Metabolic shifts	
Estrogen, androgen receptors	Hormone receptor analysis
Use of glucose for energy	Staining for glycogen
Secretion of abnormal proteins	
α-Fetoproteins	Biochemical analysis
Prostate-specific antigen (PSA)	Radioimmunoassay
IL-6 (renal cell carcinoma)	Radioimmunoassay
Collagenase, elastase	Histochemistry

hamartoma is an excessive, focal overgrowth of mature cells in an organ of identical cells. The distinction between hamartoma and benign neoplasm is often vague; small, blood-filled, cystic foci of the skin are hamartomas (although classed as hemangiomas by some pathologists), because they may regress and disappear. Hamartomas in the lung may contain cartilage, blood vessels, and bronchiolar epithelial structures.

A **choristoma** is a focus of normal cells in an abnormal location. Choristomas are viewed as ectopic "rests" of normal tissue—for example, a nodular rest of pancreatic acinar cells in the mucosa of the intestine, or a rest of adrenal cortical cells in the kidney. Very rarely, cells of the choristoma give rise to true neoplasms, as, for example, adrenal carcinoma in the kidney.

Cancer incidence and distribution

Age is a dominant factor in cancer. The incidence of neoplasms increases with age in all species. Data on the age-specific and cumulative incidence of neoplasms are important both for clinical evaluation and cancer research. Studies on the incidence of primary lung tumors in beagles revealed an incidence of lung carcinomas of 8.8%. There was a high incidence of tumors in aged dogs, those dying after the median life span of 13.6 years. Of the 40 tumors in 398 dogs, there were 35 carcinomas: papillary adenocarcinoma, $n=20$; bronchoalveolar carcinoma, $n=9$; adenosquamous carcinoma, $n=5$; and bronchial gland carcinoma, $n=1$. The other 5 neoplasms were a malignant fibrous histiocytoma, 3 adenomas, and a fibroma.

The incidence of neoplasms may be skewed by the particular animal population in your practice. In the clinic, more tumors may be seen in middle-aged animals, because the decreasing survival of animals will cause fewer tumors to be found in aged animals even though the real incidence is increasing in the animals that survive to old age. Young animals have a particular spectrum of neoplasms that includes leukemia, embryonal nephromas, and

---

FOCUS

Enhanced Glycolysis in Tumor Cells

OTTO WARBURG ESTABLISHED in the 1920s that malignant cells have a high degree of glycolytic activity, both anaerobic and aerobic. Neoplastic cells produce large amounts of lactic acid from glucose, and this pathway is not markedly reduced in the presence of oxygen, as it is in normal tissue. Although this metabolic defect is characteristic of tumor cells, it is not present in all natural tumors.

In experimental rodent hepatomas, there is increased glucose consumption and diversion of precursors into synthesis of purines, pyrimidines, RNA, and DNA. Gluconeogenesis and the urea cycle are diminished. The enzymatic imbalance responsible for this shift involves increases in key glycolytic enzymes and decreased enzymes of gluconeogenesis. This decreased dependence of the neoplastic cell on mitochondrial respiration confers a selective advantage to begin growth in the tumor mass, a poorly vascularized, oxygen-deficient environment.

Enhanced glycolysis in tumor cells is related to overproduction of inorganic phosphorus due to a high rate of ATP hydrolysis. Another reason for excessive glycolysis may be that factors that damage genomic DNA also damage the self-replicating DNA of mitochondria. In fact, carcinogenic metabolites of benzopyrene that damage nuclear DNA have a much greater affinity for mitochondrial DNA. The ATPase that operates as a sodium pump is inefficient in some tumor cells. The excessive amount of ATP required to pump out sodium produces a large amount of ADP and inorganic phosphorus, which may then stimulate glycolysis.

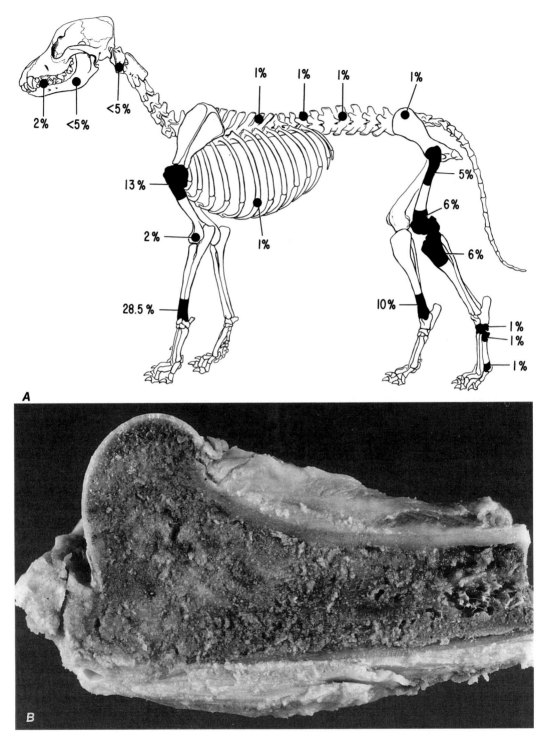

FIGURE 11.4. Osteosarcoma, dog. A. Sites of origin (data from Brodey et al., *J Am Vet Med Assoc* 143:471, 1963). B. Femur, Great Dane. This osteosarcoma has destroyed the growth plate, but there is no invasion of cartilage of the joint.

vaccination site sarcomas (in cats).

There is a strong **geographic difference** in tumor rates and types of tumors, and these differences commonly result from environmental differences—for example, the squamous cell carcinoma of the eye that develops from effects of ultraviolet radiation in white-faced cattle in subtropical zones. Neoplasms due to chemical carcinogens appear to be more common in animals exposed to industrial areas and areas with heavy chemical contamination in the environment.

Although the occurrence of tumor types is similar among species, each species has its own characteristic spectrum of tumors. The most common skin neoplasms of dogs are the mast cell tumor and cutaneous histiocytoma; in cats, mast cell tumors are common, but the cutaneous histiocytoma is never seen. The dog has a high incidence of mammary gland tumors, whereas this neoplasm is rare in the cow.

Some tumors have a characteristic distribution in the body. In dogs, the plasmacytoma has a predilection for the digits, face, mouth, pinna, and ear canal. Studies on squamous cell carcinomas in horses show that 43% occur on the head, eyes, and ocular glands; 45% on male genitalia; and 12% on female genitalia. Osteosarcomas in giant-breed dogs tend to occur on the long bones of the limbs (Fig. 11.4).

TUMOR STROMA: ANGIOGENESIS AND FIBROPLASIA

Angiogenesis

Neoplastic cells and blood vessels are interdependent. The growth of a neoplasm is dependent on concomitant growth of a supporting vascular system. Histologic analysis of blood vessels of malignant neoplasms reveals haphazard arrangements, a lack of pericyte support (present in normal blood vessels), and endothelial cells that have irregular, highly reactive surfaces. The capacity of these endothelial cells to supply oxygen, glucose, and other nutrients to the tumor is less efficient than for blood vessels in normal tissue.

Angiogenesis is activated during the early stages of development of a neoplasm, and new blood vessels grow along with the tumor. In fact, increased blood vessel density in a tumor has been shown to be a significant prognostic indicator for malignancy of human prostate and mammary tumors. The von Willebrand factor and CD31, which are pro-

teins expressed in normal endothelial cells, are used as markers of vascular density in tumors.

For the tumors to grow, populations of neoplastic cells and endothelial cells must be integrated. The mitotic index of one population depends on the other. Tumor cells stimulate endothelial cell proliferation, and vascularization has an indirect effect on neoplasm growth. The probability that a neoplastic cell will enter mitosis decreases with increasing distance from its nearest capillary. The capacity of a new neoplasm to induce angiogenesis in the normal surrounding tissue determines the growth and appearance of the neoplasm; that is, enhancement of angiogenesis is an integral component of the neoplastic cell.

Recent evidence suggests that endothelial cells of tumor capillaries are not passive bystanders in cancer—not limited to supplying nutrients and oxygen to cancer cells—but play a significant role in promoting neoplastic growth. In tumors that are known to progress through stages of increasing malignancy, an increase in neovascularization has been found in stages of hyperplasia and dysplasia, before carcinoma has developed.

Angiogenesis factors are secreted by neoplasms

New capillary growth in developing neoplasms is often vigorous, even more so than capillary bud formation in inflammation. The blood vessels in a growing tumor are a response induced in some way by the tumor itself. **Angiogenesis factor**, a humoral factor that stimulates mitotic activity in endothelial cells, has been extracted from animal neoplasms. Released from tumor cells, angiogenesis factor seeps into surrounding tissue to stimulate capillary endothelium to proliferate. Production of angiogenesis factor by the tumor cell is increased by several potent cytokines, including **vascular endothelial growth factor** (VEGF) and **fibroblast growth factor** (FGF). VEGF, a specific endothelial cell mitogen, is overexpressed in most tumors. Current research is directed to the use of anti-VEGF antiserum to treat neoplasms.

Experimentally, new capillary buds are induced in normal tissue even when tumor implants are enclosed in filter chambers. Induction of DNA synthesis in resting endothelial cells of capillaries and venules can be demonstrated within a few millimeters of an implanted tumor. Mast cells accumulate at sites of tumor formation. They release the anticoagulant heparin, which increases the migration of endothelial cells toward tumors.

Growth of a solid tumor might be deliberately arrested by the pharmacologic blockade of tumor

FOCUS

Blocking Angiogenesis

THE CONCEPT THAT cancer growth and metastasis can be prevented by blocking angiogenesis has gained popularity in the last decade. In theory, if vascularization of developing neoplastic cells can be prevented, tumors will fail to expand and invade. In 1994 it was reported that the primary tumor of a lung carcinoma model suppressed growth of metastatic lesions by releasing some unidentified angiogenesis blocking factor. In the rodent carcinoma model used for study, the primary tumor inhibited its remote metastases, and after removal of the primary tumor, metastases vascularized and grew at a greater rate. Biochemical analyses of these tumors revealed two potent angiogenesis inhibitors, angiostatin and endostatin.

Angiostatin is a fragment of plasminogen. It is cleaved from the plasminogen molecule when an enzyme present in vascular cells is activated. **Endostatin** is a small C-terminal fragment of collagen XVIII, a member of a family of perivascular collagen-like proteins that control vascular function.

Plasminogen → angiostatin

Collagen XVIII → endostatin

Angiostatin and endostatin are potent inhibitors of endothelial cells and block angiogenesis. In a seeming paradox, they are produced in large amounts by highly angiogenic tumors such as hemangiosarcomas, suggesting that their production is an exaggerated response to ineffective action in the tumor.

Angiostatin and endostatin, when given experimentally to rodents bearing small tumors, cause failure of both growth and metastasis. Analysis of tumors in treated animals shows high rates of both proliferation and programmed cell death, with no gain in tumor size. Histologically, tumor cells in the treated animal persist around remaining blood vessels.

References

Cao Y, et al. 1998. Expression of angiostatin cDNA in murine fibrosarcoma suppresses primary tumor growth and produces long dormancy of metastases. *J Clin Invest* 101:1055.

O'Reilly MS, et al. 1997. Endostatin: an endogenous inhibitor of angiogenesis and tumor growth. *Cell* 88:277.

O'Reilly MS, et al. 1994. Angiostatin: a novel angiogenesis inhibitor that mediates the suppression of metastases by a Lewis lung carcinoma. *Cell* 79:315.

angiogenesis factor production; if so, vascularization of the tumor (and its survival) might be prevented. Glucocorticoid hormones interfere with vascularization of tumors, and other hormones probably delay or facilitate tumor vascularity.

Some tumors release antiangiogenesis factors

Angiostatin, an endothelial cell inhibitor produced by some tumors, appears to restrict tumor growth by acting as an endothelial toxin. Research using experimental tumors has shown that, in the absence of angiostatin in a tumor, the programmed cell death index of the tumor is low and the mitotic index is high. The relative balance of inducers (angiogenesis factor) and inhibitors (angiostatin) of tumor angiogenesis can be regulated pharmacologically—for example, by activation of a genetic switch that turns off a tumor suppressor gene to reduce the inhibitor concentration (Table 11.4).

Endostatin, a proteolytic cleavage product of collagen XVIII (a normal component of basement membranes), has also been shown to inhibit neoplastic growth in rodents. Like angiostatin, it acts both as an angiogenesis inhibitor and as an endothelial cell toxin.

Necrosis occurs when tumors outgrow vascular supply

In highly malignant tumors, cell growth extends beyond that of the supporting vasculature, which causes **ischemic necrosis**. Hemorrhage into these foci of necrosis is common, and cross sections of these tumors may be spotted with areas of red and brown. After some time, necrotic areas will calcify, and hard, gritty granules are common in old necrotic foci in tumors. Necrosis may be accompanied by some decrease in tumor size, but the rapidly dividing malignant cells at the periphery of the necrotic area soon make up the loss.

Fibroplasia

Benign tumors often have a fibrous capsule at the periphery. Many benign tumors contain a capsule derived in part from the fibrous stroma of the surrounding normal connective tissue and in part from the tumor itself (malignant tumors are almost never encapsulated). Encapsulation tends to contain the neoplasm as a discrete, palpable mass that can easily be removed by surgery. Although a capsule is characteristic of a benign neoplasm, lack of a capsule does not make a neoplasm malignant.

Tumors can provoke fibroplasia

Fibroblast proliferation and deposition of collagen are the main components of fibromas and fibrosarcomas and in other neoplasms of connective tissue. Collagen fiber deposition also occurs in some epi-

TABLE 11.4. Balance hypothesis for angiogenesis switch

Activation (on)	Inhibition (off)
α-FGF	Thrombospondin-1 (TSP-1)
β-FGF	Interferon α and β
γ-FGF	Angiostatin; platelet factor 4 (PF4)

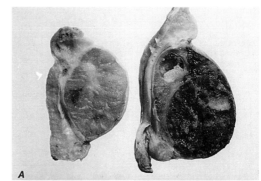

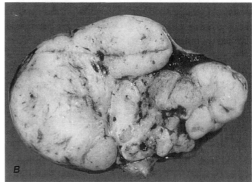

FIGURE 11.5. Testicular tumors in the dog. A. Interstitial cell tumor. The tumor is the large, dark, bean-shaped area *(right)*. Testis *(left)* is unaffected. Marked vascularity makes this tumor dark red instead of the tan/yellow usually seen in the interstitial cell tumors. B. Sertoli cell tumor with diffuse collagen formation; massive deposition of collagen makes this tumor very hard.

thelial tumors that secrete factors that stimulate fibroplasia. These fibrotic tumors are sometimes called **sclerosing** or **scirrhous** and are very firm and pale (Fig. 11.5).

Basement membranes

Neoplasms modify the interstitial ground substance in which they grow by synthesizing matrix components, stimulating adjacent normal tissue to synthesize matrix, and degrading matrix components during invasion. In any malignant tumor, all three may take place in different regions of the tumor.

Collagen and basement membrane material that are released by tumor cells usually have a normal molecular structure but fail to polymerize or aggregate properly once they are released at the tumor cell surface. Well-differentiated tumors tend to produce more of these extracellular proteins than do highly anaplastic tumors.

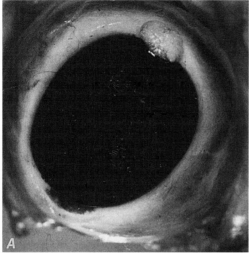

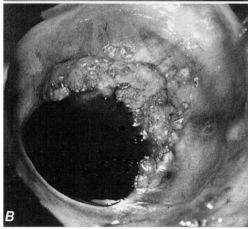

FIGURE 11.6. Squamous cell carcinoma, eye, Hereford steer. A. Early lesions. B. Advanced carcinoma.

Proteoglycans and their constituent glycosaminoglycans influence cytodifferentiation in neoplasia just as they do in normal development. They induce both proliferation and migration of cells by forming structural links between cell and interstitial components. A role of chondroitin sulfate as a growth regulator is suggested by its stimulation of tumor growth; chemical analysis of human colonic carcinomas has shown a 12-fold increase in chondroitin sulfates relative to control tissue. The source of the sulfated proteoglycan was the normal fibroblast adjacent to the tumor cells.

MAKING THE CORRECT DIAGNOSIS

Gross dissection of the tumor

After the biopsy or removal of a tumor during surgery, the surgeon and pathologist must report all changes that indicate whether a tumor is benign or malignant. This includes an examination of the size, color, location, and extent of the mass; its growth along local tissue planes; evidence for invasion of the regional arteries, veins, and lymphatics; and presence of tumor in the regional lymph nodes.

The gross appearance of the tumor mass may be described as soft, fibrotic, cystic, nodular, papillary, or encapsulated. When a neoplasm projects above a mucosal surface and into the lumen of a hollow organ, it is referred to as a **polyp**. Most polyps are found in the stomach and intestine.

- **Fibrotic** neoplasms are hard because of dense connective tissue stroma.
- **Cystic** neoplasms contain closed cavities or sacs lined by epithelium.
- **Nodular** tumors are composed of small solid nodes or nodules.
- **Papillary** neoplasms have cells that grow in fronds.

Benign epithelial neoplasms that produce warty fingerlike projections from the epithelial surface are referred to as **papillomas**. A glandular tumor that grows in papillary outgrowths is a **papillary adenoma**. Tumors of glandular origin that form large cystic masses are **cystadenomas**, and cystadenomas that contain papillary fronds of tissue into the cystic spaces of the tumor are **papillary cystadenomas**. In many organs, the small, circumscribed, and contained appearance of an early benign lesion must be evaluated with reference to the flat, multinodular, and ramifying growth of the advanced malignant tumor (Fig. 11.6).

You must be particularly attentive to evidence of **invasion** to adjacent tissue, of **implantation** along luminal or cavity surfaces, and of **metastasis** to lungs, liver, and other viscera. Invasion of tissue at the tumor margins is particularly important for the surgeon, and special techniques are used to identify the surgical margins microscopically. One of these is to place a suture in an area of particular interest. Another is "inking" of surgical margins—tumor tissue is placed in India ink for a few seconds before fixation so that when the pathologist examines the tissue section microscopically, the lines of ink are located to examine the margins for cancer cells.

Microscopic examination of tumors

The diagnosis of neoplasms requires that tissue be examined microscopically. The histologic analysis of tissue reveals the tissue of origin, establishes that the tumor is benign or malignant, and often provides, by determining a grade for the degree of malignant change, what prognosis is to be expected.

Cellular anaplasia

Cellular anaplasia and invasion of tissue are the two most reliable hallmarks of malignancy (if the tumor has metastasized, there is no doubt). Characteristics of **anaplasia** are (1) pleomorphism (differences in cell size and shape), (2) large hyperchromatic irregularly shaped nuclei, (3) increased size and number of nucleoli, and (4) decreased numbers of normal cytoplasmic organelles, with the presence of many aberrant forms. There is usually a deficiency of mitochondria, endoplasmic reticulum, and other cell work–associated organelles.

In summary, neoplastic cell function is directed to reproduction and not to cellular work and metabolic activity, and the degree of diversion from normal is a strong index of degree of malignancy. The ultrastructural analysis of anaplastic tumors may also provide clues to the degree of differentiation, such as the finding of abnormal cytoskeleton, desmosomes, intermediate filaments, and other structures typical of neoplastic tissues.

Grading of neoplasms

In order to provide a prognosis for clinical behavior, some cancers are given histologic grades that indicate the degree of malignancy. Generally, some system is used that provides simple stages—for example, grades 1 for the least and 4 for the most anaplastic. Grading is based on the extent of differentiation of the neoplastic cells and other characteristics such as the number of mitoses. In nearly all tumors, the correlation between the assigned grade and the clinical behavior in the animal is not completely accurate. A grading system for canine mast cell tumors is used:

- Grade 1 = 83% survive 4 years: compact growth, monomorphic, well granulated, no mitotic figures
- Grade 2 = 44% survive 4 years: moderate cytoplasmic granules, few mitotic figures, moderate anisokaryosis, occasional binucleated cells
- Grade 3 = <10% survive 1 year: marked anisocytosis and anisokaryosis, poorly granulated cytoplasm, 3–6 mitotic figures per 40× field, infiltrative growth

Histologic staging of neoplasms

Solid tumors can be categorized artificially into stages for use in surgical management and prognosis. Staging is based on data from appropriate studies of the correlation of histopathologic analysis and clinical outcome. The stage of a tumor is determined by the size of the primary neoplasms, the extent of spread to regional lymph nodes, and the presence of metastatic lesions.

Stage of tumor is the best predictor of survival in nearly all forms of cancer. In the following hypothetical scheme, characteristics used to formulate each stage include the appearance of the primary

FOCUS

Malignant Melanomas

MALIGNANT MELANOMAS are vicious and capricious neoplasms that occur in amphibians, reptiles, fish, birds, and mammals. They are common in dogs, in which they are found in the oral cavity, skin, and eye. Malignant melanoma cells typically have melanin granules that lead to the diagnosis. Pigmented breeds are especially affected. Non-pigmented melanomas, called amelanotic melanomas, are common in the oral cavity. Amelanotic melanomas are detected by their content of tyrosinase. Tyrosinase oxidizes dihydroxyphenylalanine (dopa), which is added to the tissue section in the histochemical test called the **dopa reaction**.

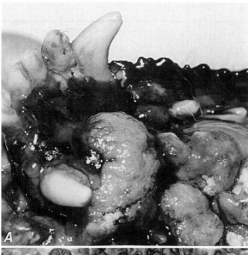

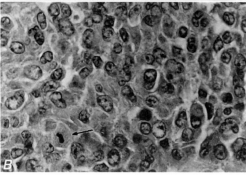

FIGURE 11.7. Malignant melanoma (amelanotic type), oral cavity, dog. A. Nodular white tumors are at the site of a biopsy of the primary tumor 3 months previously. B. Histology reveals highly undifferentiated plump cells with many mitoses *(arrow);* these are referred to as "mitotic figures."

tumor, presence of tumor in adjacent tissues, and metastasis to lymph nodes or distant sites.

Primary tumor:
T_0 = no evidence of tumor
T_1 = tumor confined to primary site
T_2 = tumor invades adjacent tissues
Lymph nodes:
N_0 = no evidence of tumor
N_1 = regional node involvement
N_2 = distant node involvement
Metastases:
M_0 = no evidence of metastasis
M_1 = tumor in same organ or cavity as primary
M_2 = distant metastases

Mitosis: counting of mitotic figures

Mitotic figures are common in malignant tumors. Microscopic examination of tumor tissue reveals an increase in the number of mitotic cells in most malignant tumors. The large cells with central aggregates of chromosomes are called **mitotic figures** (Fig. 11.7). Nucleoli and some cytoplasmic organelles may persist during mitosis of cancer cells, but they do not do this in normal cells. The mitotic process, however, resembles that in normal cells. Replication and migration of centrioles, appearance or disappearance of spindle tubules and kinetochores, and movement and replication of chromosomes are often indistinguishable from normal. The presence of mitotic figures in a tumor does not unequivocally mean malignancy, but highly malignant tumors have the greatest number and percentage of bizarre mitoses. **Tumor giant cells** with large polymorphic nuclei are a major indicator of malignancy.

Immunohistochemistry for specific tumor markers

Cytoplasmic markers

The histochemical identification of secretory products in the cytoplasm of neoplastic cells is one of the best markers for determining the cell of origin. For example, granules of melanin suggest a melanoma. In anaplastic tumors that differ so strikingly from normal tissue that they cannot be classified, specific proteins can be identified by histochemistry that may establish the tissue of origin of the tumor. Poorly differentiated, highly malignant neoplasms can be classified as sarcoma or carcinoma by staining for actin of muscle, keratin of epithelia, or other specific cytoplasmic substances found in normal cells.

Stains for secretory components such as hormones, melanin, and secretory proteins are also effective; for example, histochemical staining for casein can be used for mammary carcinomas. Other cytoplasmic markers for neoplastic tissue include **factor VIII** for identification of endothelial cells in vascular tumors, **cytokeratin** for epithelial tumors, **actin** for muscle tumors, and **glial fibrillary protein** for astrocytomas and other brain tumors.

Histochemical stains for factor VIII, or von Willebrand factor, may provide a useful measure of invasiveness because they stain both normal and neoplastic blood vessels. Clinical studies have shown that an increase in tumor microvessel density is associated with decreased disease-free survival in some forms of advanced cancer. Blood vessel density per unit of neoplastic tissue may prove to be a useful predictor of survival in addition to the stage, grade, and tumor type.

Excessive DNA

Modern techniques include the use of cell sorters and flow cytometers to produce data on tumor DNA profiles. Neoplastic cells can be digested from tissue in paraffin blocks. Nuclei are isolated, and suspensions of nuclei are applied to the flow cytometer and counted for their DNA content. Tumors that are of low malignancy will be diploid, whereas highly malignant cancers usually have evidence of aneuploidy.

Proliferation markers

Histochemical techniques to detect components involved in the cell cycle are beginning to be used as criteria for malignancy. There are many enzymes and proteins known to function in various stages of the cell cycle. Two that are detectable and that have been found to be useful in analysis of neoplasms are these: (1) **Proliferating cell nuclear antigen** (PCNA) is an accessory component of DNA polymerase δ. PCNA staining is increased in many highly malignant tumors. (2) **Protein Ki67** is a nuclear antigen that is absent in G_0 but present throughout the cell cycle. Ki67 is a better indicator of malignancy, but its detection is more capricious. Both PCNA and Ki67 have been powerful research tools but are not widely applied to tumors of animals (Fig. 11.8).

Cell death markers

Genes that induce programmed cell death (PCD) in neoplasms are important in the development of neoplasms. The presence (or absence) indicates the extent of genetic mutation that has occurred, and techniques that detect these genes or their products are used to assess the presence of PCD. The protein products of many of these genes are involved in signal transduction routes that converge into a common final pathway of cell death. The **p53 gene** encodes the protein p53, which holds cells in G_1 for repair. Protein p53 acts as a transcription factor, binding specifically to other genes and controlling their expression. Protein p53 acts as a "guardian of the genome"; it functions to block the cell cycle and stimulate DNA repair, and it also can trigger PCD. DNA damage induces the expression of p53, and the product of p53 rises in cells with DNA damage. The p53 protein acts in a second way to suppress the development of neoplasia—by initiating programmed cell death. In this process, cells are shunted into the process of cell death and are removed from the tissue by phagocytosis.

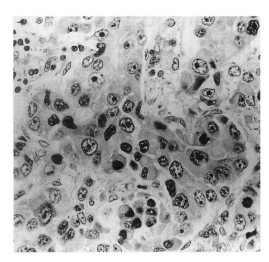

FIGURE 11.8. Cell proliferation and cell death markers in neoplastic tissue. The proliferating cell nuclear antigen, or PCNA *(top)*, detects a transcription factor that becomes elevated early in the cell cycle. The TUNEL reaction *(bottom)* detects an endonuclease that is activated to initiate cell death.

Detection of abnormal tumor cell secretions in serum

Some neoplasms, particularly those of glandular origin, secrete peptides or glycoproteins that appear in the serum of animals bearing the tumor. Detection of these products in serum samples provides another dimension for the diagnosis of these tumors. Many of these proteins are secreted by embryonic cells, but genes that direct them are shut down in the neonatal period (they are reactivated in the neoplastic cell). Hepatocellular carcinomas may secrete **α-fetoprotein**, which is not found in serum of adult animals even though it may appear in the fetus of that species.

These tests are rarely used in veterinary medicine but have wide application in human medicine. The detection of **prostate-specific antigen** (PSA) by radioimmunoassay, a major advance in human oncology, does not work with canine prostate carcinomas. Large amounts of cytokines may be secreted by some tumors, and their detection may confirm the diagnosis of some tumors; for example, some renal cell carcinomas secrete interleukin-6.

Genetic analysis

In neoplastic cells, abnormal genes (or normal genes expressed at abnormal levels) favor proliferation over differentiation. Most natural tumors arise by genetic mutation or by rearrangement of genes.

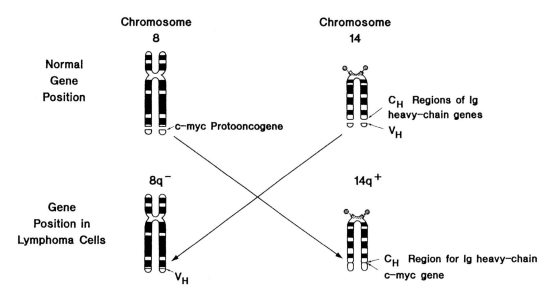

FIGURE 11.9. Staining of bands aids in studies of abnormal chromosomes. Here, in lymphocytes of a primate lymphoma, is translocation of chromosomes 8 and 14. The oncogene c-*myc* on chromosome 8 is transferred to a position adjacent to a gene for heavy chains of immunoglobulin (Ig) molecules C$_H$ and C$_V$ on chromosome 14. The breakpoint in chromosome 8 is at the terminal part of the long arm (band q24). Transfer next to the active Ig gene allows the oncogene c-*myc* to come under the influence of enhancer genes of the Ig loci. Loss of control of c-*myc* (which encodes a protein involved in growth regulation of lymphocytes) is called deregulation and is related to the abnormal growth of neoplastic lymphocytes.

The abnormal gene may produce a messenger RNA (mRNA) that directs ribosomes to begin overproduction of an abnormal gene product. The excess gene product might then diffuse throughout the cell to produce enzymatic or other reactions that lead to cellular manifestations of neoplasia. The initiating gene change could occur either as a result of direct chemical or radiation damage to DNA or by insertion of viral cancer genes into host DNA that mimic normal growth-controlling genes.

Detection of abnormal chromosomes: karyotype analysis

When examined by chromosomal analysis, malignant cells are usually **aneuploid** (having more or less than the normal diploid number) and have a variety of chromosomal rearrangements or other defects. Chromosome analysis of naturally occurring tumors commonly reveals large variations in chromosomes of individual cells, that is, a mosaic chromosomal pattern of cells with both normal and abnormal karyotypes. In some, recurrent chromosomal aberrations or rearrangements are found. Genotyping of human renal parenchymal tumors,

for example, shows that nonpapillary renal cell carcinomas have a deletion of specific chromosome 3p segments and loss of heterozygosity for loci at 3p. Pathologic karyotypes that are found in tumor cells include chromosomal deletions, translocations, and others (Fig. 11.9).

Oncogene detection: in situ polymerase chain reaction

In situ **polymerase chain reaction (PCR)** is an extremely sensitive morphological technique used to detect minute amounts of DNA or RNA that are specific for a particular gene or gene product in tissue sections or intact cells. The technique is a combination of PCR widely used by molecular biologists to amplify DNA or RNA in the test tube, and **in situ hybridization** commonly used by morphologists to detect specific sequences in cells. The combination of these two techniques enables the pinpointing of a single copy of DNA or RNA in cells and allows identification of cellular structures. It gives insight to gene mutations, gene alterations, chromosomal translocations, and low-level gene expression.

Historical Development of Oncology

Neoplasms are circumscribed atypical productions of tissue from a matrix of superabundant or erratic deposits of embryonic elements.
—Julius F. Cohnheim, 1872

EARLY STUDIES with the light microscope revealed the cellular nature of neoplasms and indicated that they grew independently. Classification schemes that were developed based on the correlation of histologic appearance and clinical behavior proved to have remarkable prognostic value.

The amazing success of microbiologists in transmitting infectious diseases at the end of the 1800s prompted similar attempts to discover a transmissible cause for neoplasms. Scattered reports of transmission occurred, but evidence pointed to accidental or fallacious interpretation; the consensus was that these attempts had failed. The singular success was that of the Russian veterinarian Novinsky, who in 1876 established the transplantability of the canine venereal tumor, one of the few truly transmissible tumors in nature. In the early 1900s, Carl O. Jensen in Denmark passed tissue suspensions of mouse mammary tumors through several generations. His careful histologic examination established that transmission was effected by transplantation and not by inciting host cells to transform.

A tumor is a new formation of cells which proliferates continuously and without control.
—F. B. Mallory, 1914

Mallory's definition went on to state that tumor cells tended to differentiate toward their cell of origin, lacked an orderly structural arrangement, and served no useful function. In the early 1900s, clues appeared that exogenous agents might cause cancer. Long-term exposures to X-irradiation and coal tar were established as carcinogenic in animals, but these models related to only a few rare instances of naturally occurring neoplasms. Two highly significant discoveries were made at this time (even though they were largely ignored). First, Ellerman and Bernhard L. F. Bang, in Denmark, showed that lymphoid neoplasms of the chicken were transmissible by cell-free filtrates. Second, at the Rockefeller Institute in New York, F. Peyton Rous readily transmitted a sarcoma of the chicken in a similar way and produced a rapidly expanding sarcoma in the recipient bird. Rous persisted for years with his chicken sarcoma and belatedly received the Nobel Prize in 1966.

ADDITIONAL READING

Classification

Alroy J, et al. 1975. Distinctive intestinal mast cell neoplasms of domestic cats. *Lab Invest* 33:159.

Darbés J, et al. 1998. Large granular lymphocyte lymphoma in six cats. *Vet Pathol* 35:370.

Hahn FF, et al. 1996. Primary lung neoplasia in a beagle colony. *Vet Pathol* 33:633.

van Garderen E, et al. 1997. Expression of growth hormone in canine mammary tissue and mammary tumors. *Am J Pathol* 150:1037.

Weinberg RA. 1996. How cancer arises. *Sci Am* 275:62.

Tumor stroma: angiogenesis and fibroplasia

Hanahan D. 1998. A flanking attack on cancer. *Nat Med* 4:13.

Hanahan D, Folkman J. 1996. Patterns and emerging mechanisms of the angiogenic switch during tumorigenesis. *Cell* 86:353.

Moses AV, et al. 1997. HIV-1 induction of CD40 on endothelial cells promotes the outgrowth of AIDS-associated B-cell lymphomas. *Nat Med* 3:1242.

Ninoyama H, Nakamura T. 1988. Vascular architecture of N-methyl nitrosourea-induced rat papillary adenoma demonstrated by scanning electron microscopy of resin casts. *Jap J Vet Sci* 50:1065.

O'Reilly MS, et al. 1997. Endostatin: an endogenous inhibitor of angiogenesis and tumor growth. *Cell* 88:277.

Skobe M, et al. 1997. Halting angiogenesis suppresses carcinoma cell invasion. *Nat Med* 3:1222.

Weidner N, et al. 1995. Intratumor microvessel density as a prognostic factor in cancer. *Am J Pathol* 147:9.

Making the diagnosis

Bratulič Z, et al. 1996. Number of nucleoli and nucleolar organizer regions per nucleus and nucleolus—prognostic value in canine mammary tumors. *Vet Pathol* 33:527.

Hahn KA, et al. 1994. Diagnostic and prognostic importance of chromosomal aberrations identified in 61 dogs with lymphosarcoma. *Vet Pathol* 31:528.

Hendrick MJ, Brooks JJ. 1994. Postvaccinal sarcomas in the cat: histology and immunohistochemistry. *Vet Pathol* 31:126.

Liu KX, et al. 1994. Antigen expression in normal and neoplastic canine tissues defined by a monoclonal antibody generated against canine mesothelioma cells. *Vet Pathol* 31:663.

Löhr CV, et al. 1997. Characterization of the proliferation state in canine mammary tumors by the standardized AgNOR method with postfixation and immunohistologic detection of Ki-67 and PCNA. *Vet Pathol* 34:212.

Moore PF, et al. 1996. Canine cutaneous histiocytoma is an epidermotropic Langerhans cell histiocytosis that expresses CD1 and specific β_2-integrin molecules. *Am J Pathol* 148:1699.

Oshimura M, et al. 1973. Chromosomal banding patterns in primary and transplanted venereal tumors in the dog. *J Natl Cancer Inst* 51:1197.

Patnaik AK, et al. 1984. Canine cutaneous mast cell tumour: morphologic grading and survival time in 83 dogs. *Vet Pathol* 21:469.

Pilling AM, et al. 1997. In situ hybridization demonstration of albumin mRNA in B6C3F1 murine liver and hepatocellular neoplasms. *Vet Pathol* 34:585.

Ritt MG, et al. 1998. Functional loss of p21/Waf-1 in a case of benign canine multicentric melanoma. *Vet Pathol* 35:94.

Sagartz KE, et al. 1996. p53 tumor suppressor protein overexpression in osteogenic tumors of dogs. *Vet Pathol* 33:213.

Sher CJ. 1996. Cancer cell cycles. *Science* 274:1672.

Simoes JPC, et al. 1994. Prognosis of canine mast cell tumors: a comparison of three methods. *Vet Pathol* 31:637.

Wolf JC, et al. 1997. Immunohistochemical detection of p53 tumor suppressor gene protein in canine epithelial colorectal tumors. *Vet Pathol* 34:394.

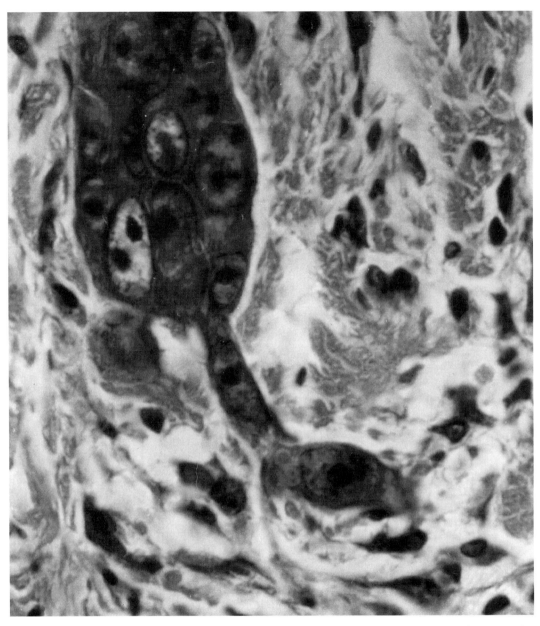

FIGURE 12.1. Invasion of a cutaneous squamous cell carcinoma into the connective tissue stroma.

CHAPTER 12

Host Responses to Neoplasms

THE SPREAD OF NEOPLASMS

Invasion and metastasis are the hallmarks of cancer. Neoplastic cells spread in the animal in different ways: by invasion through connective tissue stroma, by dissemination through the vascular system, and by implantation on new surfaces (particularly on serosal surfaces of the thoracic and abdominal cavities). In some cases, neoplastic cells erode veins and, in rare cases, arteries. Neoplastic cells also invade lymphatics and disseminate through lymphatic vessels to regional lymph nodes. In order for a neoplastic cell to detach from its site of origin, to move within connective tissue stroma, and to invade the bloodstream, it acquires unique characteristics. These phenotypic changes, endowed by somatic mutation, determine the degree of malignancy of a neoplastic cell.

Invasion

The capacity to invade host tissue is an intrinsic property of the neoplastic cell. Changes in the cell surface and subsurface cytoskeleton promote extension of pseudopodia below basement membranes and between connective tissue planes (Fig. 12.1). Mutations that result in altered surface receptors, adhesion molecules, enzymes, and glycoproteins secreted at the surface enhance the capacity of the neoplastic cell to dissect its way through normal tissues. Adhesion of neoplastic cells to the extracellular matrix is critical in invasion.

Release of enzymes that degrade connective tissue

Carcinomas typically invade tissue by elaborating enzymes that degrade connective tissue. Some squamous cell carcinomas are directly collageno-

lytic; that is, they produce a **collagenase** that specifically degrades collagen. Neoplastic cells can secrete proteases with more general specificity, and they lyse a large spectrum of proteins.

Some tumors produce factors that cause the host cells to release **proteolytic enzymes**. Squamous cell carcinomas in rodents indicate that cathepsin B, a cysteine protease that degrades both collagen and proteoglycans, is stimulated in host fibroblasts by a factor released by the neoplastic squamous cell.

Enzymes from neoplastic cells kill host cells

Enzymes secreted into connective tissues by invading neoplastic cells enhance tumor cell migratory capacity by killing some of the host cells. Release of lysosomal hydrolases has been shown to be correlated with highly invasive mammary gland adenocarcinomas. The increased capacity of a transplantable melanoma of mice to metastasize has also been shown to be related to lysosomal enzymes of the tumor cell. Contact of the tumor with normal cells may result in release of lysosomal enzymes and killing of host cells. In some cases, there is lysis of the tumor cells with liberation of massive amounts of lysosomal enzymes.

Metastasis

Metastasis is the unequivocal index of malignancy. All neoplasms that metastasize are malignant, although not all malignant neoplasms metastasize. Highly malignant cells have relatively little tendency to adhere to one another. As they invade stroma, malignant cells enter lymph vessels. They then pass into regional lymph nodes and from there into the thoracic duct. Neoplastic cells also directly invade capillaries to enter the bloodstream and may even erode vascular walls (Fig. 12.2).

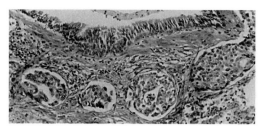

FIGURE 12.2. Collections of metastatic mammary adenocarcinoma cells in peribronchial veins and lymphatic vessels of the lung.

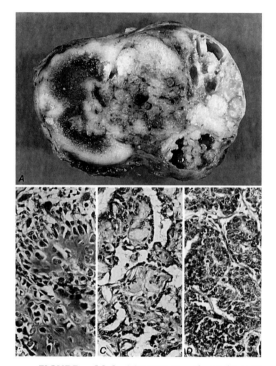

FIGURE 12.3. Metastases of malignant mixed mammary gland tumor of a dog to the regional lymph node (superficial inguinal). A. Cross section of lymph nodes with areas that correspond to differing histologic appearance of the tumor. B. Osteoid production. C. Cystic. D. Solid.

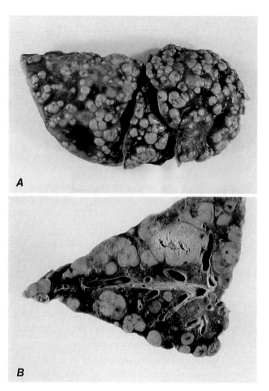

FIGURE 12.4. Metastases of hepatocellular carcinoma to the lungs. A. Large solid metastases in all lobes. B. Cut surface, caudal lobe, of the same lung.

many carcinomas. In Misdorp's collection of 56 canine mammary gland carcinomas, metastatic foci were 86% to lymph nodes, 72% to lungs, and 10–12% each to adrenals, kidneys, liver, and bone. In dogs, adenocarcinomas of the most caudal mammary glands tend to be found in the inguinal lymph nodes; tumors in the cranial mammary gland drain to axillary nodes.

Although many metastasizing cancer cells pass from lymphatic vessels to the bloodstream, the reverse also occurs. Carcinoma cells injected intravenously in rats show that within 1 hour tumor cells can be recovered from lymph. Thus, cells not trapped in the first capillary bed through which they pass may escape into the lymphatic system, probably in lymph nodes.

Cancer cells that lodge and grow in the regional lymph node usually resemble the cells of the primary tumor, although this is not always true. The remarkable variation that sometimes occurs may be due to formation of new clones of cells. The malignant mixed mammary gland tumor of dogs clearly contains both glandular and connective tissue components, and its metastases may be segregated

Metastasizing tumors may have a selective organ tropism based on receptors on the tumor cell surface. These receptors have specificity for ligands in different organs that will attract these tumors to a greater degree.

Regional lymph nodes trap malignant cells

Lymphatic drainage to regional lymph nodes provides a common pathway for metastatic spread of

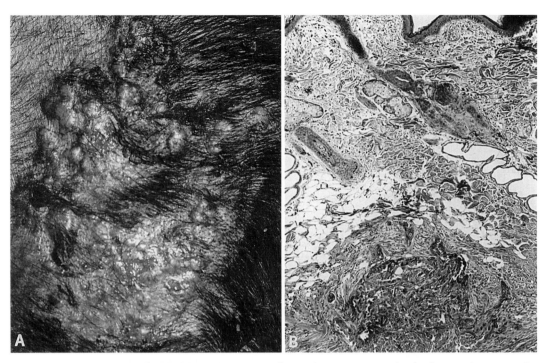

FIGURE 12.5. Metastases of a canine mammary gland adenocarcinoma to the skin. A. Massive nodular areas on the abdominal skin. B. Histology: small tumor mass in the subcutis *(bottom).*

in the draining lymph node into solid epithelial, cystic, and cartilaginous components (Fig. 12.3).

Lungs trap neoplastic cells in the bloodstream

The distribution of secondary (metastatic) neoplastic foci is determined largely by the anatomic characteristics of veins and lymphatic vessels draining the primary tumor site. In animals, many malignant tumors metastasize to the lung. Lung metastases occur because of the immense flow of blood through this organ and its large network of capillaries, through which circulation is slowed. The pulmonary capillary bed serves as a filter for aggregates of tumor cells that lodge in the vascular tree, insert pseudopodia between endothelial cells, and emigrate into the lung parenchyma. Metastatic foci in the lungs of some cancers tend to localize around bronchioles (Fig. 12.4).

Liver traps neoplastic cells in portal veins

The liver is highly vulnerable to metastases, particularly by carcinomas arising in tissues drained by the portal venous system. For example, metastases from carcinoma of the intestine are commonly found in the liver. Some tumors enter the liver via the hepatic artery, a route that is associated with tertiary seeding from metastatic tumors lodged in the lungs.

Other sites of metastasis

Other organs where metastases are common include kidney, brain, and bone. Circulation is not the sole determining factor, because some tumors have surface receptors that bind to tissue-specific ligands. For example, human prostate carcinomas thrive in bone because prostate carcinoma cells contain receptors that bind tightly to bone cells. In highly anaplastic tumors, any organ may develop metastatic lesions. Skin may be affected by carcinomas that enter the lymphatic system and creep along the subcutaneous lymphatics (Fig. 12.5).

Implantation

Because of their lack of cohesiveness, highly malignant cancer cells are prone to be shed into the surrounding spaces. **Exfoliation** of cells into fluids of the body cavities and respiratory and urogenital tracts is the basis for the cytologic examination of these fluids for cancer cells. Implantation is most serious along serosal surfaces of the thoracic and

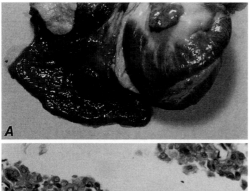

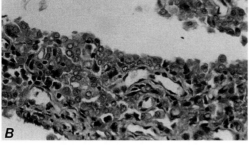

FIGURE 12.6. Carcinomatosis. Implantation of malignant cells of an aortic body carcinoma onto the serosal surface of the mediastinum of a dog. A. Dark, hyperemic, velvety coat of neoplastic cells covers the mediastinal pleura *(bottom left)*. Marked dilatation of the right ventricles of the heart. B. Fronds of tumor, composed of vascular and connective tissue, support tumor cell proliferation. There is infiltration of lymphoid cells into the interstitium.

abdominal cavities. This can lead to massive implantation and development of immense numbers of cancer cells on serosal surfaces.

Diffuse implantation of neoplastic tissue along serosal surfaces is called **carcinomatosis** and is characteristic of ovarian, pancreatic, and some other adenocarcinomas. Pancreatic adenocarcinomas may seed through the peritoneal cavity to grow along peritoneal surfaces; these lesions are referred to as **peritoneal carcinomatosis**. When the cavity is opened, massive growth of neoplastic cells may present the misleading appearance of an acute fibrinous peritonitis (Fig. 12.6). Tumor cell localization on the peritoneal membranes is enhanced when serosal surfaces are injured. Tumor cells adhere on exposed collagen fibrils and grow more rapidly. Peritoneal lymph drainage is blocked in carcinomatosis, and ascites is a common clinical sign.

Transplantation of neoplastic cells from contaminated surgical instruments and gloves is a significant potential hazard during cancer surgery. Although rarely reported, this is a well-documented sequel to cancer surgery.

Survival of metastatic cells

As malignant neoplasms expand, cancer cells are released into lymph or blood continuously. Studies of experimentally induced mammary gland tumors in mice show that when tumors reach the size of a few grams, they release several million cells daily into the circulation. The majority die quickly; only a few survive the hostile nature of the bloodstream.

In patients, it is also true that most cancer cells that enter the bloodstream die without initiating new metastatic foci. Factors that influence whether tumor cells initiate new growths at sites distant from the primary tumor include (1) the way in which metastasis occurs, whether from single cells or tumor emboli; (2) the intrinsic capacity of the malignant cells to lodge in and attach to host endothelial cells; and (3) the tissue environment at localization sites.

Survival in the bloodstream is enhanced by several conditions. Clumps of tumor cells, called **tumor emboli**, have a greater tendency to form metastases than do single cells. Thus tumor cells that adhere to each other because their surface properties and secretions have been changed are particularly dangerous. Furthermore, the larger the tumor cell clump, the more likely it is to be trapped in capillaries and form new colonies.

Systemic changes in the host that have been shown experimentally to enhance metastases include physical stress, extensive surgery, and halothane anesthesia. Tissue damage in an organ vulnerable to metastases may increase the deposition of tumor emboli. Clinical treatment with the antineoplastic drug cyclophosphamide or with radiation, which may have overriding antitumor beneficial effects, has been shown in some studies also to increase the number of metastatic lesions in some tumors. For example, marked irradiation of the thorax of dogs with osteosarcomas has been shown to increase the incidence of metastases to the lungs.

Some metastatic cells secrete procoagulant factors

Procoagulant factors secreted by neoplastic cells may cause fibrinogen to polymerize on the tumor embolus. Some cancer cells activate the clotting cascade by shedding plasma membrane vesicles that carry procoagulant activity. The mesh of fibrin tends to protect the malignant cells from destruction, enabling them to proliferate.

Fibrin can often be seen histologically in tumor emboli, but it is quickly lysed by the fibrinolytic system and disappears during late stages of embolization. Some types of malignant cells grown in

FOCUS

Transplantable Tumors

TRANSPLANTABLE MELANOMAS of mice have contributed much to our understanding of metastasis of malignant tumors. Melanoma S91 arose from the tail of a mouse at the Jackson Laboratory. It is strain specific, and subcutaneous implants kill the host within 12 weeks, after metastasizing to the lungs and other viscera. S91 produces large amounts of melanin via the tyrosinase–dopa oxidase enzyme complex, and tumor cells are filled with melanosomes.

Studies in this model indicate that few tumor cells that metastasize will survive. Experiments in which radioactively labeled mouse melanoma cells were injected intravenously showed that within minutes most cells were trapped in the lung. Only 1% remained alive after 1 day, and after 2 weeks, when metastatic lesions could be seen grossly, only 0.1% of the original cells were still alive.

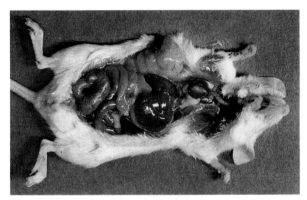

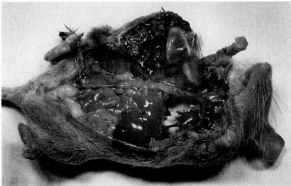

Transplanted tumors in mice.

The B16 melanoma, which arose in a strain of black mice, is transplantable and produces pigmented metastases in lungs of recipient mice, with occasional tumor foci in ovaries, liver, and brain.

▶

After 10 cycles of experimental selection of cells from lung metastases, a variant malignant cell line was established that actually seeks lung tissue. When injected into the tail vein, the cells were first trapped in lungs. When injected downstream from the lung, they were trapped in other tissues but then detached and recirculated until they lodged in the more desired lung environment. Specificity was shown more clearly when it was established that lung-prone tumor was less likely to metastasize to brain or ovary. Other variant lines were established that prefer brain or ovary rather than lung. The reason for preferences resides in the plasma membrane. Each of the three variant lines shows different patterns of specific surface proteins.

culture show increased production of **plasminogen activators**, which enhance the effectiveness of the fibrinolytic system. Although this prevents the growth-promoting stabilizing effects of fibrin during metastasis and invasion, fibrinolysis enhances tumor growth in tissue once the metastatic focus is established.

Neoplastic cells lodge at new sites by attaching to **fibronectin** and other extracellular matrix proteins. Attachment occurs on the fibronectin molecule at a unique sequence of three amino acids, arginine-glycine–aspartic acid (designated the RGD sequence). Even artificial tripeptides will bind cells to their RGD sequences, acting like a decoy to bind cellular receptors for fibronectin and thus to block the cells from attaching to the extracellular matrix.

Platelets may enhance survival of circulating cancer cells

Some neoplastic cells contain surface materials that cause them to attach to platelets and to induce platelet aggregation. Within the platelet–neoplastic cell mass, platelets support the growth of the neoplastic cell and facilitate its attachment to endothelium. Platelets contain a rich supply of growth factors, and these factors enhance cancer cell survival and growth within the blood. The clinical use of anticoagulant and antiplatelet therapy to reduce metastases has given inconclusive results. However, in studies with experimental melanomas, prostacyclin remarkably decreased the number of metastases to lungs, presumably through its potent inhibiting effect on platelet aggregation.

Cancer cells attach to endothelium

Once trapped in venules and capillaries, malignant cells adhere to endothelium and cause striking changes in adhesion of endothelial cells to their underlying matrix. Endothelial cells retract, leaving spaces through which the tumor cells can migrate in the tissue. Once in the interstitium, the neoplastic cells must induce alterations that promote further survival and replication. Again, fibrin deposited around the neoplastic cells provides a matrix for further development. Within normal stroma, neoplastic cells respond to chemotactic factors, but the role of these substances in metastasis is not clear.

Metastatic cells send false signals

To survive in a new tissue environment, the metastatic cell must develop new strategies. One of these is the expression of increased surface adhesion molecules for attachment to other cells and to the extracellular matrix. Cell-to-cell and cell-to-matrix adherence prevents migration of both normal and abnormal cells. Normal epithelial cells are said to be anchorage dependent. That is, if they fail to attach to neighboring cells or to their basal connective tissue matrix, signals go from the cell surface to the nucleus to block mitosis and to initiate programmed cell death, the mechanism whereby abnormal cells are destroyed. In cancer cells, certain products from oncogenes can convey a false message to the nucleus that the cell is properly attached when it is not, thereby blocking programmed cell death and allowing the abnormally detached cell to continue into the cell cycle and mitosis.

CLINICAL EFFECTS OF NEOPLASMS

Malignant neoplasms kill the host through a variety of effects. As neoplasms expand, they exert **pressure** on surrounding normal tissues to cause pain, interruption of vascular supplies, and lymphatic blockade. The squamous cell carcinoma in Figure 11.2 caused dyspnea and hypoxia by obstructing the pharynx, diminished saliva production due to neoplastic infiltration into the salivary gland, and anorexia from pain in the muscles of mastication. Local expansion of tumors can contribute to weight loss, especially large tumors of the limbs, which prevent foraging and cause inanition.

Ductal systems and lumens of the lungs, intestines, and brain are especially susceptible to obstruction, usually with dire consequences. Obstructions of the urinary tract and biliary ducts also contribute to death.

Invasion of vascular structures is a significant cause of death in advanced cancer. Highly malignant tumors invade and grow within the walls of veins and arteries and, by obstructing the vascular channel, cause local infarcts. Some of these tumors shed small fragments into their veins, and these emboli are carried to the lungs and into the arterial system to cause infarction of other organs. Progressive growth in the lumens of blood vessels will slowly compromise functions of the heart, lungs, liver, and other major organs (Fig. 12.7).

In the absence of overt causes of death, animals with cancer still progressively lose weight and die. Often, the mass of the neoplasm cannot fully explain death in mechanical terms. One must then turn to more subtle mechanisms that play major roles in killing the cancer patient by one or a combination of the systemic effects of neoplastic disease.

Cachexia

In neoplastic disease, animals develop **anorexia** (loss of appetite), lose weight, and become lethargic. **Cachexia** is due in part to anorexia brought on by depression of appetite centers in the brain. Many tumor-bearing animals are anorectic yet have tumors too small to affect appetite directly. In these cases, weight loss is due to cytokines and other factors released by the tumor cells.

Cytokines mobilize fat cell triglycerides

Weight loss can be associated with humoral factors secreted by tumor cells or by macrophages (indirectly affected by the neoplasm). Mobilization of triglycerides in adipocytes is associated with **tumor necrosis factor α** (also called **TNF-α**, or **cachectin**), a cytokine produced by macrophages. TNF-α causes decreased synthesis of lipogenic enzymes in adipocytes by suppressing a gene for enzymes that catalyze fat deposition.

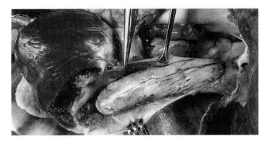

FIGURE 12.7. Growth of the adrenal cortical adenocarcinoma through the wall of the posterior vena cava, with extensive growth within the vein to reach the origin of the right atrium of the heart.

Neoplastic cells act as an amino acid trap

By virtue of tumor cell enzymes, neoplastic cells can irreversibly drain the host of essential amino acids. Skeletal muscles of animals with widespread metastatic cancer are thus in double jeopardy. They become atrophic, partially through **disuse of lethargy** but also because of **metabolic defectiveness**. Spotty dropout of muscle fibers occurs. Later, muscle cells develop decreases in glucose uptake, insulin sensitivity, and activities of enzymes for energy production. The diminished glucose assimilation compounds the amino acid drain by the tumor mass. Secondary to the amino acid drain effect, the liver, pancreas, and other organs regress in terminal cancer. Hepatocytes become small, and their enzymatic composition more undifferentiated, so that they resemble immature hepatocytes.

Anemia

Anemia is common in metastatic neoplastic disease and is often responsible for a significant part of the clinical illness of the terminally ill patient. Important causes of anemia in cancerous animals include the following:

- **Iron-deficiency anemia** associated with inflammatory disease
- **Anticancer chemotherapy**, a cause of nonregenerative anemia
- **Autoimmune anemia** in association with lymphoproliferative neoplasms
- **Suppression of erythropoietin synthesis** in the kidney
- **Activation of the monocyte-macrophage system** with excessive removal of erythrocytes from circulation

Other causes of anemia in cancer are (1) **hemorrhage** from erosion of normal tissues by the invading tumor (a common cause of death); (2) **decreased erythropoiesis** from invasion of bone marrow by the tumor and destruction of erythropoietic tissue; and (3) **erythrocyte fragmentation** as the cells pass through abnormal blood vessels of the tumor.

Highly vascular tumors are most likely to cause anemia by destruction of erythrocytes. In hemangiosarcomas of dogs, an **erythrocyte fragmentation syndrome** arises from microangiopathic hemolytic anemia. Fibrin erodes erythrocyte surfaces, and the acantholytic erythrocytes are then sequestered in vascular spaces of the tumor.

In contrast to the suppression of erythrocyte production, tumor cells may produce **polycythemia** by secreting erythropoietin, although this has been reported only in human renal neoplasms.

Coagulation defects

Fibrin is a frequent finding in tumor stroma but in most cases has no clinical significance. Histologically, fibrin is found on surfaces of tumor-associated macrophages and endothelial cells. **Tissue factor** appears to be the major procoagulant in tumors, although several other procoagulants have been found that generate thrombin (and thrombin-catalyzed fibrin). There is evidence that tissue factor regulates synthesis of **vascular endothelial growth factor** (VEGF) by tumor cells, an important growth factor in the angiogenesis that is required to support tumor growth.

Thrombosis occurs in large tumors

Local thrombosis is common in solid tumors. Thrombin arises from the combined effects of tumor-induced platelet adhesions and aggregation, incomplete endothelialization of tumor capillaries, and release of procoagulant materials by the neoplastic cells. In rare cases, tumors that release large amounts of procoagulants cause **disseminated intravascular coagulation** with thrombotic obstruction of pulmonary capillaries or renal glomeruli.

Any increase in viscosity of the blood promotes thrombosis. Cells of the plasmacytoma (multiple myeloma) secrete globulins causing **hyperglobulinemia**. In dogs the clinical features secondary to plasmacytoma are a monoclonal immunoglobulin spike in serum, lytic bone lesions (sometimes with hypercalcemia), and fragments of globulin chains (Bence Jones proteins) in urine. This is associated with a stasis syndrome in which thrombosis is promoted.

Abnormal platelet function and thrombocytopenia

Abnormalities of platelets are common in terminal neoplastic disease. Platelet survival is reduced in nearly 40% of all dogs bearing local tumors and in 80% of dogs with metastatic tumors. Fibrinogen concentrations are increased in most of these dogs. Thrombocyte production is diminished in the viral leukemias and lymphoproliferative syndromes as a result of bone marrow suppression.

Hypercalcemia

Hypercalcemia is a complication in many cancers and is lethal in some. It may arise by two mechanisms:

- **Tumor cell secretion** of peptides that mimic parathyroid hormone
- **Osteolytic metastases** of neoplasms with bone resorption and Ca^{2+} release

Tumors producing humoral factors that stimulate osteoclasts or parathyroid-like responses often produce complications in terminal neoplastic disease. In contrast, although osteolytic metastases may stimulate bone resorption and release of calcium that exceeds homeostatic capacity, this mechanism rarely produces serious disease.

Hypercalcemia of malignancy

Hypercalcemia of malignancy results from secretion of peptides with parathyroid hormone activity. There is persistent hypercalcemia and hyperphosphatemia, hyperplasia of thyroid C cells, and atrophy of parathyroids (in response to hypercalcemia). Radiographically, only mild skeletal demineralization occurs, in contrast to severe bone changes in primary and secondary hyperparathyroidism of renal or nutritional origin. Diagnosis requires that there be no parathyroid tumor (or other parathyroid lesions) or bone metastases of other tumors.

Pseudohyperparathyroidism occurs in dogs and cats and has been associated with mammary gland carcinomas, fibrosarcomas, lymphosarcomas, and various adenocarcinomas. Gastric carcinomas in horses induce this syndrome.

Pseudohyperparathyroidism is associated with adenocarcinomas arising from the anal sac apocrine glands in dogs. This syndrome occurs predominantly in aged females. The tumors develop as masses in the perirectal area ventrolateral to the anus and in close association with the anal sac (they are distinct from the more common perianal gland tumor).

Ectopic hormone syndromes

Nearly all cancer cells synthesize proteins that, when released, can cause some systemic sign of disease. When peptides are secreted with biologically active fragments that mimic hormones or neuropeptides, syndromes of clinical importance appear. These peptides are synthesized as large chains

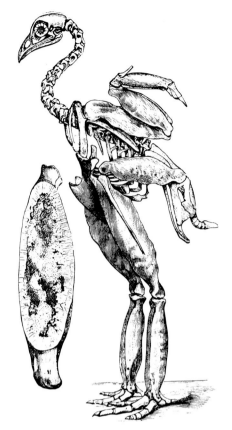

FIGURE 12.8. Avian osteopetrosis, skeleton of a chicken showing massive proliferation of bone. (Illustration: *J Comp Med Surg* 10:28, 1898)

bearing several hormone segments that must be cleaved away before release and activation. Similarly, tumor peptides may be large and abnormal and yet contain fragments resembling normal hormones closely enough to stimulate target tissues.

At least 20 hormones or their precursors have been identified in neoplasms. These vary from pituitary tumors that secrete adrenocorticotropic hormone (ACTH) to renal juxtaglomerular tumors that secrete renin. In the latter, increased renin in plasma leads to hypertension, hyperkalemia, and hyperaldosteronism. Small cell carcinomas of human lungs have been shown to secrete the neuropeptide bombesin, which in turn releases an array of gastrointestinal hormones.

Hypergastrinemia

The **Zollinger-Ellison syndrome** is associated with non–β cell tumors of the pancreas. Tumor cells secrete a polypeptide with activity similar to that of **gastrin**, which is normally secreted by "gastrin cells" of the gastric antrum and duodenal mucosae. Clinical signs involve diarrhea, vomiting, weight loss, hypersecretion of gastric acid, and **hypergastrinemia**. The spectrum of changes associated with these tumors includes ulcers in the stomach and esophagus, enteritis with villous atrophy, hypertrophy of gastric mucosa, and proliferation of C cells in the thyroid. Most of these tumors in dogs are malignant, and metastases are found in regional lymph nodes and in liver.

Diarrhea

Diarrhea in terminal cancer commonly results from intestinal bacterial and protozoal infections, particularly those that complicate antineoplastic therapy that is also immunosuppressive. Prolonged diarrhea unresponsive to routine therapy and not associated with known microbial causes may also occur in disseminated neoplasia. In rare primary tumors of the intestine, diarrhea may be linked to secretions of the neoplastic cells, although this is unusual. Even rarer is a syndrome of diarrhea that accompanies some neurogenic tumors. **Vasoactive intestinal peptides** secreted by the tumor cells are diarrheogenic and lead to a life-threatening loss of fluids and electrolytes.

Hypoglycemia

Hypoglycemia commonly occurs in the late stages of disseminated neoplasia but also can occur early as part of the initial clinical syndrome. Clinical signs of hypoglycemia, which are related directly to glucose deficits in the brain and adrenergic effects, include restlessness, weakness, tremors, and episodes of collapse and seizures.

Hypoglycemia (blood glucose <70 mg/dl) is characteristic of tumors of the pancreatic islet cells, which produce insulin. Hypoglycemia also has been reported to occur in animals bearing various epithelial, mesenchymal, and hematopoietic neoplasms. In dogs, hepatic tumors are most often responsible, although hemangiosarcomas, melanomas, and salivary gland tumors have been accompanied by low blood sugar.

Bone disease

Neoplastic tissue growing directly in bone marrow leads to severe pain and often to bone fracture. Neoplasms in bone marrow can contribute to anemia and other manifestations of systemic neoplasia. Two other abnormalities of bone are associated with special neoplasms. **Osteopetrosis** occurs in avian species as a direct effect of avian leukosis virus growth directly in osteoblasts (Fig. 12.8). **Pulmonary hypertrophic osteopathy**, a proliferative disorder of bones of the limbs, results from growth of certain neoplasms in the lungs.

Fever

Some tumor cells release **pyrogens**, and tumor-induced fever may complicate advanced stages of cancer. In the early 1900s, fever was viewed as a natural antineoplastic mechanism. Fever is indeed common in animals with advanced metastatic neo-plasms, but in most cases it is likely to result from complicating inflammatory or bacterial disease rather than a humoral factor of tumor origin. The causes of fever in neoplasia include TNF, IL-1, IFN-γ, and other cytokines.

FOCUS

Pulmonary Hypertrophic Osteopathy

A RARE AND CURIOUS DISEASE, pulmonary hypertrophic osteopathy involves new bone formation beneath the periosteum that progressively thickens and deforms long bones. Beginning at the distal ends of the limb bones, new bone grows outward in an interrupted manner, producing irregular and rough bony masses. The initial lesion is an overgrowth of subperiosteal vascular tissue that leads directly to osteoblast proliferation and bone formation. Treatment to correct this rapid increase in blood flow to the limb bones causes the lesion to regress. The case illustrated below was reported by Freddy Coignoul (*Ann Med Vet* 128:545, 1984).

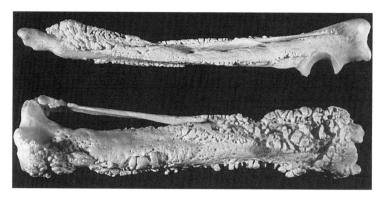

The adjective **pulmonary** indicates the unexplained association of bone lesions of the lungs. Thoracic neoplasms, pulmonary tuberculosis, granulomas of the esophagus, and lung abscesses have all been responsible. In a study of 60 canine cases, 58 dogs had intrathoracic lesions (36 secondary neoplasms, 18 primary neoplasms, 2 inflammatory lesions, and 1 case of dirofilariasis). Of the 2 dogs without thoracic lesions, one had bacterial endocarditis and one a sarcoma of the urinary bladder (Brody, *J Am Vet Med Assoc* 159:1242, 1971).

When the thoracic lesion that underlies the periosteal change is removed surgically, the bone lesions of hypertrophic osteoarthropathy regress. Improvement correlates with the correction of increased blood flow to the bones. **Chronic anoxia** has been implicated as causal, yet the magnitude of the pulmonary lesions is rarely of such extent that mechanical obstruction of the airways can explain the bone lesions. Vagotomy has been shown to suppress the bone lesions in both dogs and humans.

RESTRAINT OF NEOPLASTIC GROWTH

Malignant neoplasms grow progressively over a long period of time. There are, however, many factors that interact to restrain cancerous growth. These include endocrine secretions, intercurrent inflammatory disease, and immunologic reactions. By the use of combined strategies, clinicians hope to retard and, in rare cases, to cure neoplastic disease.

Nonspecific lysis and phagocytosis

In most tumors, malignant cells are continuously removed by inflammatory cells. The advancing edge of the squamous cell carcinoma in Figure 11.2 is surrounded by a zone of fibrovascular reactive tissue that contains monocytes and neutrophils. It is clear that these cells have not controlled the tumor and were probably functioning only to remove cells dying because of rapid growth in an environment of limited nourishment. Experimental studies, however, show that macrophages and even neutrophils can actively destroy neoplastic cells.

Activated macrophages release several soluble factors, some of which have been shown to produce antitumor activity experimentally. **Tumor necrosis factor α (TNF-α)** is the prototype of a family of antitumor factors. Secreted by macrophages, TNF-α causes necrosis in tumors by killing neoplastic cells. Although it has striking effects on

---

FOCUS

Nonspecific Macrophage Activity May Inhibit Tumor Growth

FOR A CENTURY, it has been suspected that natural tumors are suppressed by intercurrent inflammation, especially in lymph nodes and other tissues of the monocyte-macrophage system. In the late 1800s William Coley, a New York surgeon, developed mixed bacterial "vaccines" that produced fever and chills and induced substantial regression of tumors in a few human patients. "Coley's toxins" acted as an immunopotentiator to enhance an otherwise inadequate host response. Experiments in this era showed that filtrates of gram-negative bacterial cultures produced striking hemorrhage and necrosis in experimental tumors.

Long overshadowed by other methods of treatment, new variants of this type of therapy are now used in hope that spread of tumors will be inhibited by stimulating macrophages nonspecifically. *Corynebacterium parvum* and an avirulent tubercle bacillus (bacille Calmette-Guérin, BCG) are potent immunizing agents that are used as nonspecific adjuvants to stimulate the monocyte-macrophage system. In some animal tumor models, macrophages so stimulated aggressively attack and cause degeneration of target tumor cells. Cows with ocular squamous cell carcinoma treated by intratumor injection of BCG vaccines had 71% regression; the untreated controls all developed progressive tumor growth with lymph node metastases. This treatment activates macrophages to delete susceptible and aged tumor cells and also potentiates tumor-specific immunity; their effect is to enhance the production of antitumor antibodies and lymphocytes. The potent cytokines TNF-α and IL-1 appear to mediate much of the macrophage activity. Unfortunately, macrophage function is depressed in the early phases of rapid tumor growth in natural neoplastic disease, possibly by some factor released by the tumor. BCG vaccine is now being used in human leukemias and melanomas but is credited with only limited success.

some experimental neoplasms, TNF-α has not proven to be clinically useful. It is probable that the lack of specificity prevents macrophages from being effective.

Natural killer (NK) cells, a population of immature lymphocytes, arise in the late neonatal periods and wane with advancing age. Bearing Fc surface receptors, NK cells cause lysis of neoplastic cells in vitro. Experimentally, there is a close correlation between NK cell activity and cytotoxicity. It is assumed that NK cells play some role in preventing the early expansion of tumors.

Specific immunologic suppression of neoplasia

Neoplastic cells develop new proteins on their surfaces that function as tumor antigens. These proteins can evoke both antitumor antibodies and cytotoxic lymphocytes. In some cases, cytotoxic T lymphocytes appear to inhibit tumor growth. However, effective tumor immunosuppression is clouded by the capricious and elusive nature of immune mechanisms against tumors, and the difficulty of making them operable in animals.

We know that neoplastic cells inherently resist immunologic recognition and therefore killing; that is, they do not have surface components that differentiate sufficiently so that the host animals can attack them as foreign. Evidence exists that neoplastic cells also actively resist immunologic killing. Melanoma cells bear on their surfaces a molecule that drives T cells into programmed cell death.

An important killing mechanism of cytotoxic T lymphocytes is via Fas protein–Fas ligand (FasL) interaction. Activated T cells bearing large numbers of FasL on their surface bind to Fas molecules on target cells, and the Fas-FasL interaction signals programmed cell death in the target cell. Some melanoma cells, however, can use this same mechanism to kill invading T lymphocytes. Recently it has been reported that malignant melanoma cells can actually kill the cytotoxic T lymphocytes that attempt to attack and lyse them. Although cytotoxic T lymphocytes have FasL on their surfaces, they also have Fas, which makes them vulnerable to being killed by FasL-bearing melanoma cells. When melanoma cell FasL attaches to lymphocyte Fas, binding triggers the caspase cascade and cell death in the lymphocyte.

Identification of genes that encode cancer antigens opens new possibilities for treatment. For example, genes that code for melanoma-associated antigens are involved in rejection of melanoma cells. Synthetic peptides designed to increase binding and immunologic reactivity have been used as cancer vaccines to treat patients with metastatic melanoma. However, cancer vaccination strategies do not induce an efficient antigen-specific response for tumor eradication.

Why doesn't tumor immunotherapy work?

The immunoreactivity induced by a tumor is probably quantitatively insufficient to inhibit an already rapidly growing tumor. By continual antigen shedding, very large tumors could provide tumor antigens that would combine with immune cells or antibody sufficient to prevent them from reacting with neoplastic cells. There are several other theories about ineffective immunotherapy: (1) There is a close relation between oncogenesis and immunosuppression, and it may be that tumors develop in an already immunodefective host. (2) Humoral antibodies may even enhance tumor growth. It is proposed that they combine on the tumor cell surface and block the effect of more potent immunotoxic mechanisms. Antigens on the cell surface may also be blocked by mucosubstances. (3) Prolonged exposure to tumor antigens may induce a partial state of tolerance in the host, in which immunoreactivity is ineffective.

CANCER IS A GENETIC DISEASE

Every naturally occurring tumor that has been studied in depth has been found to have multiple defects in genes that in some way enhance cellular replication or growth. Genetic instability and mutation underlie the sequential acquisition of biologic characteristics of neoplasia. Mutation in a previously normal cell may provide a selective growth advantage over adjacent cells. Although most mutants die, because of metabolic or immunologic disadvantage, some of these cells survive. The surviving cell population has a higher frequency of mitotic error and other genetic changes, and each cell division carries an increased risk of variation. When mutations are acquired in genes that govern the cell cycle, neoplastic proliferation proceeds as a result of uncontrolled mitosis in the expanding tumor cell population.

Tumor progression

The phenotypic attributes of a malignant neoplasm are uncontrolled mitoses, cell surface changes that promote invasion and metastasis, production of embryonic proteins, and abnormal metabolism. They are due to multiple genetic mutations and are acquired in a stepwise manner. This is known as **tu-**

mor progression, and it occurs as an accumulation of multiple genetic lesions in the tumor cell.

Most malignant tumors develop from the **clonal expansion** of a single progenitor cell bearing a genetic mutation. Nonlethal mutations are acquired in somatic cells by chemicals, radiation, or oncogenic viruses.

Genes of cancer

Three classes of normal regulatory genes are the targets of genetic damage in neoplastic disease:

- **Oncogenes**—mutants of normal genes that code for growth
- **Tumor suppressor genes**—mutants of normal genes that suppress growth
- **Genes that govern DNA repair**

The first class, known as oncogenes, stimulate the cell cycle and lead to mitosis. **Oncogenes** (the normal gene is referred to as a **proto-oncogene**) produce a "mutant" protein that is created from the mutant oncogene code. The abnormal protein may differ from the normal protein product in only one amino acid, yet it may have the capacity to alter cell growth greatly. As the mutant proteins flood the cell, they may have access to enzymes and other target proteins that are unavailable to the normal protein.

A **tumor suppressor gene** acts by normally suppressing some phase of growth; deletion of the gene leads to uncontrolled growth (Table 12.1). Mutations in **genes that govern DNA repair** lead to a genetic lesion that makes DNA repair inefficient. By permitting the propagation of genetic error, they move the cell toward neoplasia.

CONSTRUCTING THE CANCER CELL

From the information we have on the characteristics of neoplasms and on the types of genes that are known to cause neoplasia, we are able to devise a strategy that will produce a hypothetical cancer cell. Genetic changes in multiple cell systems are required to develop a highly malignant cell (Fig. 12.9). We know that naturally occurring cancers have multiple genetic defects that are inherited from one somatic cell to another and that influence a wide spectrum of cellular events. To begin a program for perpetual mitosis, we need genes that will give the cell an unstable genome and the machinery to support uncontrolled growth, changes that will be the basis for the extensive array of genetic change needed for the cell to become truly neoplastic. We will need to create mutant genes that promote abnormal growth and differentiation, genes that cause the cell to become disengaged from its neighbor, and genes that cause the cell to replicate uncontrollably and become immortal. The design must include mutant genes that lead to loss of control of the cell cycle. It is important that you, as a student, grasp these concepts. Future diagnostic techniques and treatment modalities will be constructed based on this knowledge of neoplastic cell behavior.

TABLE 12.1. Mutations in normal genes for mitosis and growth regulation that are found in cancer

	Oncoprotein	Oncogene	Effect	Overexpressed in . . .
Growth-promoting genes[a]				
Growth factor	PDGF-β	sis	Increased expression	Glioma
Epidermal growth factor receptor	EGFr	erbB	Increased expression	Lung carcinoma
Signal transducing protein[b]	GTP binding	ras	Point mutation	Many cancers
	Ras blocked	src	Point mutation	Sarcomas
Nuclear regulator protein[c]	TA	myc	Translocation	Lymphoma
Repressor genes[d]				
Transcription factor	Protein p53	p53	No blocked cycle	Many cancers
Cyclin blocker	p21, p53 proteins	p21, p53	Cyclin inactivation	p53, p21
Binds and inactivates	Protein Rb	Rb	Unsuppressed	Retinoblastoma
Cell death genes[e]				
Blocks cell cycle	Bcl-1 protein	Bcl-1	Blocks cell cycle	Mammary tumors
Blocks cell death	Bcl-2 protein	Bcl-2	Blocks cell death	Lymphoma

Abbreviations: PDGF-β = platelet-derived growth factor–beta; TA = transcription activator.

[a]Proto-oncogenes code for proteins that stimulate cell division; mutated forms, oncogenes, cause stimulatory proteins to be overactive.

[b]Cytoplasmic relays in stimulation of signal pathways.

[c]Transcription factors that activate growth-promoting genes.

[d]Tumor suppressor genes ("anti-oncogenes") code for proteins that inhibit cell division. Mutations cause protein to be inactivated and deprives cells of restraints on proliferation.

[e]Programmed cell death genes depress normal mechanisms of cell death.

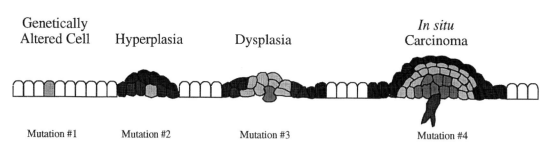

FIGURE 12.9. Progression of steps in carcinoma formation (hypothetical) on an epithelial surface. 1. An initial mutation leads to a mutant cell that appears normal but replicates to form a lesion of **hyperplastic epithelium**. 2. Within the hyperplastic focus, a second mutation develops that leads to **dysplasia**. 3. Mutation number 3 in the focus of dysplasia causes anaplastic changes in the cell that proliferate to form **carcinoma in situ**, a lesion that is not malignant but develops cancer with a greater incidence than the previous lesions. 4. Within the carcinoma in situ develops a fourth mutation that gives cells the capacity to invade and metastasize, making the lesion a **carcinoma**.

Increased signals for cell growth

Mutant genes for growth factor receptors

Increasing the number of **growth factor receptors** that are expressed on the surface of the cell will enhance the autocrine growth signal processes. This will not directly create a cancer cell but will put into motion the cellular processes that lead to growth and replication. If, for example, we increase the number of receptors for **epidermal growth factor** (EGF), the cell will be continuously instructed to grow. The production of a mutant growth factor receptor by a neoplastic cell is apt to cause the receptor to be inappropriately active on the cell itself; that is, the signal acts in an autocrine manner to self-start the cell for growth.

The EGF family of growth factors is known to be altered in cancer. For example, v-*erbB* is the transforming oncogene of avian myeloblastosis, a retroviral-induced disease of chickens; the gene encodes a mutant EGF receptor that acts via autocrine stimulation in the cancer cell. EGF receptor genes are overexpressed in up to 80% of squamous cell carcinomas of the human lung. In some cases, the detection of c-*erbB* histochemically in the tumor indicates an extreme sensitivity to growth factors, an aggressive cancer cell phenotype, and a poor prognosis for the animal.

Excessive growth factors

Activation of genes that increase the expression of growth factors is a common finding in many natural cancers. The new growth factors might be normal but produced in excessive amounts. They might act in an autocrine manner to self-stimulate the cancer cell of our exercise, or the action might be paracrine, to be released and to stimulate neighboring cells. One of the most potent growth factors known and one with widespread effects in the body is the **platelet-derived growth factor** (PDGF). We know that the proto-oncogene *sis* encodes the β chain of PDGF-β, and elevations of PDGF-β are found in osteosarcomas, astrocytomas, and several other human tumors. **Fibroblast growth factor** (FGF) is another potent growth factor. Activation of the proto-oncogene *hst* causes overproduction of FGFs in melanomas and in cancers of the stomach, bladder, and mammary gland. In these tumors, *sis* and *hst* are not mutated but are kept active through excessive stimulation by inappropriate signaling. In most cases, dysfunctional growth factor production is related to a defect in the growth factor signaling pathway.

Mutation in growth factor signal molecules

Perhaps the most ingenious way to increase synthesis of growth factors is by locking some components of the growth signal pathway permanently in the "on" position. In fact, the best-known cancer-causing mutation occurs in the *ras* gene, one of the genes in the signaling pathway for growth factors. The mutated *ras* gene encodes for the Ras protein, which floods the cell, thereby creating the permanent "on" signal for cell growth. Ras protein normally behaves as a relay switch in the signal pathway that receives signals from outside the cell (e.g., when a growth factor binds to its receptor on the cell surface) and activates the pathway to stimulate the cell to grow or undergo mitosis. Unless it receives outside prompting, the Ras protein remains turned "off," thereby blocking the signal pathway that activates the cell cycle. In neoplastic cells, however, the mutant Ras protein is incomplete, and when it attaches to the inner surface of the cell's plasma membrane to interact with growth factor receptors and other signal proteins, it behaves like a switch stuck in the "on" position, continuously signaling the cell to divide.

The NF-1 gene product is a GTPase-acting protein (GAP) that binds to active *ras* and greatly augments its GTPase activity. This interaction terminates signal transduction by the rapid hydrolysis of GTP to GDP. With loss of NF-1, *ras* is trapped in its active, signal-transmitting state.

Alteration of cell surfaces for migration

The cancer cell needs several attributes for cell movement, changes that will be important for invasion and metastasis. First, we need to alter the expression of proteins that make up intercellular junctions and function to keep the cell stable in its relation to other cells and to the extracellular matrix. Genes for the proteins of desmosomes, adherence plaques, and gap junctions are targets for mutation because they keep the cell in close contact and communication with its neighbors. Second, the secretion of a collagenase or elastase will remove connective tissue barriers that will impede movement of the neoplastic cell during invasion. Third, the capacity for invasion by the neoplastic cell will be enhanced if we can increase certain adhesion molecules on the cell surface—molecules that will cause the cell to adhere to endothelial cells in organs distant from the primary site (to enhance the capacity for metastatic localization).

We know that cell-cell adhesiveness is reduced in many cancers. Some loss of adhesion is associated with defects in cadherins, surface molecules that mediate a calcium-dependent cell-to-cell adhesiveness. The E-cadherin ("E" for "epithelial") system in cancer cells has been shown to be inactivated by multiple mechanisms, and transcriptional inactivation of E-cadherin expression occurs frequently in tumor progression.

The normal cellular *src* gene, called c-*src*, controls intercellular adhesion. It codes for a tyrosine-specific protein kinase that is attached to the cytoplasmic face of the plasma membrane. The viral mutant form of this gene, called v-*src*, was first identified in a fibrosarcoma of chickens. The mutated v-*src* is inserted into the host-cell genome and can be passed for generations before being activated to cause neoplastic change.

When activated, v-*src* causes the fibroblast to produce an mRNA that initiates ribosomal production of the *src* oncoprotein, pp60$^{v\text{-}src}$, a kinase that phosphorylates proteins to a high degree. Although the *src* gene product is present in small amounts, it floods the cytoplasm to reach substrates that normal cell enzymes do not. By phosphorylating several proteins, this one mutant enzyme can vastly alter cell function. It might stimulate DNA synthesis, enhance mitosis, or render ATP inefficient. We now know that the *src* protein binds to the plasma membrane and phosphorylates a tyrosine unit in **vinculin**, a protein in adhesion plaques at the cell surface. In this way it influences the ability of neoplastic cells to become invasive and break away from normal cellular relationships.

The cancer cell requires a high level of growth factors that will enhance the effectiveness of the Src oncoprotein to cause cancer. In experimental fibrosarcomas in chickens, Rous sarcoma virus (RSV) oncogenicity is limited to fibroblasts at the site where RSV is injected. However, wounding of skin at any site in viremic chicks leads to tumor development in 100% of wound sites (that would otherwise remain free of tumor). This effect appears to be mediated by transforming growth factor β (but not other growth factors), which itself will mimic the tumorigenic effects of wounding.

Blockade of DNA repair

By suppressing DNA repair, we will not directly cause neoplastic change, but we will increase the number of cells that have unrepaired mutations. In order to enhance the chances for genetic mutations, a defect in one of the genes that control DNA repair will lead to production of a defective transcription factor or other protein that controls the cell cycle, and this in turn will increase the chances for neoplasia. In fact, naturally occurring tumor cells frequently have defects in their DNA repair processes; e.g., up to 20% of human colon carcinomas have mutations in *MLH1*, *MSH3*, *PMSH2*, or other genes whose protein repairs DNA. Other genes indirectly play a role in DNA repair. The "checkpoint genes," which monitor the cell cycle, prevent the next stage of the cycle.

Evidence that DNA damage leads to neoplastic change comes from mice with artificially induced defects in the DNA repair enzymes. These mice are extraordinarily susceptible to tumors. Clinical evidence of the importance of DNA repair in neoplasia comes from the human genetic disease **xeroderma pigmentosum**. Because of defects in enzymes required for DNA repair, patients with the disease are extremely sensitive to sunlight and are susceptible to ultraviolet light–induced squamous cell carcinomas and other kinds of cutaneous neoplasms in childhood.

Uncontrolled mitosis

All positive and negative signals for control of nuclear transcription converge on the nucleus, where mechanisms for mitosis are present, and it is here that the products of both oncogenes and tumor suppressor genes are found. For cancer, we need genetic changes that will grease the slide into mitosis. The first candidates are those that act in nuclei to control the cell cycle, and thus we look for factors that accumulate in the nucleus of proliferating cells. Signals that arrest the cycle usually act at the G_1 control point, just before entry into S phase (this checkpoint prevents the cell from replicating damaged DNA).

The key families of proteins, the cyclin-dependent protein kinases (Cdks), which induce downstream processes by phosphorylating serine and threonine molecules of selected proteins, and the cyclins, which bind to Cdk molecules and control their ability to phosphorylate targets, may originate from genes that are defective. The mitotic cyclins, which bind to Cdk molecules during G_2, are required for entry into mitosis. The G_1 cyclins, which bind to Cdk molecules during G_1 (and are required for entry into S phase), associate successively with different cyclins to trigger successive phases of the cycle. Mitotic cyclin accumulates gradually during G_2 and binds to Cdk to form M-phase promoting factor (MPF), a complex that triggers mitosis. The ultimate activation of MPF is explosive—the MPF concentration builds to a critical flash point whereupon a flood of active MPF triggers events that propel the cell to mitosis. Normal proteolytic degradation of active mitotic cyclins by ubiquitinization and hydrolysis in the proteasome is disrupted by some viral genes. Mutations that prevent pro-

---

FOCUS

Rous Sarcoma, Retroviruses, and Cancer

IN 1911 A FIBROSARCOMA in the breast muscle of a chicken was shown to be transmissible. The virus was isolated by Peyton Rous at the Rockefeller Institute, and the Rous sarcoma virus (RSV) became the first virus that was accepted to cause tumors in animals. In the 1970s it was shown that this grandfather-of-all-tumor-viruses carries four viral genes that enter cells of the chicken, its natural host. Three genes direct the production of new infectious viruses, but the fourth, the *src* gene (for **sar**coma), induces fibrosarcomas.

The *src* gene was recognized as the first viral **oncogene** and was later shown to be a mutated form of a related gene, *c-src,* found to be part of the normal genome of many vertebrates, including humans. This suggested the hypothesis that retroviral oncogenes are derived from related genes of host cells. In fact, in the decade that followed, normal cells of many species were found to contain retrovirus-related DNA sequences.

The *src* gene is inserted into the host cell genome and can be passed for generations. When activated, it causes the host fibroblast to produce an mRNA that initiates ribosomal production of the **src gene product**, a peptide kinase that can phosphorylate proteins such as vinculin to a high degree. Disruption of the vinculin in adhesion plaques at the fibroblast surface contributes to the ability of the new neoplastic cell to break away and metastasize. Although the **src** gene product is present in small amounts, it floods the cytoplasm to reach substrates that normal cell enzymes cannot.

teasome degradation may lead to neoplasia; for example, papillomaviruses induce tumors by stimulating ubiquitin-mediated degradation of the tumor suppressor p53.

Oncogenes

Many oncogenes are known to act on the cell cycle. The gene *myc*, a nuclear regulator protein, has been found to be translocated in several neoplasms. The c-*myc* proto-oncogene produces a phosphoprotein in the nucleus that has DNA-binding capacity. This protein product of the c-*myc* gene has been found in human B- and T-cell lymphomas and in some carcinomas and sarcomas. It accumulates in proliferating cells and is believed to mediate the action of growth factors in cells, thereby facilitating cells to enter proliferation cycles; c-*myc* expression confers proliferation competence to cells and is switched off during terminal differentiation in normal cells. The precise molecular mechanism of action is unknown, but the c-*myc* protein heterodimerizes and cooperates with MAX, a protein that binds specifically to a core DNA sequence, CAC(G/A)TG.

The c-*myc* gene is highly conserved and has been identified in many species. This prototype of the *myc*-related family includes N-*myc*, found to have amplified copy numbers in human neuroblastomas, and L-*myc*, which is highly expressed in human small cell carcinomas of the lungs. In mouse embryos, the level of c-*myc* expression depends on the stage of embryonic development. Not expressed in normal adults, the gene is again turned on during growth disturbances and has been detected in liver tumors and in polycystic renal disease.

The *myb* gene is found in chickens infected with the retrovirus that causes avian myeloblastosis (thus is called v-*myb*). Its normal cellular homolog, or c-*myb*, regulates hematopoietic cell proliferation (and perhaps differentiation); that is, c-*myb* is preferentially expressed in primitive hematopoietic cells, and as cells mature, c-*myb* expression declines. Experimentally, the c-*myb* gene product is required for formation of human hematopoietic colonies of myeloid, erythroid, and megakaryocyte lineages in vitro. When normal hematopoietic cells in culture are exposed to c-*myb* sense and antisense synthetic oligodeoxynucleotides, they are blocked or stimulated appropriately.

Tumor suppressor genes

Tumor suppressor genes, when defective, have been shown to play a major role in the development of tumors. When working properly, the protein products of tumor suppressor genes suppress the development of neoplastic change. The absence of tumor suppressor genes is detected by the absence of their protein products in malignant cells. The best-known tumor suppressor genes act directly to inhibit the progression of cells through the cell cycle. Mutation of the normal **retinoblastoma**, or *Rb*, gene was the first human suppressor gene to be discovered. Loss of pRb leads to the uncontrolled

---

FOCUS

The Retinoblastoma Tumor Suppressor Gene

MUTATION OF THE RETINOBLASTOMA, or *Rb*, gene is the basis for an inherited form of **retinoblastoma** in children. Affected patients have one inherited mutant allele and then suffer a second somatic mutation in the normal allele, which gives rise to the retinoblastoma. The mutation is a small deletion in the chromosome 13 (13q14). If Rb protein, one of the targets of the cyclin-Cdk complexes, is not phosphorylated extensively, it binds to two transcription factors called E2F and DP1, and binding keeps these molecules inactive. Phosphorylation of Rb protein releases E2F and DP1, which are then able to transcribe genes that encode proteins that synthesize nucleotide precursors of DNA and enzymes that duplicate DNA—referred to as S-phase genes. Loss of Rb function deletes the regulatory control mechanism. Loss of pRB leads to uncontrolled E2F activation and markedly increased cellular proliferation.

activation of control proteins and rampant cellular proliferation. The other gene known to have suppressor function is that which produces the p53 protein.

The pRb mutations involve a change in the transcription factor binding domain, and uncontrolled cell cycling occurs because the activated transcription factor cannot be regulated. In the resting cell in G_0, pRb prevents cell replication by binding and holding transcription factors, including the c-*myc* protein and the *E2F* protein. Growth factor stimulation causes cycle-dependent kinases to phosphorylate pRb, causing it to release the transcription factors. (Factors that inhibit cell growth, such as transforming factor β, have the opposite effect—they maintain the active form of pRb by preventing its phosphorylation.)

A **transcription factor** gene called *p53* plays a vital role in stopping the cell cycle for DNA repair. By inducing either G_1 arrest or **programmed cell death (PCD)**, it prevents the cell from duplicating itself defectively, thus keeping watch over the integrity of the genome and reducing the chance for DNA mutation and development of neoplastic disease. The *p53* gene, acting through its protein product, suppresses the transition from G_1 to S phase in the cell cycle.

In response to DNA damage, the level of p53 protein rises in the cell. This protein is a transcription factor that recognizes specific DNA sequences adjacent to several different genes that control the cell cycle. By binding at these sites, p53 can regulate these genes, such as *p21,* which induces a protein that binds Cdks and inhibits the cyclin-dependent phosphorylation of their targets, including Rb protein. Expression of *p21* gives the cell time to repair the DNA damage and reduces the chance of mutation that might occur during DNA replication. When the damage has been repaired, p53 levels fall, p21 is no longer synthesized, and the cyclin-Cdk complexes can then phosphorylate Rb to signal entry into the S phase.

A protein called MDM2 can bind to p53 and block its ability to act as a transcription factor—a mechanism that appears to prevent the dangerous effect of overzealous cell cycle arrest or stimulation of PCD. MDM2 proteins prevent p53 from turning on the *p21* gene mRNA and may reverse the G_1 arrest mediated by p21's effect on the cyclin-dependent kinases. However, MDM2 has been shown to be an oncogene—thus the p53 protein can be inactivated either by mutation of the *p53* gene or by amplification of the *MDM2* gene and overexpression of its protein.

Blockade of programmed cell death

Signals for **programmed cell death** in mutant cells remove these cells and protect the host. Blockade of programmed cell death in mutants, by permitting survival, enhances the capacity for neoplastic change. Programmed cell death—death under genetic control and induced by appropriate signals—is required for normal embryologic development. Cells are shunted into a process of death and are removed from tissue by phagocytosis.

Recently, it has been shown that programmed cell death plays a major role in the development of neoplasia. Signals for programmed cell death in mutant cells remove these cells and protect the host. Blockade of programmed cell death in mutants, by permitting survival, enhances the capacity for neoplastic change.

Several genes modulate programmed cell death in neoplasms, and techniques that detect these genes or their gene products are used to assess the presence of programmed cell death. The protein products of many of these genes are involved in signal transduction routes that converge into a common final pathway of cell death. The *p53* gene encodes the protein p53, which holds cells in G_1 for repair. Protein p53 acts as a transcription factor, binding specifically to other genes and controlling their expression. Protein p53 acts as a guardian of the genome. It functions to block the cell cycle; it also can trigger programmed cell death and stimulate DNA repair. DNA damage induces the expression of *p53,* and the amount of its product rises in cells with DNA damage. The p53 protein acts in a second way to suppress the development of neoplasia—by initiating programmed cell death. Cells are shunted into the process of cell death and are removed from the tissue by phagocytosis.

The mammalian *bcl-2* gene encodes a death repressor molecule, a 25-kd integral membrane protein localized to mitochondria, nuclear envelope, and endoplasmic reticulum. The bcl-2 product prevents programmed cell death. The gene *bcl-2* was discovered as an oncogene in human follicular B-cell lymphoma, which carries the chromosomal translocation (14;18)(q32;q21). In the translocation, *bcl-2* sequences are juxtaposed to Ig heavy chains on chromosome 14, leading to marked overexpression of *bcl-2* (allowing its protein to be discovered).

The *Fas* gene product is a membrane-spanning protein, which, when cross-linked to antibodies, induces programmed cell death. Fas and the Fas ligand (FasL) act to suppress T cell–mediated cytotoxicity and certain T cell–mediated immune reactions. FasL, a cell surface molecule of the tumor necrosis factor (TNF) family, binds to Fas, its receptor, and induces death in Fas-bearing cells. FasL is expressed chiefly in activated T cells, whereas many cells express Fas. Abnormal Fas systems are associated with lymphoproliferative disorders and acceleration of autoimmune disease.

Blockade of protein synthesis

To continue our exercise, the investment of energy in cell work, that is, in protein synthesis and secretion of cellular products, needs to be blocked so that the cell can shift its resources to mitosis and cell growth. Restricting functions of the nucleolus, ribosome, and endoplasmic reticulum to functions related to replication and growth increases the capacity for malignant growth.

Shift of energy production

Neoplastic cells appear to grow more efficiently by shifting energy production of oxidative phosphorylation in mitochondria to glycosylation. Although not as efficient as oxidative phosphorylation, glycolysis is more primitive and uses the readily available substrate glucose. By shifting energy production to use glucose, the cancer cell becomes less dependent on intricate metabolic pathways—the shift to glycolysis becomes, in effect, a survival kit

for passage through the wilderness of the vascular system (Fig. 12.10).

CHEMICAL CARCINOGENESIS

Many chemical agents cause genetic change and somatic mutation and are implicated as direct etiologic agents of cancer. In cancer, however, the neoplastic process is multifactorial, and even though a primary cause is identified, there are always promoting factors that influence cancer development. For example, the multiple genetic defectiveness of naturally occurring neoplasms commonly arises from the combined effects of oncogenes and chronic tissue injury.

The wide range of chemical carcinogens proven in laboratory rodents must be kept distinct from those agents actually shown to cause naturally occurring cancer in animals. For chemical carcinogenesis (as in toxic cell injury), dosage and timing are critical. The use of massive doses of chemicals to test carcinogenicity renders some experimental results highly artificial, and such models should be placed in proper perspective.

One of the earliest reports on a cause of cancer was the finding by Sir Percivall Pott in the 1700s that English chimney sweeps suffered a high inci-

FOCUS

Gene Translocation and Neoplasia

ANTIBODY GENES are translocated to chromosomes with genes for growth in some tumors. Recent techniques using radiolabeled DNA probes are attempting to demonstrate this phenomenon. These attempts have been successful in cultured cells of human Burkitt's lymphoma, a neoplasm associated with infection with an oncogenic herpesvirus that transforms B lymphocytes. In about 90% of these patients, chromosomes 8 and 14 are abnormal and have translocated pieces of their long arms. In the process, DNA gene segments coding for the heavy-chain variable regions are moved from their normal position on chromosome 14 to number 8.

Other gene probes have shown this to be the location of another misplaced gene, designated *myc* (because it is similar to the *myc* gene of lymphoid leukosis of chickens). In avian B-cell lymphosarcoma, an oncogenic viral sequence becomes integrated near a cellular *myc* gene, which then becomes activated. The expression of the *myc* gene underlies neoplastic transformation in many mammalian tumors.

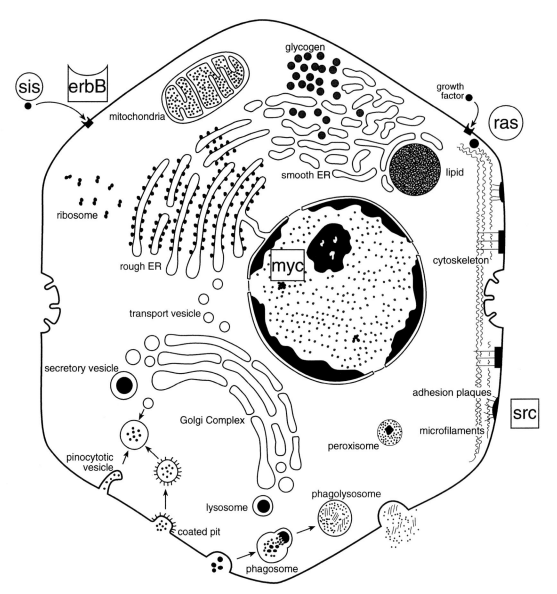

FIGURE 12.10. The cancer cell. Diagram of pathways affected by known oncogenes. Products of the following growth-promoting oncogenes are shown at the site
of cellular function that is affected: *sis* codes for a growth factor similar to platelet-
derived growth factor–β; *erbB* codes for a protein that acts as a growth factor receptor; *ras* codes for a signal-transducing protein that acts as a GTP-binding molecule;
and *myc* codes for a transcriptional activator that enhances replication. The oncogene *src* codes for a tyrosine-specific protein kinase that alters many cellular functions; one of the more important is to decrease normal cell-to-cell attachments by
affecting adhesion plaques of the plasma membrane.

dence of carcinoma of the scrotum because of continual exposure to substances in soot. Although it
was soon obvious that an oncogenic factor involved in scrotal cancer was present in soot, the
substance was not identified for nearly 150 years. In
1915, Yamagiwa reproduced a squamous cell carci-

noma similar to that in chimney sweeps by painting rabbits' ears with coal tar. The precise chemical
carcinogen, dibenzanthracene (DBA), a polycyclic
aromatic hydrocarbon, was identified in 1930 as
the first known chemical carcinogen.

The polycyclic hydrocarbons, the most powerful

chemical carcinogens known, are present in tobacco smoke and in the urban atmosphere. DBA, 3-methylcholanthrene (MC), and 7,12-dimethyl-benzanthracene (DMBA) have been widely used experimentally. By painting these carcinogens on skin of laboratory rodents, it is possible to produce epidermal carcinomas.

A clear picture of chemical oncogenesis comes from studies done in mice and rats in the 1960s that involved the chronic application of carcinogens to skin. Polycyclic hydrocarbons, after being painted on skin, accumulated in hair follicles and sebaceous glands and produced a necrotizing effect. After death of random cells, a transient hyperplastic reaction developed. Cells immediately above the germinal layer were enlarged and had large nuclei and nucleoli. Hyperplastic foci disappeared within several days unless the carcinogen was repeatedly applied. With each successive application, the epidermal cells showed an increasing resistance to the toxic effect of the chemical, but hyperplasia became more intense. In time, anaplastic cells appeared, and the tumor progressed to malignancy even when the carcinogen was no longer applied to the skin.

Initiation and promotion

The concept that multiple mechanisms are involved in the chemical induction of cancer has given rise to a **two-stage theory of carcinogenesis**. Although the carcinogenic **initiator** induces an irreversible transformation in some of the epidermal cells, their neoplastic characteristics may remain unexpressed for the life span of the animal. The subsequent presence of a **promoter** will determine whether the neoplastic characteristic is expressed. That is, initiation involves mutation; promotion leads to stability of the mutant in cell proliferation.

In the rabbit–coal tar model, benign tumors induced in ears disappeared if painting was discontinued early. Rous could enhance carcinogenicity by punching holes with a cork borer in the ears of rabbits having received this minimal painting. After wounding, tumors began to grow along the edge of the wound. Thus tar **initiated** and wounding **promoted** tumor growth. Chronic inflammation may be a critical factor in promotion of natural tumors, and experimental promoters are often inducers of inflammation (Table 12.2).

Mechanisms of chemical carcinogenesis

Chemical carcinogens induce cancer by altering DNA. Although some produce direct damage, most carcinogens require enzymatic conversion to strongly electrophilic reactants, which are the ultimate carcinogenic molecules (Table 12.3). This conversion is accomplished by soluble transferases in the **smooth endoplasmic reticulum**. For example, oxidases in the endoplasmic reticulum catalyze benzopyrene to products that bind covalently to DNA. The carcinogenic potency of this and other polycyclic hydrocarbons correlates with the extent of their binding to DNA.

Mutation may lead to mRNA template instability

Loss of differentiation may depend on a defect in messenger RNA template stability—that is, an altered capacity of mRNA to express the cellular proteins for differentiation faithfully. A new, altered set of mRNA templates for peptide production leads to anaplasia. Instability of mRNA is often first manifest in the loss of control of enzyme synthesis. Some of the azo dyes are potent carcinogens of this type. **N-methyl-aminoazobenzene** (MAB, or butter yellow) was used as a hepatic carcinogen in rats in the 1960s. MAB requires conversion, during detoxification in the hepatocyte, to the oncogenic metabolite N-hydroxy-MAB, which induces foci of hyperplasia in the liver that progressively change to adenoma and, subsequently, to adenocarcinoma.

Progression in carcinogenesis

Primary tumors of the liver usually occur in older animals with nodules of hyperplasia or other evidence of chronic liver injury (Fig. 12.11). Hepatic cancer has been linked to ingestion of toxic chemicals because of the liver's association with the portal venous system that drains the intestine, and the important role of the liver in detoxification.

Chemical carcinogenesis develops in progressive stages

Experimental feeding of carcinogens such as dimethylnitrosamine leads to formation of **hyperplastic nodules** (regenerating nodules) in the liver. These hepatic nodules are viewed as preneoplastic lesions. In a very small number of nodules, additional mutations develop that lead to **hepatocellular carcinoma**. Experimentally, the incidence of carcinoma is increased by prolonged feeding of dimethylnitrosamine. If the carcinogenic diet ceases, hyperplastic nodules disappear, and the cells are remodeled to become part of normal liver structure.

Enzyme cytochemistry detects the initial change

Within 6 weeks after the start of a dimethylnitrosamine diet, small foci of hepatocytes with specific enzyme deficiencies develop. Affected cells appear normal by standard hematoxylin-eosin

TABLE 12.2. Causes of naturally occurring neoplasms

Organ	Tumor	Species	Agent and exposure
Liver	Hepatocellular carcinoma	Trout, human	Aflatoxin B_2 (contaminated feed)
		Human	Hepatitis B virus (chronic infection)
		Rat	*Taenia taeniaeformis* (liver infection)
		Human	*Clonorchis sinensis* (chronic infection)
	Bile duct carcinoma Angiosarcoma	Human	Vinyl chloride gas (aerosol, plastic industry)
Kidney	Renal cell carcinoma	Frog	Herpesvirus (infected water, via urine)
Bladder	Carcinoma	Cow	Bracken fern toxin (feeding)
		Human	Azo dye, or naphthalene (dye manufacturing)
			Schistosoma haematobium (contaminated water)
Vagina	Adenocarcinoma	Human	Diethylstilbestrol (exposure of fetus)
Lung	Mesothelioma	Human	Asbestos (industrial worker inhalation)
	Carcinoma	Human	Cigarette smoke
			Nickel, or crystalline Ni_3S_2 (refinery worker inhalation)
Skin	Carcinoma	Human	Soot, or benzopyrene (chimney sweeping, scrotum)
		Many species	Ultraviolet irradiation (sunlight)
Mammary gland	Adenocarcinoma	Mouse	Oncornavirus (nursing, milk)
Tongue	Carcinoma	Human	Radiation from radium (licking contaminated brushes in watchmaking)
Esophagus	Sarcoma	Dog	*Spirocerca lupi*
		Human	Aflatoxins
Rumen	Carcinoma	Cow	Bracken fern toxin (feeding)
Thyroid	Carcinoma	Human	Radiation from X rays (therapeutic radiation)
Hematopoietic	Granulocytic leukemia	Human	Benzene
	Malignant lymphoma	Chicken, mouse, cat, cow	Leukemia viruses
Connective tissue	Sarcoma	Human	Nickel subsulfide, or Ni_3S_2 (refinery workers)

staining but fail to stain for glucose-6-phosphatase (in the Golgi complex) or ATPase (in hepatic canaliculi), as do normal cells. Hepatocytes in these foci have a higher rate of DNA synthesis than do normal hepatocytes. Furthermore, small groups of cells develop with extremely high rates of DNA synthesis and structures resembling those of carcinoma; they may be classified as carcinoma in situ.

Carcinogens in food

Many chemicals are intentionally added to foods during processing. Carcinogens have been identified in antioxidants, preservatives, dyes, and flavoring agents that are added to processed foods. Carcinogens may be in food grains as unrecognized natural toxic plant contaminants or as spoilage molds on feed. Food grains can be contaminated by chemicals during growth and processing. These include carcinogenic agricultural chemicals, pesticides, and mycotoxins. Contamination may be direct or may involve residues in plants and water supplies.

Regulatory action to ban chemicals in food is based on tests to detect carcinogenesis in laboratory rodents. Thioacetamide and thiourea, used as fungicides on fruit, produce hepatomas in rats. Aramite, used to control mites on fruit trees, induces hepatomas in several species. The herbicide aminotriazole, for control of weeds in cranberry bogs, produced thyroid adenomas in rats. Release of this information to the press at the height of the holiday sales season produced disastrous results in the marketing of cranberries in the 1970s. The political furor that results from events of this kind can in turn adversely affect appropriate decisions based on real scientific evidence concerning the danger of carcinogens. Careless exploitation by journalists makes it difficult to place the valid scientific data of the biological danger of these chemicals in perspective.

TABLE 12.3. Models of initiation and promotion in experimental carcinogenesis

Initiator	Promoter	Tissue	Tumor produced
Benzopyrene	Croton oil	Mouse skin	Squamous cell carcinoma
2-Acetamidofluorene	Phenobarbital	Rat liver	Hepatocellular carcinoma
Methylnitrosourea	Saccharin	Rat bladder	Transitional carcinoma
Aflatoxin B$_1$	Methylsterculate	Trout liver	Hepatocellular carcinoma

Aflatoxin and hepatic carcinoma

Hepatomas were found to be widespread in fish farms and hatcheries in 1960. The cause was commercially pelleted cottonseed meal fish feed that contained the aflatoxins of *Aspergillus flavus*. Experiments promptly established that aflatoxin B$_1$ was the specific cause. Most species of trout were susceptible, but tumors developed more rapidly in fish reared commercially in water of higher temperature. Dietary aflatoxin B$_1$ at 1–20 ppb induced hepatomas in trout in 3–6 months. When aflatoxin levels were high (1–15 mg/kg), fish died of acute hepatic necrosis and hemorrhage. Hepatomas also have occurred in turkeys fed on feed contaminated with aflatoxin.

Epidemiological evidence has incriminated aflatoxins as contaminants of peanuts and other feed grains in human hepatocarcinogenesis. Chronic aflatoxicosis is one factor in the high incidence of human hepatocellular carcinomas in Africa and Asia. Aflatoxin induces conversion of guanine to thymine bases (in DNA), a mutation seen in *p53* genes from human cancers. Mutation in the *p53* gene developed in the liver of 13 of 26 liver cancers from patients in Qidong, China, and in South Africa, areas where hepatic cancer is especially common.

Aflatoxins require activation by cellular enzymes to be carcinogenic. Activation causes neoplasia by the formation of chemically bound **adducts** that lead to mutations (if they are not repaired). Aflatoxin also forms adducts with albumin and other proteins, adducts that can be used for diagnosis when present in urine or blood. Adduct formation has been useful in diagnosis of other types of cancer. Adducts between hemoglobin and 4-aminobiphenyl, a chemical in cigarette smoke, have been found in bladder cancer. Adduct formation by the DNA of white blood cells reflects the occupation exposures of iron foundry workers in Finland and coke oven workers in Poland to polycyclic aromatic hydrocarbons, which are powerful carcinogens.

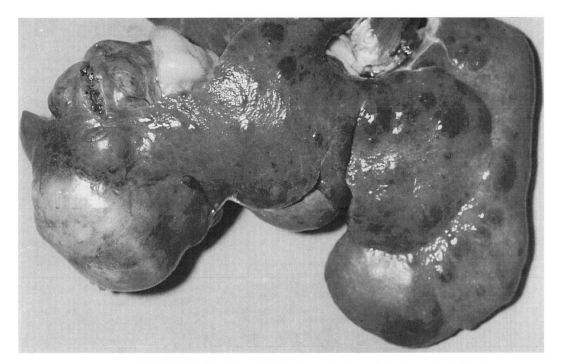

FIGURE 12.11. Liver. Multiple hyperplastic nodules throughout the liver are associated with a single, large hepatocellular carcinoma *(lower left)*, aged dog.

Bracken fern and bovine bladder tumors

Bovine enzootic hematuria is a disease of grazing cattle largely confined to woods and areas containing bracken fern. This disease has been shown to be accompanied by carcinomas of the bladder in cattle and water buffalo. Bladder tumors have been reproduced experimentally by feeding dried bracken fern. Tumors indistinguishable from natural lesions developed in cows that survived more than 3 years of feeding.

Natural grazing of bracken fern in upland areas of Scotland has been known to promote carcinogenesis in viral papillomas of the alimentary tract. The chemical carcinogen in the fern is not characterized but is believed to be a metabolic breakdown product of a fern toxin. Experimentally, these toxins extracted from ferns produce intestinal and urinary tumors in rats, aplastic anemia in cattle, and leukemia and pulmonary tumors in mice.

Cycasid nuts and liver tumors

Nuts of the plant *Cycas circinalis* contain cycasin, a carcinogenic glycoside. When flour from these nuts is fed to rodents, they develop renal, intestinal, and hepatic carcinomas. Methylazoxymethanol, an aglycone moiety of cycasin, is cleaved away by intestinal flora that possess a β-glucosidase and is the active carcinogen. Experimentally, methylazoxymethanol causes inhibition of DNA synthesis, which, in turn, blocks protein synthesis and leads to an increased incidence of mutation.

Other carcinogens

Environmental or societal habits associated with cancer in humans include betel nut chewing and lip cancer; blood fluke (*Schistosoma* sp.) infections and bladder carcinoma; and cigarette smoking and lung carcinoma. Carcinomas of the human esophagus, which have a high incidence in certain provinces of China, are ascribed to the combined effects

---

FOCUS

Telomeres and Microsatellite Instability

TELOMERES, DNA SEGMENTS at the ends of chromosomes, are part of a mechanism used to count the number of mitoses in the cell. Telomere caps on the ends of chromosomes protect these structures from damage. The telomere shortens slightly every time chromosomes are replicated during the S phase of the cell cycle. Once a critical telomere shortness is reached, the cell is instructed to enter senescence. Shortened telomeres cause chromosomes to fuse with one another or to break, creating genetic chaos that is fatal.

The rapid doubling of chromosomes in cancer cells should quickly lead to changes that drive the cell into senescence and programmed cell death. In neoplastic cells, however, this cellular defense is overcome by activation of a gene that codes for the enzyme **telomerase**. Absent from normal cells, telomerase is active in cancer cells, progressively replacing telomeric segments that are normally trimmed during each mitosis. This telomeric activity enables cells to continue to replicate, and the result is to enhance the neoplastic process.

Microsatellite instability, which is associated with defects in DNA repair, contributes to neoplastic change by diminishing chromosomal stability. Microsatellites are DNA segments consisting of a few bases repeated over and over. Abnormalities are a common result of defective mismatch DNA repair (the pathway that repairs damage that occurs when DNA is being copied and one strand slips relative to the other). These defects increase as the mitotic rate of the neoplasm increases.

of dietary nitrosamines and fungal metabolites. *Candida* spp., found in metaplastic premalignant lesions in the esophagus, release metabolites that reduce the pH of esophageal surfaces to induce production of carcinogenic nitrosamines.

Dietary fat and cancer

Epidemiologic studies implicate high dietary fat as a cofactor in several human cancers. In some rodents, addition of unsaturated fatty acids to the diet significantly enhances the incidence of chemically induced tumors. Rats are more susceptible to aflatoxin carcinogenesis when fed high-fat diets deficient in lipotropes such as methionine and choline. These deficiencies depress hepatic enzymes required for aflatoxin catabolism. In contrast, dietary antioxidants such as vitamin E decrease tumor incidence, probably by regulation of hepatic enzyme levels. In addition to these effects on detoxification, other dietary deficiencies may lead to biochemical malfunctions that promote neoplasia.

Endocrine-related cancers

Quantitative biochemical assays for estrogen receptors in extracts of mammary carcinomas have proven useful in predicting estrogenic dependency in tumors. Steroid receptor molecules that bind estradiol have been found in the cytoplasmic fractions of extracts of mammary gland and perianal gland tumors of dogs. Hormone receptors have also been localized in canine mammary tumors histochemically. In preneoplastic lesions of canine mammary gland, hormone secretions are dependent on estrogens, but growth of cells is not.

The canine **perianal gland tumor** is androgen dependent. Males show more than a five-fold increased risk over females, and estrogens and castration have been used in treatment therapy for this tumor. Normal perianal glands are small at birth and enlarge until senility. Treatment of puppies with androgen induces adult-sized perianal glands in two weeks.

Carcinomas of the prostate, in most species, are enhanced and inhibited by testosterone and estrogen, respectively. The canine prostatic carcinoma is not as androgen dependent as its human counterpart; neoplastic cells are more refractory to castration, because of a shift from a reductive to an oxidative pathway of steroid metabolism to reach an androgen-independent state.

Mammary tumors of dogs increase with advancing age and are clearly endocrine driven. Ovariectomy at an early age exerts a protective effect, and progestins given to dogs lead to dose-dependent mammary tumor development. How ovarian steroids promote mammary tumorigeneses in the bitch is not known. It has been proposed that growth hormone, produced in mammary tissue under the influence of progestins, acts as an autocrine (or paracrine) mechanism to initiate aberrant growth. Synthesis of growth hormone (mammary epithelial cells) was proven by demonstrating the presence of growth hormone–containing secretory granules by immunoelectron microscopy. Growth hormone probably promotes tumorigenesis by stimulating proliferation of epithelial cells genetically altered by other mechanisms.

VIRAL ONCOGENESIS

Retroviruses

Retroviruses cause malignant tumors in mammals, birds, and reptiles. The retroviral genetic code is carried on RNA and is transcribed "backward" into DNA. In the infected cell, this new viral DNA is integrated into the host chromosome in a sequence of units called a **provirus**. Later, the cell transcribes the proviral genes, and synthesizes the proteins they encode, which are assembled into new virions.

Retroviruses bearing oncogenes can rapidly produce tumors in animals, and most can also transform cells in culture. Viral oncogenes are designated by the prefix v- plus a three-letter word that relates the oncogene to the virus from which it came. The viral oncogene in **f**eline sarcoma is v-*fes;* that in **si**mian sarcoma, v-*sis*. The *src* gene of Rous sarcoma virus is a prototype oncogene. If the gene segment bearing *src* is isolated and transferred to cells in culture, it can cause transformation.

Other retroviruses, such as avian leukosis virus, lack oncogenes but carry a viral RNA segment called a **long terminal repeat (LTR)** sequence at the end of the viral genome. The LTR sequence contains segments called **promoters** and **enhancers** that activate transcription of viral genes into mRNA. Viruses that lack oncogenes produce tumors more slowly in animals and do not transform cells in culture. Some retroviruses transform cells by **transactivation**; that is, they contain proteins with the ability to increase the expression of genes attached to viral control sequences, whether or not these genes are integrated into the cell genome (Table 12.4).

In many cases retroviral infection is innocuous. Virions are produced and leave the cell without damaging it. This partnership goes awry when an oncogene is selectively activated (as in Rous sarcomas) or when a **provirus** is inserted into the chromosome and activates an adjacent normal cell growth gene. Avian leukosis virus does not carry its own oncogene, for example, but the provirus is in-

TABLE 12.4. Viruses that cause or are associated with neoplasia

Virus family	Virus	Tumor produced
Papovaviridae	Papillomavirus	Squamous carcinoma[a]
Herpesviridae	Human herpesvirus 6	Kaposi's sarcoma
	Frog cytomegalovirus	Renal carcinoma
	Marek's disease virus	Lymphoma
Hepadnaviridae	Hepatitis B virus	Hepatocellular carcinoma
	Woodchuck hepatitis virus	Hepatocellular carcinoma
	Duck hepatitis virus	Hepatocellular carcinoma
Retroviridae		
Subfamily Oncovirinae		
HTLV-related group	Bovine leukemia virus	Lymphoma
	Simian T-cell lymphotrophic virus	Lymphoma
MLV-related group[b]	Feline sarcoma/leukemia viruses	Leukemia et al.[c]
	Murine sarcoma/leukemia viruses	Leukemia et al.[c]
AVL-related group	Avian sarcoma/leukemia group	Leukemia et al.[c]
Mammalian type B group	Mouse mammary tumor virus	Mammary gland carcinoma
Mammalian type D group[d]	Pulmonary adenomatosis virus	Bronchioloalveolar carcinoma
		Nasal ethmoid carcinoma
Subfamily Lentivirus	Human immunosuppressive viruses	Lymphoma
	Simian immunosuppressive viruses	Lymphoma
	Feline immunosuppressive viruses	Lymphoma
	Bovine immunosuppressive viruses	None
	Equine infectious anemia virus	None

[a]Papillomas are common; carcinomas that develop from them are very rare.
[b]Group includes viruses of monkeys, pigs, baboons, mink, gibbon apes, guinea pigs, rats.
[c]Virus causes a wide range of neoplastic disorders and proliferative syndromes.
[d]Group contains many viruses of nonhuman primates.

serted in the vicinity of another gene known as *myc,* which is then greatly amplified and plays a role in the neoplastic change.

Retroviruses native to the host, called **endogenous** retroviruses, are detectable in the DNA of animals by determination of nucleic acid sequences and by detection of RNA in normal tissue expressed by these viral genes. Even though infectious viruses cannot be isolated, the transcription of their gene information can be detected.

Retrovirus-induced lymphoma

One of the most common malignant neoplasms in the animal kingdom, **lymphosarcoma** (also called **malignant lymphoma**), evolves by the neoplastic transformation of lymphocytes. Lymphosarcomas appear as solid, fleshy, white masses that destroy the architecture of lymphoid organs and develop in the parenchyma of spleen, liver, kidney, and other viscera (Fig. 12.12).

The malignant cells vary from small, normal-appearing lymphocytes to large blastic cells (Fig. 12.13). When lymphoma cells disseminate throughout the bloodstream, the disease is called **lymphoid leukemia**. The white blood cell counts

of leukemic animals may exceed 100,000 WBC/mm³. Some animals with large masses of lymphoma throughout their body never become leukemic. In contrast, some lymphoid tumors are leukemic, even though defined space-occupying masses are not found.

Lymphosarcoma and lymphoid leukemia in cats and cows are caused by retroviruses. Feline leukemia virus (FeLV) causes several neoplastic and non-neoplastic syndromes in cats (Table 12.5). Persistent viremia precedes clinical evidence of disease, and FeLV antigens can be detected in circulating leukocytes with an indirect immunofluorescent antibody test. Cats showing antigens in their tissues may be healthy or may have any of the FeLV-associated diseases. Resistance to and recovery from FeLV infection depends on two separate responses of the host: one toward the infecting virus, because antibodies to viral envelope antigens prevent viremia; and one toward tumor antigens, because antibodies against the **feline oncornavirus-associated cell membrane antigen** (FOCMA) correlate with resistance to oncogenicity.

FeLV is most active in immunosuppressed cats. Induction of leukemia is related both to FeLV and

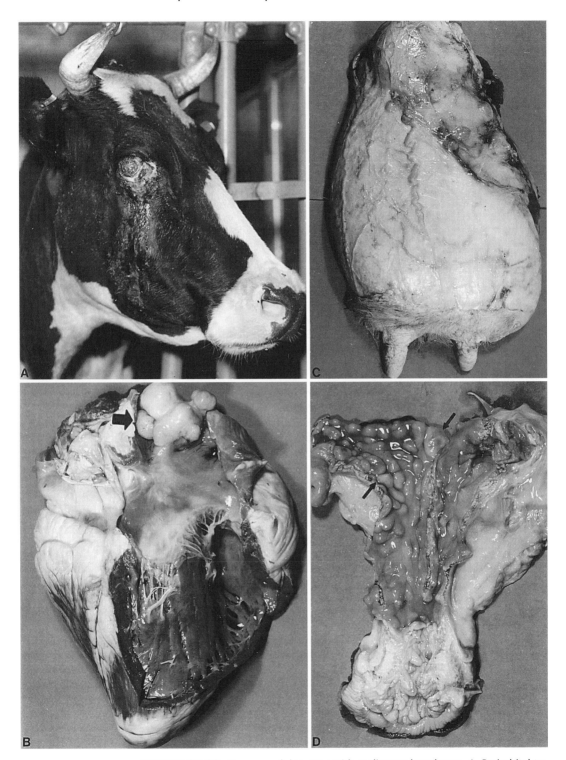

FIGURE 12.12. Tumor nodules, cow with malignant lymphoma. A. Periorbital tumor tissue with marked panophthalmitis. B. Tumors in atrial wall *(arrow)*. C. Supramammary lymph node with tumors *(top)* and lymph stasis in afferent lymphatics. D. Tumor invasion of placentome *(arrows)*, uterus.

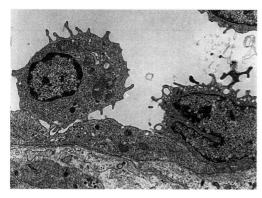

FIGURE 12.13. Emigration of neoplastic cells in the liver. Separation of hepatic sinusoidal endothelium by a malignant lymphocyte. Other lymphocytes are in intersinusoidal spaces *(bottom left)*.

TABLE 12.5. Diseases associated with feline leukemia virus

Neoplastic diseases	Nonneoplastic diseases
Lymphosarcoma	Immunodeficiency
Erythroleukemia	Anemia (nonregenerative)
Erythremic myelosis	Glomerulopathy
Myelogenous leukemia	Abortion/fetal resorption
	Panleukopenia syndrome

mechanisms to keep these enzymes active and not turned off, as they are in the normal process of keratinocyte differentiation.

Oncogenic papillomaviruses are integrated into the genome of the cell. The site of integration into the host cell genome is random, but in papilloma-associated cancers, it is within the E1/E2 reading frame of the viral genome. Because the E2 region of viral DNA represses transcription of the E6 and E7 early viral genes, its interruption causes overexpression of E6 and E7 proteins. E6 binds to and facilitates degradation of p53 protein, causing the loss of its capacity to block the cell cycle at the G_1-S checkpoint in order to prevent abnormal DNA from being produced. E7 protein binds the unphosphorylated form of pRb (retinoblastoma susceptibility protein), and with its binding sites filled, pRb cannot function (recall the roles of pRb and p53 in cell cycle regulation). In early G_1, pRb sequesters transcription factors into inactive complexes, preventing them from up-regulating the promotion of genes for cyclins and DNA polymerases, which are required for entering into and progressing through the S phase of the cell cycle.

Although papillomaviruses play a role in oncogenesis, they do not do so alone. Even with these genetic abnormalities in p53 and pRb, oncogenic papillomaviruses appear to require *ras* or some other oncogene to initiate carcinogenesis.

Bovine papillomavirus (BPV) causes cutaneous fibropapillomas in cattle, unique because of the massive subepithelial fibroblastic proliferative masses. This virus will cause meningiomas when injected into the brain of calves and chondromas when placed next to cartilage in rodents. When bovine papillomavirus infects the limbs of horses, it causes a fibroma called **equine sarcoid**. Equine sarcoids can be produced experimentally by injecting bovine papillomavirus subcutaneously in young horses. DNA sequences of BPV have been shown in tumor cells isolated from naturally occurring sarcoids.

Polyomavirus simiae, which causes a natural infection of monkeys, is oncogenic in laboratory

to immunologic deficiency. When kittens are inoculated with FeLV, radiation increases the percentage of animals that develop lymphosarcoma. Predisposing factors involved in natural disease are those associated with immunosuppressive diseases that occur in kittenhood.

FeLV is itself immunosuppressive. This attribute is necessary in the prodromal stages of infection for lymphosarcoma to develop. The marked depression of T-lymphocyte activity that occurs during FeLV viremia is caused by activity of an envelope protein of the virion called p15E. FeLV-induced immunosuppression also renders kittens susceptible to other infections. Cats with lymphosarcoma have a much higher incidence of anemia induced by *Haemobartonella felis* than do non-FeLV-bearing cats. In the preneoplastic phases of experimental disease, significant depression of cell-mediated immunoreactivity occurs, and thymic atrophy is prominent.

Oncogenic papovaviruses

Papillomaviruses

Benign squamous papillomas (warts, verrucae) are virus-induced hyperplastic lesions of skin and oral mucosa. They are not neoplasms, and they regress naturally because of specific cell-mediated mechanisms of immunity. However, a small number of papillomas, when accompanied by appropriate cofactors, provide the cellular basis for malignant transformation into squamous cell carcinomas. The role of specific strains of canine, bovine, and human papillomaviruses in development of squamous cell carcinomas has been clearly established. These viruses require host cell DNA polymerases and cyclins to replicate and have developed unique rodents and has been widely studied as a model of viral oncogenesis. It is considered a potential human oncogenic virus.

Polyomavirus maccacae, which causes lytic infection in susceptible rhesus monkey cells in vitro, causes stable transformation in cells that are incompetent for viral replication. Transformation is linked to the activation of the large T antigen (T_{ag}), which induces cell cycle progression to S phase and DNA synthesis. Induction of the S phase is due in part to interaction or binding of SV40 T_{ag} with two tumor suppressor gene products, the *Rb* gene products p110 and p53.

Hepadnaviruses

The hepadnaviruses are hepatotropic DNA viruses that cause acute and chronic liver disease in ducks, woodchucks, chimpanzees, and humans (hepatitis B virus). By causing hepatocellular necrosis and **regeneration** (which occurs as a consequence of necrosis), the hepadnaviruses expand the pool of cells at risk for genetic damage. In the mitotically active hepatocytes, mutations arise spontaneously at a higher rate. Mutational activation of *p53* is found in humans in geographical areas where hepatitis B virus and aflatoxicosis are endemic. In the hepadnavirus-related liver cell cancers, viral DNA is integrated into the host cell genome, and tumor cells bearing these insertions are clonal. Tumor development is multifactorial, and viral oncogenic effects are indirect.

The hepatitis viruses of ducks and woodchucks have been widely studied as models of human hepatitis B infection. There is a strong correlation between the presence of hepadnaviral antigens and incidence of hepatocellular carcinoma in these animals. Viral antigens have been demonstrated in tumor cells, and integration of duck hepatitis virus into carcinoma cells has been established. In a study of 15 woodchucks infected with woodchuck hepatitis virus, all 15 had chronic hepatitis, and 13 of them had a primary hepatocellular carcinoma.

Hepadnaviruses typically do not encode for oncoproteins, and there is no integration of the viral genome in the vicinity of any known proto-oncogene. However, hepatitis B virus encodes a regulatory element, **HBx protein**, which disrupts growth control by transcriptional activation of several proto-oncogenes and can affect several signal transduction pathways.

Oncogenic herpesviruses

Oncogenic herpesviruses include Marek's disease herpesvirus of chickens, the frog renal carcinoma herpesvirus, Herpesvirus saimiri of nonhuman primates, the human Epstein-Barr virus (lymphosarcoma), and human herpesvirus 6, associated with human Kaposi's sarcoma.

Herpesvirus saimiri is indigenous and noncytopathic in squirrel monkeys (*Saimiri sciureus*). When injected into other New World monkey species, a rapidly progressive T-cell lymphosarcoma develops. This neoplasm produces extensive invasion of many organs. The fundamental change is proliferation and invasion of tissue by neoplastic reticulum cells.

Avian herpesviral lymphosarcoma

In 1907, Josef Marek described a disease of chickens in which the peripheral and central nervous systems were infiltrated by lymphocytes. Designating the disease **polyneuritis**, he also recognized a concurrent second form, **malignant lymphoma**. A herpesvirus, Marek's disease virus (MDV), causes a disease of major economic importance in the poultry industry. When injected experimentally, this virus first causes lymphoid necrosis and then infects epithelium of feather follicles, producing large herpes inclusions. Virus is transmitted from bird to bird by skin flakes in dust aerosols. Persistence in lymphoid tissues leads to progressive neoplastic change, ending in malignant lymphoma with tumors developing in the liver and other parenchymal organs.

Adenoviruses

For three decades, some adenoviruses have been suspected of being oncogenic. In rodent models, particularly hamsters, injection of certain viral strains will induce sarcomas. The mechanism involves specific activities of viral components—for example, adenoviral *EIB* gene product binds to and inhibits activation of *bax* to suppress programmed cell death. However, the role of adenoviruses in clinical neoplasia is not clearly established.

PHYSICAL AGENTS ASSOCIATED WITH NEOPLASIA

Solar radiation

Cancer of the skin occurs in lightly pigmented animals exposed to intense sunlight for long periods. Squamous cell carcinoma of the eye develops in white-faced Hereford cattle in the southern United States; the incidence of these tumors in black Angus cattle is lower. Carcinomas first appear at the corneal periphery in the medial and lateral aspects of the eyeball, areas not covered by the eyelid when the eyes are open. Bovine ocular squamous cell carcinomas arise from nonmalignant precursor plaques.

Solar radiation induces neoplasia by causing damage to DNA. The relation between solar radiation and carcinoma induction has been proven experimentally, and the carcinogenic effect has been shown to be in the ultraviolet spectrum between rays of 2800 and 3200 Å. Ultraviolet radiation reaching the earth on sunny days generates pyrimidine dimers in DNA of exposed skin cells by linking adjacent thymine and cytosine. Once injured, DNA is repaired in normal cells by excision repair. Repair is never totally efficient, and some cells die. Others survive with DNA scars left by the process of mutation.

Evidence that DNA damage is a direct cause of squamous cell carcinoma comes from the human genetic disease **xeroderma pigmentosum**. Because of defects in enzymes required for DNA repair, patients with this disease are extremely sensitive to sunlight and are susceptible to various kinds of skin neoplasms in childhood. It has been reported that excessive ultraviolet radiation stimulates suppressor T lymphocytes, and that this may activate oncogenic viruses or directly suppress host antitumor activity.

FOCUS

Bacteria and Parasites Cause or Enhance Carcinogenesis

INFECTIOUS AGENTS have been shown to enhance carcinogenesis induced by toxic carcinogens. *Helicobacter hepaticus*, which colonizes the lower intestinal tract and biliary system of mice, causes progressive, chronic hepatitis that leads to hepatocellular carcinoma. Bacterial infection is associated with simulation of cyclin D expression and the subsequent acceleration of the development of liver tumors.

Gastric infections in ferrets associated with the spirochete *Helicobacter mustelae* are associated with an increased incidence of gastric carcinoma. This follows the pattern of human gastric infections by *H. pylori*, which has also been linked to gastric adenocarcinoma. This bacterium appears to enhance hepatocarcinogenesis; for example, N-methyl-N'-nitro-N-nitrosoguanidine induced gastric carcinoma in nearly 100% of ferrets infected with *H. mustelae*. A similar promotion of bile duct cancers in hamsters has been reported by liver fluke infection.

The parasite *Spirocirca lupi* encysts and causes granulomatous lesions near the esophagus in dogs. In a small number of cases, a sarcoma develops in these lesions. In a similar model in rats, liver sarcomas are caused by larvae of *Taenia taeniaeformis*. Secretions of this cestode cause fibroblastic hyperplasia of the liver, and in rare cases sarcomas develop.

References

Diwan BA, et al. 1997. Promotion of *Helicobacter hepaticus*–induced hepatitis of hepatic tumors initiated by N-nitrosodimethylamine in male A/JCr mice. *Toxicol Pathol* 25:597.

Ward JM, et al. 1994. Chronic active hepatitis and associated liver tumors in mice caused by a persistent bacterial infection with a novel *Helicobacter* species. *J Natl Cancer Inst* 86:1222.

Ward JM, et al. 1996. Autoimmunity in chronic active *Helicobacter* hepatitis of mice. *Am J Pathol* 148:509.

X-irradiation

Since the early days of the use of X rays, it has been known that they can induce cancer. Pioneers in radiology were often affected by carcinomas of the skin overlying the hands and arms, the areas most exposed to radiation. The primary event in radiation-induced oncogenesis is direct damage to DNA. There is production of specific genetic alterations, that is, **somatic mutation**.

Dose, rate, and quality of radiation influence the frequency of mutation. Enhancing factors in radiation mutagenesis include damage to the cellular mitotic apparatus, damage to non-DNA chromosomal components, and damage to other enzymes of DNA repair and detoxification. Additionally, activation of latent oncogenic viruses may play a role in some forms of radiation-induced neoplastic change.

Whole-body radiation increases incidence of neoplasms

Epidemiologic studies show that even small doses of radiation delivered to the entire body increase the risk of neoplastic disease. Beagles given low-dose, whole-body, Co^{60} γ-radiation had an increased incidence of hyperplastic nodules of the liver (which are common in aged dogs) and a few cases of hepatocellular carcinoma. When dogs or other mammals receive **large doses** of whole-body radiation, a spectrum of neoplasms occurs in ensuing years, including lymphosarcoma, reticulum cell sarcoma, and myeloid leukemia.

Oncogenic changes resulting from whole-body radiation have been clearly illustrated in studies on human survivors of bomb fallout in Hiroshima and Nagasaki (Fig. 12.14). Leukemia was more common in these populations, and the incidence of solid tumors also increased slightly. Fallout of I^{131} caused adenomatous changes in thyroid of exposed humans.

Inhalation of radionuclides produces tumors in organs of deposition. Inhaled Sr^{90} goes to the skeleton, where bone sarcomas evolve. Ce^{144} deposits in lung, liver, and spleen and causes carcinomas; hemangiosarcomas are common in some species. Long-range β-radiation emitters are more apt to produce neoplasms than are radionuclides that emit shorter radiation.

Trauma

Development of neoplasms at sites of tissue injury has been reported very rarely in dogs and humans, usually on the limbs. Burn scar neoplasms are predominantly squamous cell carcinomas, although basal cell carcinomas and sarcomas have been re-

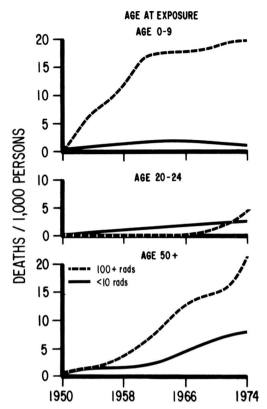

FIGURE 12.14. Incidence of radiation-associated leukemia in humans among exposures to atomic radiation in Japan. Data (from Beebe, *Am Sci* 70:35, 1982) are cumulative leukemia deaths from 1950 to 1974. Development of leukemia is associated with both young and old populations.

ported. Anaplastic sarcomas have been reported in the eyes of cats several years after trauma to the affected eyes.

In large breeds of dogs, osteosarcomas may develop at healed fracture lines of long bones. Fracture-associated sarcomas differ from other osteosarcomas in being diaphyseal rather than metaphyseal in location. The mean interval between fracture and tumor diagnosis is about 8 years.

Carcinomas at vaccination sites

Sarcomas at sites used for vaccination for rabies and feline leukemia virus occur in cats. Sarcomas are more common when multiple vaccines are given in a single site. Sarcomas develop 3 months to 3 years after vaccination, most often in sites in interscapular and caudal thigh regions. Most are fibrosarcomas, and the cells arise from fibroblasts or myofibroblast lineages. They are locally invasive and often recur, but rarely metastasize.

Vaccination site sarcomas are typically invasive tumors of spindle cells, multinucleated giant cells, and pleomorphic macrophages or polygonal cells. They often infiltrate by inflammatory cells, multinucleated giant cells, and fibrous or granulomatous tissue. Macrophages may contain cytoplasmic material that originated in the adjuvants of the vaccine. Rare vaccine-induced tumors that have also been reported include malignant histiocytomas, rhabdomyosarcomas, osteosarcomas, chondrosarcomas, and myofibroblastic sarcomas.

In very rare instances, other neoplasms have been reported at sites where vaccines were given. Cutaneous squamous cell carcinomas develop at sites of papilloma vaccine injection and have been reported in scars of poxvirus vaccination of primates. Suspicious cases of muscle tumors in other species have been reported at sites where vaccines were given intramuscularly.

ADDITIONAL READING

Spread of neoplasms

Agrawal B, et al. 1998. Cancer-associated MUC1 mucin inhibits human T-cell proliferation, which is reversible by IL-2. *Nat Med* 4:43.

Durham SK, Dietze AE. 1986. Prostatic adenocarcinoma with and without metastases to bone in dogs. *J Am Vet Med Assoc* 188:1432.

Hahne M, et al. 1996. Melanoma cell expression of Fas (Apo-1/CD95) ligand: implications for tumor escape. *Science* 274:1363.

Clinical effects of neoplasms

Germolec DR, et al. 1998. Arsenic enhancement of skin neoplasia by chronic stimulation of growth factors. *Am J Pathol* 153:1775.

Hall GA, et al. 1972. Thymoma with myasthenia gravis in a dog. *J Pathol* 108:177.

Leifer CE, et al. 1985. Hypoglycemia associated with nonislet cell tumors in 13 dogs. *J Am Vet Med Assoc* 186:53.

Marini RP, et al. 1993. Functional islet cell tumor in six ferrets. *J Am Vet Med Assoc* 202:430.

Meuten DJ, et al. 1983. Hypercalcemia in dogs with lymphosarcoma. *Lab Invest* 49:553.

Shoji M, et al. 1998. Activation of coagulation and angiogenesis in cancer. *Am J Pathol* 152:399.

van Garderen E, et al. 1997. Expression of growth hormone in canine mammary tissue and mammary tumors. *Am J Pathol* 150:1037.

Van Keulen LJM, et al. 1996. Diabetes mellitus in a dog with a growth hormone producing acidophilic adenoma of the adenohypophysis. *Vet Pathol* 33:451.

Restraint of neoplastic growth

Oliff A, et al. 1996. New molecular targets for cancer therapy. *Sci Am* 275:144.

Timmeran JM, Levy R. 1998. Melanoma vaccines. *Nat Med* 4:269.

Williams N. 1996. Tumor cells fight back to beat immune system. *Science* 274:1302.

Cancer is a genetic disease

Cordon-Cardo C. 1995. Mutation of cell cycle regulators. *Am J Pathol* 147:545.

Enomoto A, et al. 1998. Interactive effects of c-*myc* and transforming growth factor α transgenes on liver tumor development in simian virus 40T antigen transgenic mice. *Vet Pathol* 35:283.

Hartwell LH, Kasten MB. 1994. Cell cycle control and cancer. *Science* 266:1821.

Hirohashi S. 1998. Inactivation of the E-cadherin–mediated cell adhesion system in human cancers. *Am J Pathol* 153:333.

Pennisi E. 1998. How a growth control path takes a wrong turn to cancer. *Science* 281:1438.

Wright EG. 1999. Inherited and inducible chromosomal instability: a fragile bridge between genome integrity mechanisms and tumourigenesis. *J Pathol* 187:19-27.

Chemical carcinogenesis

Jarrett WFH. 1978. Transformation of warts to malignancy in alimentary carcinoma. *Bull Cancer* 65:1914.

Leffell DJ, Brasch DE. 1996. Sunlight and skin cancer. *Sci Am* 275:52.

Pamukcu AM, et al. 1972. Lymphatic leukemia and pulmonary tumors in female Swiss mice fed bracken fern *(Pteris aquilina)*. *Cancer Res* 32:1442.

Viral oncogenesis

Callanan JJ, et al. 1996. Histologic classification and immunophenotype of lymphosarcomas in cats with naturally and experimentally acquired feline immunodeficiency virus infections. *Vet Pathol* 33:264.

Caniatti M, et al. 1996. Canine lymphoma: immunocytochemical analysis of fine-needle aspiration biopsy. *Vet Pathol* 33:204.

Chiba T, et al. 1995. Immunohistologic studies on subpopulations of lymphocytes in cattle with enzootic bovine leukosis. *Vet Pathol* 32:513.

Fox JG, et al. 1997. *Helicobacter mustelae*–associated gastric adenocarcinoma in ferrets *(Mustela putorius furo)*. *Vet Pathol* 34:225.

Hendrick MJ, et al. 1994. Comparison of fibrosarcomas that developed at vaccination sites and at nonvaccination sites in cats: 239 cases (1991–1992). *J Am Vet Med Assoc* 205:1425.

Moses AV, et al. 1997. HIV-1 induction of CD40 on endothelial cells promotes the outgrowth of AIDS-associated B-cell lymphomas. *Nature Med* 3:1242.

Patey N, et al. 1996. Intercellular adhesion molecule-3 on endothelial cells. Expression in tumors but not inflammatory responses. *Am J Pathol* 148:465.

Rudmann DG, et al. 1996. Pulmonary and mediastinal metastases of a vaccination-site sarcoma in a cat. *Vet Pathol* 33:466.

Index

329